Praise f
BURSTING WITH ENERGY

"Dr. Shallenberger's book is bursting with compelling new insights into health and longevity."

—Wendy Whitworth, Executive Producer, *Larry King Live*

"*Bursting With Energy* is also bursting with practical information for the layperson and for the busy practitioner. With mathematical precision, this book adds up to a true set of rules for health and healthy living. Some books you buy and never read; this one you will read and reread for the easy flow of ideas, the proven guidelines for staying young, and the clear answers about how and why they work."

—Richard Kunin, MD, Author of *Mega-Nutrition*

"Well written and thorough. This innovative book provides very practical methods for increasing your energy production at any age."

—Hyla Cass, MD, author of *All About Herbs, Supplement Your Prescription,* and other popular health books

"This book provides dramatic information on stuffing yourself with oxygen, the single greatest preventer of chronic and degenerative disease."

—Robert Rowen, MD

BURSTING WITH ENERGY

THE BREAKTHROUGH METHOD TO RENEW YOUTHFUL ENERGY *and* RESTORE HEALTH

2ND EDITION

FRANK SHALLENBERGER, MD, H.M.D.

Foreword by **JONATHAN WRIGHT**, MD

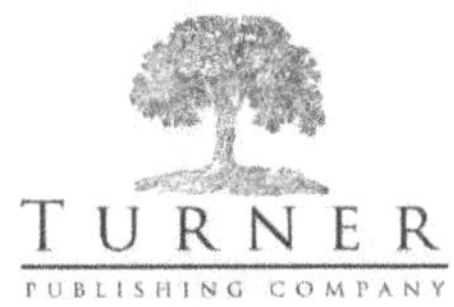

Turner Publishing Company
Nashville, TN
www.turnerpublishing.com

Bursting with Energy, 2nd edition

Cover design by Pete Garceau
Book design by Gary A. Rosenberg

Library of Congress Cataloging-in-Publication Data
Names: Shallenberger, Frank, author.
Title: Bursting with energy : the breakthrough method to renew youthful energy and restore health / Frank Shallenberger, M.D., H.M.D. ; foreword by Jonathan Wright, M.D.
Description: Revised second edition. | Nashville, Tennessee : Turner Publishing Company, [2022] | Includes bibliographical references and index.
Identifiers: LCCN 2021025578 (print) | LCCN 2021025579 (ebook) | ISBN 9781591201274 (paperback) | ISBN 9781681627045 (hardcover) | ISBN 9781591205661 (ebook)
Subjects: LCSH: Longevity. | Energy metabolism. | Fatigue.
Classification: LCC RA776.75 .S455 2022 (print) | LCC RA776.75 (ebook) | DDC 613--dc23
LC record available at https://lccn.loc.gov/2021025578
LC ebook record available at https://lccn.loc.gov/2021025579

Printed in the United States of America

To my patients, the most wonderful group of people a doctor could ever hope to serve.

You have allowed me to practice on you for years.

You have given your trust and often bared your souls.

You have faced the uncertainty of sickness and the certainty of death with great strength and courage.

You have given me support when I needed it most, and have taught me more about life and medicine than all my medical books and training.

In you, I have often been privileged to see the beauty and magnificence that humans are capable of. I feel humbled and honored in your presence.

This book is also dedicated to my wife and children, who have had to endure everything from coffee enemas to soyburgers as part of my particular search for truth.

CONTENTS

APPENDICES

*

FOREWORD

Natural health care and natural medicine really aren't hard. We just need to read our human blueprints and follow them. It's simple common sense. We do this if we're trying to maintain or repair anything else. Find the original plans, the original specifications, and work with or duplicate them. To repair broken equipment, we find parts identical to the damaged ones, put them in place just as the original plan specifies, and the equipment works again. No big deal. Maintenance is done like this all the time, everywhere.

Unless you're a doctor.

If you're a doctor, you try to repair humans with parts never, ever found in the original blueprints. Where the human biochemical plan calls for a protein or an amino acid, you use a patent medicine (pharmaceutical drug). Where the plan specifies a vitamin, you use a patent medicine. Where the plan calls for a combination of essential fatty acids, zinc, and vitamin A, you use . . . a patent medicine.

Is it any wonder that more than 100,000 of us in the US reportedly die of adverse reactions to patent medicines every year? The real surprise is that patent medicines do any good at all, since they're simply not part of our original design.

It's as if an entire country's auto mechanics insisted on fixing cars with airplane parts: it wouldn't make any sense. Customers would be screaming at them to follow the original plan. "Use automobile parts for automobiles, and never mind whether the Federal Automobile Administration approves or not," the customers would demand. It's just common sense.

Dr. Frank Shallenberger is a very unusual doctor. He follows the original human blueprint, even though he, too, was educated to use parts that have never, ever been part of the blueprint of human malfunction repair. For his first several years in practice, he recommended patent medicines as he'd been taught in medical school. After observing that using airplane parts to fix automobiles didn't work, he did something very unusual (for a doctor): he decided to figure out for himself what would really work, and in this book he shares his discoveries with us.

Dr. Shallenberger went back to basic principles. He decided to apply the factors that have supported human life for literally hundreds of thousands of years (not one of them a patent medicine), and . . . they *worked.*

- Water
- Rest
- Sunlight
- Food (real food, please)
- Exercise
- Breathing (healthfully)

Simple things, but things we all need to *re*learn in the twenty-first century. Come to think of it, humans have needed to relearn them for several centuries, since our way of life has strayed so far from that of original humanity.

But Dr. Shallenberger doesn't expect or want us to live as original, primitive humans. He blends the factors that have helped keep humans healthy over thousands of generations with real improvements that modern scientific knowledge has brought to health care:

- Supplements (no one ever knew about vitamins a century ago)
- Natural (not synthetic or horse) hormone replacement
- An advanced knowledge of human biochemistry that allows for a much more accurate diagnosis and treatment

In addition, he's put together a testing system that, logically enough, measures your body's basic air intake and output to gauge how efficiently your body works. Even though his system is quite innovative, it's just common sense (again). It's just like testing automobile exhaust to determine how efficiently the engine works. Even better, if a malfunction is found, he can tell us how to fix it.

Please don't think I am unappreciative of some of the tremendous advances made in medicine over the last century. Dr Shallenberger and I agree that if you get run over by a truck, it doesn't matter whether the truck carried whole, natural, organic, or junk food. Either way, you will benefit greatly from skilled surgeons using the latest techniques guided by the most up-to-date diagnostic equipment. These areas of medicine are the best ever. It's just those patent medicines we have a big problem with.

The focus of this book isn't only health. It's health with plenty of energy to do whatever it is we want to do while we're here. And *bursting with energy* doesn't come from surgery or the latest diagnostic equipment. Energy comes from applying the basic principles taught in this book.

When I'm at a convention for natural medicine (original human blueprint) doctors, I'm always happy and never disappointed when Dr. Shallenberger speaks to us. I always learn something from his insights.

I'm sure you will too!

Jonathan V. Wright, MD
Tahoma Clinic
Renton, Washington
www.tahoma-clinic.com

Author: *Why Stomach Acid Is Good for You, Maximize Your Vitality and Potency for Men Over 40, Natural Hormone Replacement for Women Over 45* (All written with Lane Lenard, PhD)

INTRODUCTION

It's been fifteen years now since the first edition of *Bursting with Energy* was published. It was the first book to bring attention to the overriding importance of mitochondrial function to aging. Since then, it is now commonplace for doctors and scientists to further validate what the book stated: that mitochondrial function is the single most important factor in the aging process.

That is so much so, that any person with optimal mitochondrial function, no matter what their age, is practically immune to all the diseases of aging, including cancer, atherosclerosis, diabetes, macular degeneration, Parkinson's, Alzheimer's, weakness, and frailty. These are all mitochondrial diseases, and people with optimal mitochondrial function are highly unlikely to get them.

A ruling principle in medicine is that if it's not measured, it's not considered. This is exactly why it is so critical to measure mitochondrial function. *Bursting with Energy* was also the first book to describe a patented, reproducible, and accurate way to easily determine mitochondrial function using pulmonary gas analysis. I call the system, Bio-Energy Testing®. To date, it is the only system available that can accurately measure mitochondrial function.

Since I wrote the first version of *Bursting With Energy,* more and more doctors are starting to see how incredibly important it is to measure the mitochondrial function of their patients using Bio-Energy Testing.

In this second edition and update of *Bursting With Energy,* I have not only added in new information that validates the importance of measuring and optimizing mitochondrial function, but I also provide new therapies designed to maximize mitochondrial function.

After close to fifty years of seeing and treating patients, I can say without a doubt that there is nothing more important for health, longevity, and disease prevention than measuring and optimizing mitochondrial function. I look forward to the day when every doctor recognizes this and acts on it.

Frank Shallenberger, MD, HMD

My Story—The Emergence of a Renegade Physician

I've been practicing medicine for almost fifty years, the last forty of which have been devoted to researching and developing alternative medical strategies to increase the length and quality of my patients' lives.

Frequently, my patients ask why I decided to pursue alternative medicine. It's a good question. Especially since, when I first began to investigate this field, there was a stigma attached to it. Most doctors regarded it as quackery. The softer terms, *complementary medicine* and *alternative medicine,* had not yet been coined.

Times have certainly changed. Now there is an Office of Alternative Medicine at the National Institutes of Health. Hundreds of books have been written about alternative medicine. And even the *Journal of the American Medical Association,* a leading voice of mainstream medicine, has dedicated whole issues to the subject.

Many states have even passed legislation protecting doctors who use alternative medicine from unfair persecution by medical boards. But the climate was totally different, and actually hostile, back in the late seventies when I first became enamored with the idea of working with natural remedies to treat and prevent disease.

Symptoms Improved—But Not Patients

After I graduated from medical school in 1973, I received training in surgery and specialized in emergency medicine. I worked in this very exciting field for the next five years and then decided I needed a change.

I chose to open a general-medicine practice across the street from the hospital emergency room where I had been working. I naïvely hung up my shingle and prepared to begin a new medical career. Boy, did I have a few lessons to learn.

Within six months, I began to make the rather unsettling observation that none of my patients with chronic diseases were getting well. The ones with acute disorders—broken legs, colds, cuts, flu, and sprains—all got well, often regardless of my treatments. But my patients with chronic conditions, such as arthritis, diabetes, and heart disease, never showed any real improvement at all. Of course, with the proper medication I was able to help their symptoms. They would feel better. Their medical tests would improve. Yet the same disease process was still present.

Not only that, but many of them developed serious side effects and secondary medical conditions from the drugs I was giving them. Was I causing more problems than I was solving? Years later, statistics would become available showing that more than 100,000 people die annually as a result of *properly* administered medical therapy. But back then I was just barely beginning to appreciate the depth of this problem.

Treat the Cause, Stupid

My years in the emergency room had made me completely naïve about how day-to-day medicine was being practiced on people with chronic conditions. In the emergency room, if a person was brought in with a knife protruding from his head (as actually happened once), we didn't just give him some pain medication for the symptoms and send him home. First, we treated the cause of his symptoms by removing the knife and repairing the injuries. Then we sent him home.

Likewise, when a desperate patient reported that he could not breathe, we quickly determined the cause and then fixed it. We didn't just send him home with oxygen.

Emergency-medicine specialists directly treat the cause of the problem, not just the symptoms. I had become used to treating the causes of the symptoms that my patients had, and I just assumed that doctors treating chronic diseases had the same approach. But I was wrong.

A few months after I launched my general-medicine practice, one of my arthritis patients developed an ulcer, the result of taking a standard medication that I had prescribed. The incident alarmed me greatly. I felt that I had failed this person. I decided to discuss the situation with one of the best physicians in the community at the time, a person I held in great esteem. I compared notes on how he treated various diseases and how I treated the same conditions. What I learned surprised my innocent brain.

What he told me was: "Frank, you're doing just fine. When it comes to the treatment of chronic diseases, you have to accept the fact that at this point in time we can't treat causes, because nobody knows what the causes are. The best we can do is simply make our patients feel better, and try to avoid complications with the intelligent and judicious use of medication."

Could it be, I thought, that the reason mainstream medicine doesn't know what causes the various diseases it is treating is that *it is not bothering to ask the question?* This started me wondering just what kinds of factors could cause chronic disease. In medical school, we looked at the *results* of chronic disease, the pathology. But no time was spent on the possible *causes* of the pathology.

It was around this time that I happened to pull out an old publication on vitamins that my dad, a physician himself, had received from a drug company back in the early fifties. I started to read it and found myself devouring the information. I recall looking under the symptoms of deficiencies of different vitamins and seeing anxiety, arthritis, cancer, colitis, depression, diabetes, heart disease, hypothyroidism, rashes, and virtually every other chronic illness for which there was no known cause.

In the one hour of study that my medical school had dedicated to nutrition, we had been taught that these kinds of deficiencies only occurred in serious starvation situations. They certainly did not exist among average Americans. I now began to wonder about that assumption.

The Linus Pauling Approach

In the summer of 1980, I learned about an Orthomolecular Medicine conference in San Francisco. The conference was organized by physicians who had been influenced by two-time Nobel Prize winner Linus Pauling, PhD. Pauling believed that diseases were caused by delicate imbalances in the body's biochemistry, and that these diseases could be prevented and often reversed simply by correcting these imbalances. He called the concept *orthomolecular* because it involved restoring the right (ortho) molecule to the body at the right time.

I anxiously went to the conference, hoping to gain insight into the questions I had been pondering. I was not disappointed.

I heard about reversing—and even curing—anxiety, arthritis, gout, headaches, heart disease, hypertension, and schizophrenia merely through the scientific use of vitamins and minerals. Better yet, I learned how many of these conditions could be *prevented* using the same concepts.

I listened to medical pioneers who had been successfully using these treatments for years. I was especially happy to hear that none of these doctors were making their patients worse by creating other disorders from the side effects of pharmaceuticals. While the rest of medicine was busy pursuing the use of treatments that routinely caused death and injury from side effects, these physicians were looking for safe and effective alternatives. Although at the time I hadn't been sure where I was going in my medical career, I knew then and there that I wanted to go wherever these doctors were headed.

It's All About Energy

Back then, except for an occasional conference, there was no place to learn how to proceed with this approach. There were very few books available. So I developed a set of criteria for the application of unproven, alternative techniques.

First, I reasoned, they must be inherently safe. Second, they must either have a record of effectiveness, or at least be theoretically reasonable. And third, they must be inexpensive. Using these criteria as my guide, I began to take myself and my patients down an exciting and rewarding path.

Forty years later, I can honestly say that I made the right decision to follow this path. I have been able to help thousands of people in ways I couldn't possibly have done using only my conventional medical education.

I have learned that many natural treatments actually correct the cause of disease. I have learned that many diseases still considered incurable are, in fact, curable when the cause is recognized and treated. I have learned that virtually all the diseases that are so common today are easily preventable. Even aging itself is very treatable. What's the secret? In a word: *energy*.

I have learned that a decrease in energy production is the primary cause of all diseases, allergies, fatigue, infections, obesity—and even the very process of aging. And that's what this book is all about. If you can just keep your energy production at optimal levels throughout your life, you will live longer and be healthier—and the chances are good that you will never become ill.

Optimizing Energy Production

So, by now you are probably ready to go out to the local health-food store and buy a lifetime supply of energy. Doesn't really matter what it costs. How can you go wrong by taking a substance that is so critical to your health and well-being? The only problem is, you can't buy it. And even if you could, you couldn't swallow the pills fast enough to make a difference.

You can't buy energy—you have to *make* it. And you make it by converting oxygen to carbon dioxide and water. Sound complex? It's not really. In the pages to follow, you will learn exactly how your body uses this process to harness the sun's energy and make it your own.

You will learn what you can do to maximize energy production in the most efficient way possible. You will also learn about some very common bad habits that can seriously impair energy production. Knowledge is power. And you will discover firsthand the power of having maximum energy.

Bio-Energy Testing®

And here's the key to the whole program. Thanks to new technical advances in oxygen uptake and carbon dioxide production measurements, your ability to make energy can be measured right in your doctor's office. This is done with a new testing method called Bio-Energy Testing. As of this writing, there are fifteen centers right here in the United States that are offering Bio-Energy Testing, and five others internationally. Using this technology, in about forty minutes you can determine if your lifestyle is effectively working with your genetics to produce optimal energy levels.

Not only that: if it turns out that your energy production is less than perfect, the Bio-Energy-Testing Report can often pinpoint where you are going wrong. If you are struggling with an illness, you need to maximize your energy production to get well again. And if you are fortunate enough to still be free of disease, optimizing your energy production is critical to staying that way. An entire chapter of this book is devoted to this exciting new medical advancement.

Using this new form of energy measurement, I've been able to establish optimum values related to your maximal energy production, your resting metabolism, your fat-burning ability, and other key markers that can help you home in on optimal energy production.

How This Book Works

In Part One, I'll explain in detail how Bio-Energy Testing works. I will also show how the primary cause of all chronic disease, and even the process of aging itself, is decreased energy production. Chronic disease almost never happens in people with optimal energy production. I'll explain how decreased energy production is also the cause of our obesity epidemic.

With the Bio-Energy Testing method, I have been able to quantify and confirm the effects of all the age-defying, energy-enhancing secrets in this book. It offers the most complete and exact measurement of health and aging I have ever encountered in all my years of practicing preventive and anti-aging medicine.

In Part Two, I will sequentially unfold these clinical secrets with you. There are eight of them. They involve lifestyle changes—some very simple, and some involving a bit of effort on your part, but all hugely rewarding. These secrets have the potential to raise your energy to a level you may have experienced only in your younger days, or, in many cases, to a height you never imagined possible. The goal is to be *bursting with energy* for a long, long time.

The Future Is Here, Now

Anti-aging research has demonstrated that the human equivalent of living a fully functional life for a hundred and fifty years can be achieved in animals. Not surprisingly, the secret is energy production. In one particular study, those animals with the highest levels of energy production lived 46 percent longer than those with the lowest levels. Even more important than living longer, the quality of their lives was much better. They were free of disease, and of course they had much more energy.

The new medical specialty of anti-aging medicine is now spurring this research on and making it an increasing reality for humans. The American Academy of Anti-Aging Medicine was formed in 1993 in response to growing interest among physicians and researchers. There are now hundreds of physicians all over the world who are board-certified specialists in Anti-Aging Medicine.

Ronald Klatz, MD, president of the organization, predicted in 1999 that a full "50 percent of all baby boomers alive and well today will celebrate their 100th birthday with physical and mental faculties intact." The question is, if you are a boomer, will you be among them? And if you are, how will you feel? To maximize your chances, maximize your energy. Please read on to see just how you can do that.

✴ PART ONE ✴

YOU ARE YOUR ENERGY LEVEL

✳ 1 ✳

ENERGY PRODUCTION—THE REAL GENERATION GAP

Harry, Before

Five years ago, Harry was seventy-seven. He went to his doctor complaining of fatigue; insomnia; lack of stamina; stiff, achy joints and muscles; weakness; and a decreased interest and enjoyment in life.

His doctor ran the usual battery of tests and told Harry the one thing he really didn't want to hear: "You are perfectly healthy for your age." Harry knew better. He knew that "perfectly healthy" did not describe him. He left the doctor's office feeling depressed. If this was what it was like to feel perfectly healthy for his age now, what did the future bode?

Harry was a man of action, and always had been. He wanted more out of life, no matter what age he was. Drawing on an inherently resilient nature, he shoved aside the depression, discarded the doctor's verdict, and came to me for help, telling me in his first visit that he was setting out to recharge his battery.

Harry, After

Today, Harry is eighty-two, and his batteries are definitely recharged. Using the data supplied by his Bio-Energy Testing, it was easy to pinpoint where the problems were and what to do about them. Today, Harry's energy production resembles that of someone thirty years younger rather than someone his own age. He exercises daily and has 18 percent body fat and good musculature. His balance is good. He still backpacks up the same trails that he trekked more than half a century before. He cycles, roller-skates, and skis with ease.

He sleeps well, averaging eight hours of good sleep a night. He wakes up feeling fresh and full of vigor. His mood is exceptional. His mental-function tests reveal a fully functional brain with scores almost as good as those of a twenty-two-year-old. He has passion for life and is always keen to engage and solve new problems.

He has full sexual function, and his muscles and joints are flexible and free of the pain and stiffness that so many of his contemporaries experience. In short, Harry is living his life at an optimum level.

Caroline, Before

Caroline was pretty messed up when she came to see me. She had just passed her forty-sixth birthday, and for the previous five years she had been plagued with depression, fatigue, insomnia, menstrual disorders, and all sorts of aches and pains. She had gained thirty pounds for no apparent reason, and couldn't lose weight even with exercise and a good diet.

She had seen several different specialists who variously diagnosed her with chronic fatigue syndrome, depression, fibromyalgia, and hypothyroidism. More than once she had been told to remember that she was not getting any younger, and that for her age she wasn't really all that bad.

Caroline's symptoms were different from Harry's, but the doctors were giving her the same age-related nonsense. They prescribed antidepressants, pain pills, and sleeping pills, but never gave her any hope for curing or reversing her problems. In fact, they didn't even seem to know what was causing her problems in the first place.

Like Harry, she found herself depressed by her medical treatments. What kind of future did she have, she wondered, if she was already feeling this bad before turning fifty?

When I first tested Caroline, her energy production was equivalent to that of a ninety-two-year-old. "No wonder I feel like an old lady," she lamented. "From all functional aspects, I am."

But that was then.

Caroline, After

Today, Caroline, like Harry, has remade herself. First, I confirmed her low-energy status with Bio-Energy Testing. Then, using the test results, I identified the problems causing it, and designed a program to correct them. Her many problems included a deficiency of adrenal and thyroid hormones, along with improper breathing, poor fitness, and too much stress.

Caroline lacked the energy to fight off an ordinarily benign virus, the Epstein-Barr virus, EBV for short. This bug is often cited as the culprit in chronic fatigue states. Her previous physicians had focused on ridding her body of the virus rather than the cause of her real problem—an energy deficit that weakened her immune system. The EBV was only causing a problem because her body did not have the energy it needed to contain it.

Caroline's thyroid function was low, which, unfortunately, had not been recognized by her doctors. They missed the diagnosis because, as is often the case, they failed to rely on the time-honored practice of taking a history and performing a physical examination along with the kind of metabolic testing that Bio-Energy Testing provides. Instead, they relied exclusively on blood tests, which are often inaccurate when it comes to thyroid function. Caroline's test results fell in the normal range, despite the fact that her symptoms, physical findings, and metabolic tests confirmed that she had hypothyroidism (low thyroid). But, as with most complicated cases, that was not all.

When the body is under stress, the adrenal glands produce special hormones that help it deal with the stress. And, as long as the adrenal gland is working effectively, the body can hold up well in the face of all kinds of stress. But when it is under stress for a prolonged period of time, as it is with a chronic illness, the adrenal glands cannot produce enough of the hormones, and the stress takes over. We call this adrenal exhaustion. Like most sick people I see, Caroline was experiencing adrenal exhaustion.

Within six weeks of instituting a program that treated all these abnormalities, she began feeling energetic for the first time in many years. And, after another three months, her repeat Bio-Energy Testing scores were 80 percent better.

Six months later, Caroline had lost thirty pounds and was back to working full-time. Her energy production was now that of a forty-three-year-old, and she had developed an entirely fresh and enthusiastic attitude toward life.

Age-Related Symptoms

Before she remade herself, Caroline was a relatively young person with the energy level of a much older person. And after he remade himself, Harry was an older person with the energy production of a much younger person. Many of you reading this book right now may be able to identify with their so-called age-related symptoms.

Harry and Caroline's symptoms are collectively known as age-related because they result solely from the aging process itself. In other words, age-related symptoms are not caused by any disease or psychological condition.

Another way of putting it is that in conventional medicine, you can have all these symptoms and be considered perfectly healthy for your age.

Common age-related symptoms include the following:

* Anxiety and depression
* Decreased balance
* Decreased clarity, memory, and mental speed
* Decreased concentration or focus
* Decreased energy levels
* Decreased immune function
* Decreased sexual desire and function
* Digestive disturbances
* Dry, loose, wrinkled skin, and age spots
* Hair loss
* Increased joint and muscle pain
* Insomnia
* Urinary and bladder disorders
* Vision and hearing impairment
* Weakness, fatigue, and decreased stamina
* Weight gain and increased body fat

For some of us, the onset of these symptoms can begin as early as age thirty-five. For most people, they begin later. Lifestyle factors, such as diet, exercise, and smoking, have a significant influence on when the symptoms show up. But remember this. Long before you actually see the first signs of aging, the process has already been going on, and your age-related symptoms are on the way. It's not a case of *if;* it's simply a case of *when*.

What's Your E.Q.?

Caroline, Harry, and every other person with age-related symptoms, no matter what their age, all have one thing in common—*decreased energy production*. That decrease in energy production stems from a loss in the efficiency with which the body produces energy from oxygen.

My term, Energy Quotient (E.Q.), refers to your body's ability to produce energy from oxygen. A high E.Q. means you are doing this very efficiently and have a lot of cellular energy. A low E.Q., on the other hand, represents a real energy crisis.

High E.Q. and Low E.Q.

A high E.Q. means you are producing energy from oxygen very efficiently. A low E.Q. means your energy production is inefficient and represents a real energy crisis. Just as you want your I.Q. (intelligence quotient) to be high, you also want a high E.Q.—the higher it is, the healthier you are.

If you'd like a dramatic insight into what a low E.Q. feels like, just hold your breath while reading the next few sentences. Since efficient energy production is 100 percent dependent on the presence of oxygen, you will very quickly feel the effects of a low E.Q.

Of course, decreased energy production from a decreased E.Q. is not quite as drastic as holding your breath. It is much more subtle. Sometimes my patients with a modestly decreased E.Q. feel fine. Often, they are even able to exercise, and only in the severest cases do they complain about being short of breath. If the oxygen levels of their blood and tissue are tested, the results are almost always normal, and yet their cells may be slowly starving for the basic energy requirements that can only be met by an optimal E.Q.

To understand how this can occur, you will first need to learn four things:

* How the body uses oxygen to make energy
* What factors interfere with this process
* What happens when this process becomes inefficient
* How to improve and optimize the process

This book will give you this vital information.

Live Old—Die Young

The consideration of decreased energy production as a cause of aging and of the symptoms of aging is overlooked in medical practice today. Even in geriatrics, the specialty that focuses on older people, the main emphasis is simply on treatment of symptoms. It is primarily only among physicians like myself, who are interested in anti-aging concepts, that you will find any recognition and application of this concept.

Twenty-five years ago, when I first became interested in preventive medicine, nobody had much of a clue about this. I vividly remember my dad, who practiced medicine for more than half a century, telling me "Your patients are going to die anyway. The only thing you are going to accomplish is that they are going to die in better shape." "That's precisely the point," I replied.

Of course, many of us in the anti-aging field are interested in increasing the length of our lives. Life is much too precious to throw away even a day. But we should never lose sight of the fact that it is much more important to live well than to live long.

I personally hope to do both. I envision myself passing away in great shape. Free from the diseases, incapacity, and limitations that so frequently affect the older population.

Science is clearly showing us that this goal can only be accomplished by maintaining the energy-production efficiency we had in our youth, even as we grow very old. It is true that the younger you are when you first start making the changes, the more effectively they will work for you. I tell everyone not to wait until they are dragging before they decide to improve their energy production. Of course, even if you start very late in life, it will help. But the earlier you start, the more substantial your results will be. So, don't put it off. You should have your first Bio-Energy Testing on your fortieth birthday.

Feeling young is a lifetime endeavor. Make it habitual, and you will live longer. More importantly, you will enjoy your life more. The purpose of this book is to help you do exactly that.

What This Book Can Do for You

If you are currently healthy, vigorous, and operating on all cylinders, you might be tempted to think you have a pretty good E.Q. But the only way to really know is to check it. To the degree that your E.Q. is optimal, you are in fact bursting with energy. In that case, the information on these pages can help you function even better and keep you at that optimum level for many years to come.

But what if your E.Q. is not what you supposed it to be? That happens a lot, because in many people, especially young people, the E.Q. can be going down for years before the first symptoms start showing up.

And, of course, if you are less than vigorous and energetic, suffer from ill health, or are over the age of fifty and not very active, you probably won't be too surprised to discover that you have a sub-optimal E.Q. You're bursting all right, but without energy. In that case, I'm glad you found out about it sooner than later. And the information I present here can help you improve your E.Q., enhance your body's self-healing mechanisms, and give you a brighter outlook about your future health and rate of aging.

Dear readers, you won't find any of this information in another book, or in the medical library. It is based on years of working with my patients and learning the secrets that improve their energy production, health, and vigor—at all ages.

As you read through the information, you will note how the various components work together in a classic holistic sense. In other words, how you eat affects how you exercise; how you exercise affects how you sleep; how you sleep affects how you view life; and how you view life affects how you eat and exercise.

For this reason, I would like you to regard the individual secrets in this book as threads in a fabric. You are the weaver. You take the threads. You put them together and they produce a beautiful fabric. Incorporate them comfortably into your life in stages, but make sure your ultimate goal is to eventually include all of them.

It's important not to feel overwhelmed, not to think you need to adopt them all at once. You will be pleased to observe, as I guide you through one, then another, that you are steadily feeling better and better. And then you'll be hooked.

Energy can be very addictive, you see. If you follow the guidelines, I promise you'll become an energy addict. Making you one, and making you healthier and more youthful in the process, is why I have written this book.

✳ 2 ✳

HOW YOUR BODY MAKES ENERGY

Your body produces energy two ways: aerobically and anaerobically. Aerobic production refers to energy that comes from oxygen, while anaerobic production is energy created without oxygen. The two mechanisms are totally different, so take a moment to see how they work. We'll deal with aerobic first, because that's the more important process.

The Aerobic Process

Inside the trillions of cells in your body, molecules of oxygen, hydrogen, sugar, fat, vitamins, minerals, and amino acids pass through an assembly line of enzymatic processing that generates an enormous amount of energy. About 60 percent of this energy is used to produce heat. The remaining 40 percent is used to fuel every single physiological and biochemical reaction in your body. Your E.Q. is a direct measurement of how well your cells are doing this.

But poor aerobic energy production causes a decrease in energy that results in much more than simply being tired and cold. *More than any other single factor, it is the underlying cause of aging, disease, and the current obesity epidemic.*

Remember when you could easily bounce up three or four flights of stairs? Now you get winded after even one or two flights. That's because your E.Q. has decreased. As you age, your E.Q. steadily falls in a very predictable manner. This decline is a solid indicator of your functional age—the age level that your body is functioning at.

And here's a key point: anything that improves your E.Q. makes you functionally younger.

The Anaerobic Process

Anaerobic energy production is a way for the cells to get extra energy without using oxygen. It was created for emergencies, such as when trying to escape from a lion that has you in its sight for its next meal. It kicks in when a very high amount of energy is needed immediately for a short period of time.

Anaerobic energy production occurs on a limited basis as an everyday part of cellular function, and is considered completely normal and healthy. However, when aerobic energy production is decreased, as measured by a low E.Q., anaerobic production is increased to make up for the deficit. And this increased level of anaerobic energy production is what accounts for many of the aches, pains, and other infirmities doctors routinely see.

Here's how the excessive reliance on anaerobic energy production that happens when the E.Q. is low causes symptoms, chronic disease, and an increased rate of aging:

* It generates only a fraction of the energy produced by the aerobic process, and the cells become energy-poor.
* It generates a high level of free radicals, highly destructive molecules that damage cells and their genetic material. Free radicals are considered a major cause of accelerated aging.
* It also creates high levels of lactic acid. You already know what lactic acid feels like. It is a waste product of anaerobic energy production that causes the breathlessness, fatigue, and muscle pain that occurs with exercise. As your E.Q. decreases, you will begin to have these symptoms even with lower levels of exertion, because the body is simply losing its ability to produce energy aerobically and is forced to rely more on anaerobic production.

A common reason for the development of a low E.Q. and the subsequent increase in anaerobic energy production is a decreased delivery of oxygen and other nutrients to the cells. Another is a loss of function in the mitochondria, the energy-producing structures inside cells. Both situations routinely result from a number of sources, including the following:

* Deficient dietary protein
* Dehydration
* Excessive dietary carbohydrates
* Hormonal deficiencies
* Improper breathing
* Inadequate sleep
* Poor fitness
* Poor nutrition
* Sunlight deficiency

Decreased E.Q. = Increased Aging and Disease

Whether it is a brain cell sparking a thought, or a stomach cell initiating your digestion, every aspect of your physiology is 100 percent dependent on aerobic energy production. Your liver is critically dependent on it, as is your hair and skin, your sex organs, your strength, your vision—*everything*.

Nothing is as important to your health and your experience of life as the energy you produce from oxygen. Without efficient aerobic energy production, your ability to think, move, reproduce, resist infection, detoxify yourself, or make a structural protein or enzyme is compromised. *You can't do anything.*

And, not surprisingly, every disorder that people develop as they age is associated with a low E.Q. This is why I have spent the last twenty years of my life researching how to both measure and improve E.Q. What I have learned through clinical experience, research, and feedback from my patients, I am now passing on to you.

Ever wonder why young people rarely develop disease despite their typical excesses, stress, lack of sleep, the worst of diets, and even smoking? How do they manage to stay out all night long and come back for more activity the next day? The answer ultimately lies in their incredible E.Q. Once you understand the factors involved in how your body uses oxygen to make energy, you will see how it is possible to maintain a youthful E.Q. even as you grow older—and thereby avoid disease; feel and function like a young person; and slow down the aging process.

The Oxygen Odyssey

All energy production starts with the sun. Its radiant energy is picked up by plants and, through a process called photosynthesis, is used to convert carbon dioxide into oxygen. This oxygen is then released into the air. All animals inhale the oxygen and convert it back to carbon dioxide. In the process, aerobic energy is produced.

Plants keep the process of life going by continually using the sun's energy to convert the carbon dioxide that is produced back into the oxygen that is crucial to life. So, next time you feel the sun's rays, or see a tree, be sure to offer thanks because all life on earth depends on them. If it were not for the plant kingdom's recycling of the carbon dioxide back into oxygen, all living creatures would have long ago used up all the planet's oxygen and become extinct.

Depending on where you live, the air you breathe contains from 20 to 23 percent oxygen. If you live in a metropolitan area, or at a high altitude, there will be less oxygen in the atmosphere. If you live at sea level, or in a rural area with lots of trees and vegetation, oxygen will be more abundant. No matter where you live, however, your body adapts to the level of oxygen that is present.

Step 1—Your Lungs

The first step in the utilization of oxygen is taking in a breath. This draws oxygen into the lungs where it can be picked up by the blood.

In this process, oxygen atoms bind to hemoglobin, a protein present in red blood cells. The oxygen is then transported by the hemoglobin to all the cells in the body. The more hemoglobin you have, the more oxygen you can take into your body.

Cigarette smoke and other forms of atmospheric pollution bind up a percentage of the hemoglobin and interfere with its ability to take up and carry oxygen. Smoking just one cigarette, for example, significantly reduces the oxygen-carrying capability of hemoglobin for about forty-eight hours.

Lung diseases, such as asthma, bronchitis, and emphysema, decrease the blood's ability to pick up oxygen from the lungs. Additionally, improper breathing is a very common cause of decreased oxygen uptake in the lungs (more about this in chapter 13). But assuming you don't have a lung disease, don't smoke, don't live or work in a contaminated environment, and you breathe correctly, you will be able to saturate your hemoglobin with oxygen. This is the first step in assuring yourself an optimal E.Q.

Step 2—Your Heart

From the lungs, your oxygenated blood then travels to the heart, which works nonstop to pump blood throughout your body. A heart that pumps optimally helps you meet your energy needs in two ways: first, by sending your oxygen-saturated blood out to your body's tissues; and second, by returning it to the lungs to pick up another load of oxygen. The heart's stroke volume is defined as the amount of blood pumped with each beat. Obviously, the heart is going to be able to deliver oxygen more efficiently when its stroke volume is optimal. In connection with this, the more you exercise, the greater your stroke volume.

The other important factor for optimal heart efficiency is the heart rate. The faster the heart is capable of beating, the more oxygen it can deliver. Both stroke volume and maximum heart rate decline with aging and with decreased fitness. Conversely, both improve with anti-aging therapy and fitness programs—another good reason to exercise.

Step 3—Your Arteries

In this delivery system, the heart is only half of the equation. Your arteries are the other half. It is the arterial system that carries the oxygen from the heart to the tissues and cells. Although your heart is a pump, unlike a centrifugal pump, which has a constant output, it pumps in beats. For maximum efficiency, therefore, the arteries need to be flexible so they can expand to accommodate the sudden increase in pressure when the heart pushes out a volume of blood. Then, when the heart relaxes between beats, the arteries must contract back to their original shape in preparation for the next beat.

This flexibility of the arteries is just as important to adequate circulation as the heart itself. When arteries lose flexibility and become constricted due to stress, aging, and other factors, the result is an elevation of blood pressure. This is why blood pressure goes up in most people as they get older.

The degree to which your blood pressure becomes higher than it was when you were younger is important. It reflects how much flexibility your arteries have lost. And even though your readings may still be in the so-called acceptable range, your circulation is compromised if they are higher than they used to be.

Although blood-pressure readings are a good indicator, there is now a more sensitive way to measure the loss of arterial flexibility. It is called arterial-stiffness measurement. Using these measurements, decreased arterial flexibility can show up even in those who have normal blood-pressure readings.

Additionally, because their stroke volume is so low, people with poorly conditioned hearts can have a normal blood pressure even when they have significant arterial stiffness. In these cases, their blood pressure may not become elevated until they begin to exercise.

When deposits of plaque develop on arterial walls, the condition is called atherosclerosis. Atherosclerosis results in hardening and narrowing of the arteries, which further chokes the blood supply. When this condition becomes advanced, it can set the stage for deadly heart attacks or strokes.

Compromised circulation is one of the most common causes of a decreased E.Q. in the over-fifty crowd.

Step 4—2,3 DPG

Your oxygenated blood courses through many thousands of miles of arteries and arterioles (smaller arteries) until it gets to the capillaries, which are the tiniest of all the blood vessels. The capillaries are where the real action is. It is in the capillaries that the hemoglobin will release the oxygen in order for it to be taken up by the cells. And, in this process, a special enzyme called 2,3 DPG becomes critical. This enzyme forces the hemoglobin to release its tight hold on oxygen. Without enough 2,3 DPG, the hemoglobin riding aboard the red blood cells would simply cruise right on past the cells and back to the heart without giving up its oxygen payload.

People who don't exercise regularly, or who have elevated insulin levels or diabetes, have decreased levels of 2,3 DPG. This makes their cells unable to obtain enough oxygen, even in the presence of the normal functioning of their lungs, heart, and arteries. Although their blood-oxygen levels may be quite normal, this can be very misleading. Because even though the oxygen is present, it can't get into the cells. And when oxygen can't get to the cells, you might as well be holding your breath.

Step 5—Your Mitochondria

The delivery addresses for oxygen in your body are the mitochondria located in the cells of your body. These microscopic structures are the power plants of the cells. Inside them, oxygen, carbohydrates, and fats are processed by special enzymes. This complex process leads to the production of the aerobic energy I have been talking about. Besides producing energy, the mitochondria also produce water and carbon dioxide as by-products.

The mitochondria are very complex structures influenced by diet, genetics, and hormones. As people age, these cellular dynamos become especially vulnerable to damage. Anti-aging experts believe that the decrease in energy production caused by damaged mitochondria is responsible for all the diseases, frailty, and infirmities so typical of the aging process.

How Your Mitochondria Are Undermined

Because of the importance of optimal mitochondrial function to your health, I want to focus on what causes mitochondria to operate less efficiently and eventually to lead to their destruction.

Decreased Fitness

The most critical factor in mitochondrial function is an adequate delivery of oxygen. This means there needs to be plenty of iron and hemoglobin, good lungs, adequate breathing, good heart function, flexible arteries, and plenty of 2,3 DPG. The key to all these factors being optimally maintained is regular, efficient exercise.

When people are sedentary and unfit, and especially if they smoke, they are dramatically decreasing the efficiency of their mitochondria. No wonder it is so uncommon to hear a person who exercises regularly complaining of poor energy. No wonder it is so uncommon to hear about a person who is in tip-top shape come down with a disease. In chapter 13, I go into great detail about how to exercise properly.

There is no question about it: lack of proper, regular exercise is the single "best" way to decrease mitochondrial efficiency. But there are many other factors that also undermine the mitochondria. By paying attention to all these factors, you can be sure that your mitochondria will be operating just as efficiently as they did when you were young, even as you grow very old.

Hormonal Deficiency

Your body has an inner intelligence that regulates all its functions. And no body function is more important than energy production. This is where hormones play their most important role: your body uses hormones to regulate energy production.

When the body needs more energy, certain hormones called catabolic hormones turn on cellular energy production just like a light switch turns on a light. If there is a deficiency in any of these hormones, the cells do not get turned on, and every one of the body's functions becomes impaired. The most important hormones for energy production are cortisol, growth hormones, progesterone, testosterone, insulin, and thyroid hormones. In chapter 15, I will tell you how you can keep these hormone levels youthful, even into old age.

Adrenal Insufficiency

Next to lack of exercise, the most common reason for decreased mitochondrial function is due to a shortage of glucose (sugar). This deficiency occurs as the result of poorly maintained blood-glucose levels—a condition referred to as hypoglycemia, or low blood sugar. Hypoglycemia is a condition, not a disease. It exists to one degree or another in just about everyone with any medical disorder. It can even be found in healthy people, and it is the single most common cause of fatigue.

Every cell in the body has the ability to create energy from either glucose or fat. Every cell, that is, except brain cells. For the most part, brain cells can only utilize glucose. Therefore, low blood glucose affects the brain far more than it does the other organ systems, and it is a very common cause of brain dysfunction.

Because blood glucose is so important, the body is blessed with two glands which see to it that adequate glucose levels are maintained at all times. These glands are called the adrenal glands. They are located just above your kidneys on either side of your mid-back. The adrenal glands are quite small; but don't worry, they pack a very big wallop.

If you are exercising and rapidly using up your blood-glucose levels, your adrenal glands will secrete just the right amount of the hormones hydrocortisone and adrenalin. These hormones will see to it that the levels remain rock-steady. Even in conditions of starvation, your adrenal glands will make sure that your body has an adequate supply of glucose. No matter what the circumstances, through the action of hydrocortisone and adrenalin your adrenal glands will be there for you to make sure that your cells are getting as much glucose as they need. That is, until they become exhausted.

Exhausted adrenal glands is the most common disorder doctors see. When I give lectures to doctors about how to make sure their patients are producing adequate levels of energy, I ask the question "How can you tell if your patient has exhausted adrenal glands?" I then give the answer. "Because they are in your office." This is because no matter what problem their body is dealing with, most people can get by until their adrenal glands become overtaxed. Once the adrenals become exhausted, however, blood-sugar levels can no longer be maintained, and their body quickly feels the effects. It is then that they usually decide it is time to see the doctor.

Symptoms such as ADD (attention deficit disorder), anxiety, depression, headaches, hyperactivity, insomnia, low energy, moodiness, and poor mental clarity and concentration are usually just side effects of adrenal exhaustion. Unfortunately, this is a diagnosis that is too often missed by conventional physicians.

And, all too often, many of the remedies that people use to self-medicate the early symptoms of adrenal fatigue involve alcohol, coffee, or sugar. And although they do help temporarily, persistent use of them only serves to further weaken the adrenals.

The ultimate result of adrenal exhaustion is decreased energy production. This is especially noticeable when exercising. Because as long as the body is at rest, the mitochondria (in all cells except brain cells) can meet their energy needs from fat. But every cell relies heavily on glucose metabolism during exercise.

So, a hallmark of early adrenal insufficiency is normal energy at rest with a decrease in exercise tolerance. As the adrenals further weaken, however, low energy will be felt even when not exercising. Although there are many causes of fatigue, the fatigue of adrenal exhaustion can be recognized by the fact that it is much worse in the afternoon hours. This is due to the natural rhythm of adrenal function, which causes the glands to have a high level of activity in the morning that decreases as the day progresses.

Adrenal insufficiency results from chronic stress and excessive carbohydrate consumption. Let's take stress first.

Adrenal insufficiency from stress. Most physicians will tell you that, more than any other single factor, disease is caused by stress. This is because stress depletes the adrenal glands, and depleted adrenals add up to low energy production.

Stress comes from many sources and in many forms—mental and emotional, allergies, dehydration, drugs and pharmaceuticals, illness, inadequate rest, infections, injuries, nutrient deficiencies, pain, sunlight deficiency, or toxins. Thanks to the adrenal glands, the body is well equipped to deal with all these stresses. As the various stressors act to put the body into a state of imbalance, the adrenals produce hormones that put it back on track. As long as the stress load isn't too severe, or doesn't last too long, the adrenals can do their jobs. Too much stress, however, eventually results in fatigued and exhausted adrenal glands.

The late Hans Selye, MD, who pioneered the understanding of how stress contributes to disease, confirmed in experiments how prolonged stress gradually wears out the adrenals. When this happens, they are unable to produce an adequate amount of their anti-stress hormones. Since the primary function of the adrenal hormones is to maintain a healthy glucose level, the end result of chronically overworked adrenals is low blood sugar. This, in turn, results in more stress in the form of decreased energy production, further depleting the adrenals, and an exceptional craving for carbohydrates since eating carbohydrates increases blood sugar levels.

Adrenal insufficiency from diet. Unfortunately, although eating carbohydrates does act to raise the blood sugar, the adrenal glands, and hence your energy production, are compromised by a diet too high in carbohydrates. By this, I mean sugar (white and brown sugar, honey, corn syrup, molasses, etc.); food items made from grains such as corn, rice, and wheat; fruits (particularly fruit juice); tubers (beets, potatoes, yams, carrots, etc.); and to a lesser degree, beans. Carbohydrates such as these rapidly elevate your blood sugar. This is especially true when they are consumed without adequate protein and fat to decrease their blood-sugar-elevating effect.

From what I have already said about low blood sugar, you might think eating foods that raise blood sugar would be a good thing. But you'd be wrong. A rising blood sugar level causes the pancreas to secrete the hormone insulin. Insulin acts to lower the blood sugar. This stresses the adrenal glands, since in order to prevent insulin from lowering the blood sugar too much, they will now have to produce hormones to raise the blood sugar and counteract this effect of insulin. This is how a diet too high in carbohydrates, through the action of insulin, will weaken and eventually exhaust the adrenal glands.

The Wrong Fats

So far, you have learned three ways in which mitochondrial energy production can be decreased: decreased fitness, hormonal deficiency, and adrenal exhaustion. Another way is by eating the wrong kinds of fats. This is because a diet high in the wrong kinds of fats decreases the function of the cell's membranes—both the outer cell membrane and the mitochondrial membrane. Let's look at the effect of dietary fats on the outer cell membrane first.

Each cell has special gateway sites called receptors on the surface of its outer membrane. These receptors are critical to all cellular activities, including energy production. They must be working well in order for the cell to take in fat, glucose, and nutrients. They are also critical for the functioning of hormones and other messenger molecules.

Receptors are extremely complicated structures, and there is a great deal that is not yet known about how they function. One thing medical researchers do know is that they are very much affected by the kinds of fats we eat—particularly the kind of polyunsaturated fats. The polyunsaturated fats in our diet determine the makeup and function of cell membranes. And since the receptors reside on membranes, their ability to function well is dependent on the composition of the membranes.

Up until fifty or sixty years ago, our diets provided us primarily with only one kind of polyunsaturated fats, called CIS fats. These are the fats that make up healthy functioning cell membranes. The other kind are known as trans fats. Trans fats occur naturally in some foods, but only in extremely low amounts. The overwhelming amount of trans fats that are found in today's modern diets are not there naturally. They are the result of food processing.

Food processing refers to "foods" that were created in a factory by man, instead of by nature. An important part of food processing involves separating out the fats that are found in a food from the rest of the nutrients in the food. An example would be taking the CIS fat oils out of the safflower seed to produce safflower oil. The problem with doing this is that when the fats are separated from the other protective nutrients in the plant, they become very susceptible to rancidity. So susceptible that the shelf life of the products that are then manufactured from them is extremely short. In only a matter of days, the fats in the products will become rancid.

So when commercially processed foods began to proliferate in the early 1900s, manufacturers needed to find a method to protect the fats from rancidity. The method they discovered involved chemically treating the CIS fats with hydrogen, a process known as hydrogenation. The first commercial example of hydrogenated fats was Crisco. Although this treatment process completely destroyed the nutritional benefits normally derived from these fats, it did protect the fats from rancidity.

Hydrogenation offered a long shelf life, and it offered the food manufacturers who used hydrogenated fats a better bottom line.

The problem with hydrogenating fats is that in the process of doing that, as much as 45 percent of the CIS fats are converted to trans fats. And so the delicate natural balance of fats as they are found in nature—primarily CIS fats with only very little trans fats—becomes completely turned around. This dramatically affects the function of the cell's membranes, because the shift in the fat balance found in the diet causes a similar shift in the composition of the fats in the membranes. And researchers have shown that membranes contaminated with trans fats cannot function efficiently.

Unfortunately, hydrogenated trans fats have now become a major part of the American diet. The National Academy of Sciences (NAS) advises the United States and Canadian governments on nutritional science for use in public policy and product labeling programs. Their 2002 publication, the *Dietary Reference Intakes for Energy, Carbohydrate, Fiber, Fat, Fatty Acids, Cholesterol, Protein, and Amino Acids* contains their findings and recommendations regarding the consumption of trans fats. The NAS concluded that "trans fatty acids are not essential and provide no known benefit to human health." They further stated that there is no safe level for eating trans fats. This viewpoint has been supported by a 2006 *New England Journal of Medicine* scientific review that states "from a nutritional standpoint, the consumption of trans fatty acids results in considerable potential harm but no apparent benefit."

You can identify these harmful fats by looking at the ingredient label to see if it contains the words *hydrogenated* or *partially hydrogenated*—for example, hydrogenated soy oil, or partially hydrogenated safflower oil.

Trans-fatty acids are harmful to the cells in two ways. First, they undermine the integrity of membrane receptors. Nothing gets into the cells except through the action of these receptors. And the energetic effect of hormones, which is so crucial for efficient mitochondrial function, depends completely on the cell receptors. And second, because of their effects on the function of the mitochondrial membranes, trans fats block the ability of the mitochondria to produce energy. Scientists refer to this effect as "uncoupling," because it uncouples the production of energy from the metabolism of oxygen.

The bottom line? A diet containing trans fats can markedly affect how cells function, resulting in a significant decrease in mitochondrial energy production.

Inefficient Fat Utilization

For the purpose of clarity, in the remainder of this book I will refer to glucose metabolism as carbohydrate metabolism. Technically, glucose is only one example of a carbohydrate. But since all carbohydrates must be broken down to glucose before they can be absorbed and used for energy, I think it is easier to refer to carbohydrates instead of always referring to glucose.

All cells, with the major exception of brain cells, prefer burning fat rather than carbohydrate (glucose) for energy. The body was designed this way because fat is more efficiently stored, was much more available in the pre-supermarket days, and produces less acid waste than carbohydrate.

People have been led to believe that dietary fat makes body fat, but this is only half the truth. In fact, both dietary carbohydrate and dietary fat make body fat.

It works like this. When you eat, only a fraction of the food is used immediately for energy—most of it is stored as fat. That's right. If you eat carbohydrates, they get stored as fat. And if you eat fat, it gets stored as fat. Either way, your body will store the energy content of your foods as fat. And that's a good thing.

Fat storage allows us to go long times between meals and still maintain good energy production. That is, as long as the stored fat can be easily accessed.

The body can all too easily store fat. But certain factors make it hard for it to break down that stored fat to be converted to energy. The primary factor that blocks the release of stored fat for energy is carbohydrate intake. That's right: the more carbohydrate you eat, the less fat you will burn.

Another major factor is eating itself. The more often you eat, the less stored fat you will burn. So, intermittent or occasional fasting is another good way to make sure your body is burning fat efficiently. I'll talk more about that in chapter 12.

A third factor is hormonal deficiencies, particularly deficiencies of testosterone, the growth hormones, and the thyroid hormones. I will cover the importance of hormones in chapter 15.

The ability to break down stored fat and get it to the mitochondria to be burned by oxygen for energy production is referred to as fat utilization. Poor fat utilization leads to poor oxygen utilization, which ultimately results in decreased energy production. This is one of the most common causes of a decreased E.Q.

An additional problem here is that the body can only store a very small amount of carbohydrate. Carbohydrate is stored in molecules called glycogen. When stored fat cannot be adequately utilized, the body has to rely ever more on its stores of glycogen. And, because we can only store a small amount of glycogen, within a matter of hours the carbohydrate reserves become exhausted. This results in a falling blood-sugar level. When the blood-sugar level gets low enough, the adrenal glands step in to try to restore normality. If this scenario is repeated too often, it will ultimately stress the adrenal glands enough to cause the adrenal insufficiency described above.

Carnitine Deficiency

Early humans ate a diet high in meat. Very high in meat. Which meant they had an abundant intake of amino acids, the components of protein. And one of the most vital of these amino acids is carnitine. Researchers estimate that early man took in around 5,000 to 10,000 milligrams of carnitine per day. Currently, the average intake among Westerners is more like 100 milligrams.

Why? Because carnitine is found only in animal protein, and contemporary diets have shifted away from animal protein and toward carbohydrates.

In the body, carnitine is converted into an enzyme called carnitine transferase. This enzyme is responsible for transporting fats into the mitochondria for energy production. Diets low in carnitine result in low levels of carnitine transferase in the body, and a deficiency of this enzyme—common now because of carbohydrate-heavy diets—compromises fat-burning capability.

A deficiency of carnitine can result in a significant decrease in mitochondrial function. A commonly seen indicator of carnitine deficiency is the combination of fatigue, weight gain, and an elevation in the blood of certain fats called triglycerides.

Vitamin and Mineral Deficiencies

Once fat and/or glucose are introduced into the mitochondria, they enter into an assembly-line process that eventually produces energy. In what is called the Krebs cycle (also known as the citric acid cycle), hydrogen atoms are removed from the fat and glucose molecules. These hydrogen atoms are then combined with oxygen to make water and energy. In order for the Krebs cycle to function efficiently, optimum amounts of key amino acids, vitamins, and minerals are required.

The most important nutrients are the B vitamins (especially B_{12}, B_6, niacin, and riboflavin), certain amino acids, and the minerals chromium and magnesium. These nutrients can easily become depleted when the body is stressed or the diet is poor. The result is decreased energy production.

Coenzyme Q_{10} Deficiency

Coenzyme Q_{10}, CoQ_{10} for short, is a vitamin-like substance that is absolutely necessary for cellular energy production. As I mentioned above, after the Krebs cycle removes the hydrogen atoms from fat and glucose, they are combined with oxygen to form water and energy. This process is known as cellular respiration. The first enzyme in this process is CoQ_{10}. As people age, they become deficient in CoQ_{10}. Additionally, a poor diet can cause a deficiency. A deficiency of this vital enzyme will greatly limit mitochondrial function.

Mitochondrial Decay

Obviously, to the degree that the mitochondria become destroyed, the entire energy process suffers. Scientists refer to this process as mitochondrial decay. Mitochondrial decay is known to occur universally in all humans as we age.

One cause of mitochondrial decay is exposure to harmful chemicals, such as pesticides. But a more frequently occurring problem comes from the long-term impact of what are known as heavy metals. The most common heavy metals in question are aluminum, arsenic, cadmium, lead, and mercury. The level of these metals in the environment has dramatically increased in the past 150 years as a direct result of industrialization. They have crept into the water and food supply to such an extent that it is simply impossible to avoid them.

Elevated levels of mercury have crept into tuna and other fish to the extent that public health authorities in some areas of the country have warned against eating more than two fish a month because of the mercury content. Additionally, the mercury contained in silver dental fillings, the most common dental filling material, has been shown to leak into the body and accumulate.

What has now become a routine source of exposure to heavy metals is the increasing use of vaccines. Most vaccines are manufactured with and contain aluminum and/or mercury.

Arsenic, lead, and cadmium are now routinely found in the food and water supply in this country. Well water and tap water from the faucets of older high-rise buildings can be especially problematic. Even if your current water supply is clean, you may have toxic levels in your body as a result of drinking contaminated water years ago. An exposure to heavy metals will often still be present in the body many years later, because they are very poorly eliminated from the body.

But of all the factors that lead to mitochondrial decay, the most influential one is decreased energy production. Stay with me on this, because in the next chapter I'm going to do more than just explain how this can happen. I'm also going to show you that in all likelihood, unless you have been doing something about it, your own mitochondria are traveling down the road to destruction even as you read this book.

✳ 3 ✳

ENERGY AND AGING

What Is Aging?

Before I get into what causes aging, let me first define what I mean by the word. Misunderstanding the meaning behind the word *aging* often leads to a lot of confusion, even among physicians. As most people use it, the word *aging* is synonymous with getting older. In other words, it is an inevitable consequence of celebrating birthdays. You get older, you age. Simple. Using this definition, any discussion about decreasing or reversing aging becomes ludicrous.

But in the medical sense, the word *aging* takes on a slightly different meaning. Because in medicine, aging is defined as the decrease in the ability of the body to function efficiently associated with getting older. Using this definition, a person will age only to the extent that his or her body is functioning less efficiently. Let me give you an example of how this works.

Let's look at the case of a typical twenty-year-old man. Ten years later, on his thirtieth birthday, he is ten years older. People using the usual definition of aging would say that he has aged ten years. But if he is typical of most young men, no decrease in his body's ability to function efficiently has occurred. Therefore, from a medical standpoint, he has not aged at all.

Okay, so how about when he reaches forty: Will he have aged by then? Again, the functional difference between a thirty-year-old and a forty-year-old is virtually nil. And so, using the medical definition of aging, he still has not aged, even though he has now celebrated forty birthdays.

Using this functional definition of aging, you can begin to see that aging is not purely a matter of getting older. It is very possible, indeed quite common, to get older and yet show no signs of aging. But let's continue with this same example.

What about when this man reaches fifty? Surely by then he will have some measurable decrease in his body's functional efficiency. And the answer is: of course he will. I don't know of any fifty-year-old man with a body that functions every bit as well as it did when he was twenty. So, finally, by the age of fifty, we are pretty much sure to find at least some evidence of aging in all of us. Aging is certainly inevitable, provided we live long enough. We can't do much about that. But what is not inevitable is the rate at which we age. And that is what anti-aging medicine is all about.

And as we age, we will develop what are known as "age-related symptoms." These are the symptoms that result as the body begins to lose its functional efficiency. In other words, age-related symptoms are not caused by a disease or a psychological condition. Another way of putting it is that you can have all the following symptoms and be "perfectly healthy for your age."

Common age-related symptoms include vision and hearing impairment; anxiety, depression, and insomnia; weakness, fatigue, and decreased stamina; increased body fat; decreased muscle and bone; decreased sexual desire and function; dry, loose, wrinkled skin, and age spots; and decreased memory, mental speed, and clarity. In addition to these symptoms, aging also renders us significantly more susceptible to cancer, cardiovascular disease, osteoporosis, Alzheimer's, dementia, and all the other diseases that are so common as we get older.

What Causes Aging?

There have been dozens of theories attempting to explain what causes the decrease in function that defines the aging process. These include the free-radical theory, the Hayflick-limit theory, the neuro-endocrine theory, the mitochondrial-decay theory, the telomerase theory, and the wear-and-tear theory, just to mention a few. For a good descriptive synopsis of all the various theories of aging, refer to *Stopping the Clock*, an excellent book on anti-aging medicine by Drs. Ronald Klatz and Robert Goldman.

Each theory has its own special attraction and logic. And each theory leads to a particular line of therapy designed to retard or reverse aging. But a very practical problem that all theories of aging have in common is that their effects can't be measured. So there is no good way to determine whether the therapies stemming from any of these theories are actually working.

If you adhere to the free-radical theory of aging, for example, you believe that aging is caused by a certain class of molecules called free radicals. Proponents of this theory believe that by decreasing the amount of these molecules, it is possible to slow down the aging process. But since we are unable to measure the amount of free-radical damage in either an animal or a person, it's impossible to determine if any given line of therapy is actually decreasing it—and hence impossible to validate whether or not the theory actually holds water.

Similarly, those who believe in the telomerase theory have the same problem. They believe that aging is the result of accumulated damage in the end section of a chromosome called the telomere. Telomeres protect the genetic code from being altered during the cell's replication cycle. Therefore, damage to the telomeres will result in loss of genetic code, ultimately causing aging. Unfortunately, although there are laboratories that measure the telomere length of white blood cells, there is no way to know if these tests indicate the telomere length in other cells. Also, it can take years between telomere tests to see if the telomeres are actually stabilizing.

Regrettably, the sobering truth is that each and every theory of aging is plagued with the same curse: *there is no good way to determine whether or not it actually has value in the real world.*

The Energy-Deficit Theory of Aging

One of the best-studied aspects of the aging process is that the older a person is, the less capable he is of making energy. To use my terminology, the older you are, the lower your E.Q. becomes. According to the mitochondrial-decay theory of aging, this decrease in energy production is caused by the destruction of the mitochondria. In other words, as you age and you lose your mitochondria, you will not be able to produce energy as efficiently—which is to say, *aging causes low energy production.*

My research, using Bio-Energy Testing, has led me to a radical departure from this conventional assumption. The results of my experience after testing and improving the energy production of hundreds of individuals has led me to formulate an entirely new model of what causes aging, one that offers a unique perspective on aging and what can be done about it.

In short, my new model is this: The decrease in energy production that is observed in all aging animals and humans is not only a result of aging; it is also the *cause* of aging—which is to say, *low energy production causes aging* rather than the other way around. Put another way: to the extent that an individual can maintain optimum energy production as he or she grows older, that person will not age.

Take a look at how this new idea of mine, which I call the Energy-Deficit Theory, explains all the other theories of aging.

The Telomere Theory

According to the Energy-Deficit Theory, it's not that damaged telomeres result in aging and decreased energy production. Rather, it is decreased energy production that leads to damaged telomeres and aging. How? When telomeres become damaged, as they routinely do during the cell's replication cycle, they are repaired by telomerase enzymes. These enzymes are 100 percent dependent on energy production. In the absence of adequate energy production, telomerase enzymes can't be fully effective, and the result is damage to the telomere.

The Free-Radical Theory

According to the Energy-Deficit Theory, it's not free radicals that cause aging and decreased energy production; it's decreased energy production that leads to free-radical damage and aging. How? Free radicals are natural by-products of normal energy production. But when energy production becomes less efficient, free-radical production escalates dramatically. Combine this with the fact that free radicals are reduced by certain enzyme systems called antioxidant enzymes. And, as with all enzymes, the synthesis of, the maintenance of, and the function of these antioxidant enzymes are completely dependent on energy production. Therefore, when energy production is decreased, antioxidant enzyme function is decreased, and free-radical-induced tissue destruction escalates.

The Neuro-Endocrine Theory

This theory states that aging is caused by a natural decrease in the sensitivity of hormone receptors in the brain. Proponents have evidence that this results in decreased hormone production, which in turn leads to aging and decreased energy levels. But hormone receptors are 100 percent dependent on energy production in order to function. Therefore, according to the Energy-Deficit Theory, it is an initial decrease in energy production that causes the decreased receptor sensitivity, which results in the decreased hormone production that is so much a part of the aging process. So it's not the decreased receptor sensitivity of the neuro-endocrine theory of aging that leads to aging and decreased energy production; rather, it's decreased energy production that *causes* the decreased receptor sensitivity.

The Mitochondrial-Decay Theory

This theory states that the decrease in energy production seen with aging is a result of irreversible damage to the mitochondria, called mitochondrial decay. But long before there is any actual mitochondrial decay, there is already a measurable decrease in energy production. This decrease stems from a combination of all the factors discussed in the previous chapter. And, according to the Energy-Deficit Theory, it is precisely this early decrease in energy production that ultimately leads to mitochondrial decay and aging. I will describe how this happens in the next section.

A Unifying Theory of Aging

No matter what theory of aging you examine, it can invariably be explained as secondary to decreased energy production. This is one of the most compelling and attractive aspects of the Energy-Deficit Theory. It can explain *all* the phenomena that have led other investigators to arrive at each of the other theories of aging. This makes the Energy-Deficit Theory the *only* central unifying theory of aging.

The Energy Deficit Comes First

In a paper that was published in the *American Academy of Anti-Aging Medicine Yearbook* titled, "The Energy Deficit Theory of Aging and Disease," (see appendix C), I describe a condition I discovered, which I call EOMD. EOMD is short for early-onset mitochondrial dysfunction. It refers to a deterioration of mitochondrial function that leads to decreased energy production.

This condition is commonly found in young, healthy people and becomes even more prevalent with age. Deterioration of mitochondrial function is not the same as mitochondrial decay. The latter refers to the actual destruction of the mitochondria, whereas deteriorated mitochondrial function means that the mitochondria are still there and intact—they are just not producing energy efficiently.

To investigate just how common EOMD is, I reported on fifty young people between the ages of twenty and forty who were being tested at one of several clinics routinely using Bio-Energy Testing. Each person was free of disease and felt great. They were just having the test in order to make sure that their health program was working. The results were as follows:

* 54 percent (27) had normal mitochondrial function
* 46 percent (23) had EOMD (< 100 percent of predicted mitochondrial function)
* 36 percent (18) had < 90 percent of predicted mitochondrial function
* 26 percent (13) had < 80 percent of predicted mitochondrial function
* 12 percent (6) had < 60 percent of predicted mitochondrial function, and fell within the diagnostic category of severe dysfunction

The results of the study confirmed that close to half of these young people were already showing evidence of EOMD. A quarter of them had less than 80 percent of what was expected from healthy, young people. And a surprising 12 percent of them were in the diagnostic category of severe mitochondrial dysfunction.

These test subjects were much too young to have mitochondrial decay, free-radical damage, telomere damage, or any other effects of the aging process. And they were much too healthy to have cardiovascular disease—or any other disease, for that matter. Yet, an alarmingly high number of them had evidence of a measurable decrease in their mitochondrial function, leading to significant decrease in energy production.

The only conclusion that can be drawn from these data is that mitochondrial decay, free-radical damage, telomere damage, and all the other consequences of aging and degenerative disease are *preceded* by a decrease in mitochondrial function—EOMD. Furthermore, this decrease can often be severe, and can occur in the absence of any warning symptoms.

EOMD, therefore, refers more to a deterioration of mitochondrial function in the absence of true mitochondrial decay. This distinction is important because while mitochondrial decay is irreversible, the treatment of people with EOMD reveals that it is completely reversible.

And You Can Measure It

The Energy-Deficit Theory is not only a unifying theory of aging. As is shown in the study mentioned above, it is also verifiable. As a doctor who actually works with real people every day, by far the most exciting thing about this theory is that it can be routinely tested and measured. Using the Bio-Energy Testing technology (see chapter 7), doctors are now able to determine whether or not a person has EOMD without having to wait for either symptoms or disease to show up first.

This new model of thinking has led to some profound and very practical implications. Instead of breaking down all the symptoms of aging into their many tiny components, I can simply ask one question: How can I increase this person's energy production to match that of a younger person?

For example, if a certain herb is shown to increase energy production in a particular individual, then I know it will decrease his rate of aging. Similarly, if a particular practice, such as meditation or sunbathing, can increase energy production, then it will also slow down aging.

Using this newfound capability, I have been able to discover what remedies and practices increase energy production and which ones seem to have little effect. In this way, I don't have to guess if a particular diet, therapy, or practice is going to slow down an individual's aging process. If it works to increase their energy production, that's all I need to know.

Individualizing an Anti-aging Program

We are all different. We all respond differently to various diets, exercises, medications, nutrients, and other therapies. So the simple fact that a particular program works to slow down the aging process in one person doesn't necessarily mean that it will be effective in another person. We have to have a way of determining what therapies are working in each individual person. That's another reason why Bio-Energy Testing is so critical.

If I put so-and-so on a program that ultimately improves his E.Q., I know the program is working as advertised. If it doesn't increase his E.Q., then I know we are wasting our time and money, and it's on to

Plan B. When you are testing something regularly, you don't have to wait until bad things happen to realize that what you thought was going to work, in fact, did not.

The Energy-Deficit Theory in Action

I believe that mitochondrial-energy production is the single most important aspect of health, aging, and degenerative disease. But don't just take my word for it: the medical literature is loaded with proof.

Take, for example, an article that appeared in 2000, titled "Meta-analysis of the Age Associated Decline in Maximal Aerobic Capacity in Men: Relation to Training Status." This research paper dramatically demonstrates the relationship between health and mitochondrial efficiency.

In the article, using technology very similar to Bio-Energy Testing, the researchers determined the aerobic capacity in men who exercised extensively, and compared it to men who did not exercise as much. Aerobic capacity means the maximum amount of energy production that can be produced by the mitochondria. It is just another term for E.Q.

According to the authors, "Maximal aerobic capacity [a really excellent E.Q.] is an independent risk factor for cardiovascular disease, cognitive dysfunction, and all cause mortality." This is medicalese for "Your E.Q. will determine your likelihood of getting heart disease, dementia, and every other disease that can kill you." And it will determine this risk independent of any other factors including smoking, diet, cholesterol levels, or anything else. This is a very powerful statement.

Then they addressed the subject of aging in particular. According to their findings, although most aspects of aging can be reversed with physical-fitness training, "there continued to be a significant decline in aerobic capacity" even in health-conscious, endurance-trained men as they got older. In other words, there is no better assessment of aging than optimal mitochondrial efficiency as determined by E.Q. All the other measurements of aging such as insulin resistance, body-mass composition, bone density, cardiovascular function, etc., can be reversed by training. Therefore, they are simply measurements of conditioning, not of aging per se. On the other hand, a person's E.Q. cannot be trained away. And therefore, it represents the best measurement of health and aging.

In another article, using a different technique, the researchers examined the mitochondrial efficiency in twenty-nine men and women of different ages. Some of them were as young as sixteen years old. And some were in their nineties. They noticed a significant and consistent decline in mitochondrial efficiency with age. Across the board, the older a person was, the lower their E.Q was.

The scientific literature is loaded with studies like these. And every single one demonstrates the integral role that decreased mitochondrial efficiency plays in the aging process. Some of them even show how certain cell functions shut down as a result of decreased mitochondrial efficiency. These functions include the ability of the body to detoxify itself, to repair damaged tissues, to reproduce DNA, and to maintain its water balance and even its higher-order processes such as thinking and remembering.

The Proof

Two recently published studies prove that decreased mitochondrial energy production is the primary cause of aging. In the first study, the mitochondria of certain mice were genetically altered to self-destruct much faster than normal. The researchers then compared these altered mice to mice with normal mitochondria. By now you can probably guess what happened: the normal mice lived much longer than the ones with the rapidly deteriorating mitochondria. That was because their mitochondria were functioning much better. But what was even more astonishing: the altered mice not only died sooner, but they also showed all the signs of aging at a much earlier age. In other words, they were aging prematurely.

They developed all the signs of aging, such as muscle loss, hair loss, degenerated joints, anemia, osteoporosis, reduced fertility, and heart enlargement. But they developed them at a much younger age.

The authors concluded that the results of the study very clearly demonstrated how decreased mitochondrial function causes aging.

In a different study, scientists measured the resting mitochondrial function in a group of mice. They then observed the mice over the course of their lifespan. They then compared how long each mouse lived to what its mitochondrial function was. The mice with the highest mitochondrial efficiency lived 36 percent longer than the mice with the lowest.

Experiments such as these provide proof that aging and longevity are simply a matter of energy production. If you want to live a long time and be fully functional and healthy, you'd better make sure that your mitochondria are functioning optimally.

Everyone agrees that unless you die young, aging itself is inevitable. At some point in time, whenever that may be, if you live long enough, you will become feeble and then die. However, the dramatic rate and extent of aging that is commonly seen today is not inevitable.

There is no reason at all that, barring serious genetic disorders, each and every one of us can't live to be at least 110 years old and be fully functional. The secret? As you grow older, be sure that you do whatever it takes to maintain youthful mitochondrial function. More than anything else, the rate and extent of aging depends on it.

This is also true of all the diseases that occur as we get older, such as Parkinson's, Alzheimer's, diabetes, cancer, and heart disease. The literature is very clear: the single best way to prevent the diseases of aging is to maximize mitochondrial function.

But Is It Really Possible?

In June of 2000, I was invited as a speaker at the First International Learning Conference on Anti-Aging Medicine in Monte Carlo, Monaco. My subject was how to set up an anti-aging clinic.

There was a fairly large contingency of physicians from China, where the government is interested in establishing a network of such clinics. During the question-and-answer session following my talk, one of these physicians asked me if I really thought it was possible to halt, and even reverse, the aging process.

My response was that it is not only possible, but, in fact, I was already doing it in my clinic in Nevada. I then explained my theory that the single best determinant of aging is the measurement of how efficiently an individual is able to produce energy.

I went on to describe how, with proper testing, it is now possible to measure anyone's energy-production efficiency (their E.Q.) quickly, easily, and with great precision. "With this method," I told them, "I have found that many of my sixty- and seventy-year-old patients [who follow the anti-aging guidelines discussed in this book] are now producing energy as efficiently as a forty-year-old. I believe that these people have literally slowed down aging to a snail's pace."

Someone once said that as soon as you are born, you start dying. This isn't quite true, because the dying part doesn't really start until somewhere around the age of forty, but the point is well taken nonetheless. After age forty, unless something is done about it, the body's cells enter into deterioration mode, and with time, the rate of decline accelerates. This is called aging.

Have you ever asked yourself how and when you want to die? If you haven't, I think you should. The reason is this. What you are doing (or not doing) today, right now, is going to determine just that. If you want to live a long and fully functional life, the time to get going is now, *before* you experience the symptoms of aging. It is never too late to start, but sooner is better than later.

Someday I will die, but until then I want to live as healthy and vibrant a life as possible. I don't want arthritis, cancer, dementia, diabetes, or heart disease. I especially don't want the feebleness and frailty that is often considered an inevitable part of hitting the eighties and nineties. And throughout my professional life, it is this strong desire that has compelled me to discover as much as I can about the aging process. How to slow it down, and how to prevent the diseases of aging. I now know that, to a very large extent—barring an accident or an act of violence—we are able to determine not only how and when we will die, but—more importantly—how long and how well we will live.

The Golden Years?

A patient once told me that the golden years were when you needed more gold. More gold to pay for doctors, medications, and nursing homes. This concept of what it's like to get old is so universal that when I first began to discuss the idea of living longer forty-some-odd years ago, many people would say that they were just not interested.

"I'll deal with that later," they often say. "Why bother myself with that while I am still feeling well? I want to focus on the positive. And besides, no one wants to live forever."

True, no one wants to live forever. But just about everyone would like to live their golden years free of the diseases and frailties that so commonly characterize this end-of-life period. Free to feel young, be employed, serve mankind, go fishing with great-great-grandchildren, hike up a mountain, have sex, maybe even go back to school—or just be free to really enjoy another beautiful day.

It seems that Mother Nature really plays a dirty trick on everyone. She weakens and deteriorates people just when they have gained the wisdom and experience to really appreciate the beauty that life has to offer. Just as they are realizing more and more what a wonderful blessing life can be, they are rudely interrupted by a damaged heart and the need for someone to drive them to the cardiologist.

Me, 100 Years Old!?

They say you could live to be more than a hundred years old. And they're right. According to the World Health Organization, "There have been more gains in life expectancy in the last fifty years than in the previous five thousand years."

The U.S. Census Bureau has gone on record as saying that "by the year 2025 there will be two sixty-five-year-olds for every teenager in America." So the odds are looking better and better that you will live to be quite old. The question then becomes: what do you want it to be like, and what can you do about it?

Recent advances in medical research have shown that much of the mental and physical decline traditionally perceived as the inevitable consequence of aging can be delayed, prevented, and often even reversed. Many doctors are realizing that aging is a treatable condition, just like any other physical disorder.

The diseases associated with aging are preventable. So, too, is the functional decline in mental and physical ability. The disabilities that we have been so used to seeing in older people do not have to be a part of our lives.

Perhaps the best news is that achieving these benefits is becoming easier. Moreover, you don't have to be rich to make the golden years really golden.

✱ 4 ✱

ENERGY AND DISEASE

*"They always say time changes things,
but you actually have to change them yourself."*

—Andy Warhol

Einstein once said that the definition of insanity is repeating the same thing over and over again and expecting a different result. If that's the case, then our current system of internal medicine is clearly insane.

The NIH went on record years ago stating that the evidence is that 85 to 90 percent of all chronic diseases can be avoided with a healthy lifestyle. So, if they are right, if the way you live has brought you to the diagnosis of a disease, then according to Dr. Einstein it would be insane to treat the disease and expect a different result without changing the way you live. That is, unless you want to keep the disease. If you want to keep the disease, it makes good sense to keep on living the same way.

But I can't completely blame the medical system for this insanity. Much of the blame must go to human nature. Human nature makes people lazy and resistant to change. Human nature makes people want that bypass surgery, and gets them to somehow deny that unless they change the way they live, they'll be having another one in five or six years.

Human nature says, "I don't want to do anything that could make me healthier if it is not covered by insurance."

Human nature says, "Doc, just please cure me. Cut the problem out. Give me that magic pill, and don't tell me I have to change anything. I want to be healthy and still maintain the same lifestyle that made me sick in the first place."

But let's assume you are not that person. What are the various factors that go into causing disease?

Atherosclerosis

Arteriosclerosis develops when blood vessels become hard, stiff, and inflexible. If this occurs in the major arteries leading to the heart, brain, and legs, the consequences can be serious and life-threatening.

Atherosclerosis is a term adopted from the Greek words *athero* (paste) and *sclerosis* (hardness). The Greeks had it right. In this condition, plaque deposits form on the inner lining of the arteries. They are made from fat, mostly cholesterol, and then become hardened by the deposition of calcium. The result is a hardening and narrowing of the arteries and the reduction of vital blood flow.

This reduction in circulation deprives cells throughout the body of oxygen and essential nutrients. When this process becomes advanced in arteries leading to the heart, you can develop chest pain (angina) and heart attacks—the number one killer. When the process involves arteries leading to the brain, or small arteries within the brain, you can develop a stroke or senility.

Atherosclerosis is also a major contributor to premature aging, because the decrease in circulation means that less oxygen and nutrients are reaching the cells for energy production.

Scientific evidence indicates that atherosclerosis is completely preventable. *When I say completely, I mean 100 percent.*

With what we currently know, this condition—and all the diseases associated with it—can be completely eradicated. But to understand how to eliminate the problem, you must first have an understanding of what causes it.

What Causes Atherosclerosis?

When asked, most people would say that the villain is simply too much cholesterol in the blood from too much cholesterol in the diet. This answer contains but a small shred of the truth. *Cholesterol is only one of many different factors, and is, in fact, a relatively minor one at that.* It is not the Great Satan of Heart Disease, as we have been led to believe.

The beginnings of atherosclerosis occur with damage to the inner lining of the artery. The primary factor involved in this initiating injury is decreased energy production, and many of the causes for this decrease are well known. Happily, all of them are treatable. Let's examine each of them here.

Exaggerated Stress Response

Hardening of the arteries seems to be accompanied by a hardening of attitude. As people get older, they tend to react more to stress than when they were younger. This results from an accumulation of attitudes, such as inflexibility, clinging to grief, guilt, old hurts, a lost sense of purpose, regrets, decreased appreciation of beauty, and fear of death and disease. Over the years, this kind of stress wears out the adrenal glands and decreases blood flow to the cells, causing a measurable decrease in energy production. Chronic stress also causes adrenalin-induced free-radical damage, increased cholesterol, and high blood pressure, all of which damage arteries.

There are many cures for dealing with stress. Meditation. Exercise. Rest. Spending quality time with family and friends. Pursuing a hobby that unleashes unexpressed creativity within us. Good companionship. A pet. No matter how old you are, or what misfortunes have befallen you, the key is finding things in life that bring you joy and nourish the heart and mind. This is what dissolves stress.

Over the years, Dean Ornish, MD, has published amazing studies clearly demonstrating that coronary-artery disease can be reversed by stress-management techniques, such as meditation and yoga, along with proper diet and exercise.

Hormone Deficiencies

The most significant hormone deficiencies leading to atherosclerosis involve DHEA (DHEA is a hormone that your body naturally produces in the adrenal gland), estrogen, growth hormone, testosterone, and thyroid. These hormones are critical for optimal maintenance of energy production. As we get older, these hormones will become deficient. It's not a question of *if* they become deficient, it's simply a question of *when*. And as their levels start to fall, we will be at greater risk for developing atherosclerosis. Natural hormone replacement is one of the most effective ways to keep your arteries soft and pliable (see chapter 15, Secret 8).

Mineral Deficiencies

A proper diet minimizes the risk of mineral deficiency. However, due to commercial farming methods, the use of synthetic fertilizers, and the processing of food, meals often end up short of the key minerals that contribute to healthy arteries. The most common deficiencies I find among my patients are chromium, magnesium, and zinc.

Having these minerals in your body in adequate amounts is critical for optimal energy production. Chromium is especially important for fat metabolism. And zinc and magnesium are key to mitochondrial function. The medical literature is replete with studies connecting deficiencies of both chromium and magnesium to atherosclerosis.

In one study, every single person with coronary-artery disease was found to have low chromium levels, whereas only 20 percent of those without the disease had low levels. Animal studies have also demonstrated a 50-percent reduction in atherosclerotic plaques in animals given supplementary chromium.

According to an article appearing in the prestigious cardiovascular journal *Circulation*, magnesium deficiency is associated with an increased risk of coronary-artery disease, myocardial infarctions, fatal arrhythmias, and sudden cardiac death.

Using a new technology, electron-beam coronary tomography, researchers have been able to document that coronary-artery disease is directly correlated with increased levels of calcium in the coronary arteries. Magnesium supplementation has been shown to decrease the calcium content of these arteries, making them much less likely to develop atherosclerosis.

Regular supplementation that includes these minerals is critical for maintaining your health, even if you think you are eating a perfect diet.

Chronic Heavy-Metal Poisoning

In the previous chapter, I discussed the toxic effects of chronic heavy-metal exposure on our ability to produce energy. These toxic metals in the air, water, and foods can build up in the body over decades, and when they do, they poison the mitochondria. Arsenic, cadmium, and lead, in particular, contribute to arterial damage. The most common source of these metals is drinking water. This is a very good reason to make it a habit to drink only filtered water.

Once inside your body, the heavy metals get deposited in the tissues, particularly the arteries, where they accumulate and cannot be readily excreted. Because the body can't eliminate these metals efficiently, they will not be detectable using standard blood and urine tests that are used to discover acute heavy-metal poisoning. Their presence in the body can only be discovered using what is known as "provocative testing." Provocative testing is a technique offered by many practitioners of alternative medicine. The method involves the administration of chelating substances that bind to heavy metals stuck in the arteries and other tissues and promote their excretion through the urine.

By obtaining a urine specimen before and after the chelating substance is administered, it is possible to ascertain the full extent of the heavy-metal poisoning. The pre-provocative urine specimen will show few, or no, heavy metals, while the post-provocative specimen will be loaded with them. This demonstrates two principles connected with heavy metals.

1. Simply examining the blood or urine for heavy metals without using a provocative chelator is basically useless for documenting their presence.
2. Without the continuous use of chelation, the heavy metals won't be removed.

Of course, the most effective way to determine if heavy metals are poisoning you is to look at your E.Q. If it is over 100 percent, you are okay. If it is below that, you might have a problem.

Inadequate Sleep

Lack of adequate sleep is a documented cause of diabetes, hypertension, and obesity, all of which are contributors to atherosclerosis. Why? As you will see in chapter 9 (Secret 2), sleep deprivation and sleep disturbances are one sure way to markedly decrease your body's energy-producing capability.

Poor Cardiovascular Conditioning

This means insufficient exercise. Specifically, not enough of the right amount and right kind of exercise (see chapter 13, Secret 6).

One thing that Bio-Energy Testing routinely discovers is how poor the typical over-fifty heart is at providing adequate oxygen to the cells and tissues. One group of cells, the intimal cells that line the arteries, requires a very high level of oxygen to properly function. These cells cannot optimally function without adequate oxygen levels, and this makes them especially vulnerable to the various processes that cause atherosclerosis.

Regular exercise to the rescue here. Of all the measures that you can take to improve your energy production, regular exercise is by far the most effective. It can prevent—and even reverse—poor cardiovascular functioning by providing increased levels of oxygen to the intimal cells, thereby reducing atherosclerosis.

Obesity and Insulin Resistance

I lump these two together, because they are almost always found together. In the next chapter, you will learn that both of these conditions occur as a direct result of decreased energy production. You will also learn how to diagnose them, and how to treat them by increasing your body's ability to produce energy.

Elevated Homocysteine Level

Homocysteine is a naturally occurring amino acid in the body. Under normal circumstances, it is formed in the mitochondria as a part of energy production. It is ultimately cleared by the liver with the help of vitamins B_6, B_{12}, and folic acid, and by food substances known as methyl donors. However, any deficiencies of these vitamins and/or sub-optimal liver function can result in an elevated homocysteine level. And that spells trouble, because homocysteine is not only dangerous in itself; it is a marker molecule for mitochondrial function. An elevated homocysteine level indicates poor mitochondrial function and all the problems that go with it.

The excess homocysteine triggers harmful reactions that initiate damage in the arterial walls. Studies confirm that about 10 percent of all deaths from atherosclerosis occur as a result of an elevated homocysteine level.

People with a close relative who developed heart disease before the age of sixty often have elevated homocysteine levels. This buildup can be counteracted by maintaining a healthy liver and supplementing with the key vitamins listed above.

Excessive homocysteine also has damaging effects beyond the arteries. According to a study in the *Annals of the New York Academy of Sciences,* it can also cause chromosomal damage, which is a major sign of aging. Other studies have shown that people with even a moderate elevation of homocysteine have as much as a 50 percent increased risk of dying from all causes compared to those with the lowest levels. The lab reports the statistical range of homocysteine to be between 5 and 15 umol/L, but optimal levels are below 10 umol/L.

Homocysteine levels become elevated as a result of a deficiency of the metabolic process called methylation. As such, an elevated homocysteine level often means that adequate methylation is not taking place. Methylation is a process that occurs in every cell in the body. It involves the transfer of methyl groups (three hydrogen atoms attached to a carbon atom) from one molecule to another. This methylation transfer is critical for many important functions, including detoxification, mental and emotional functioning, and energy production. In terms of energy production, methylation creates all of the ADP (adenosine diphosphate) that is made in the body. Without enough ADP, energy production immediately slows down.

The process of methylation is also where another critical energy molecule called creatine phosphate is made. Besides ADP, creatine phosphate is the other way that the body can store energy once it is produced. Creatine phosphate is able to very quickly generate ATP (adenosine triphosphate). ATP is our primary energy molecule. When we need immediate energy, we get it from creatine phosphate. In the absence of enough creatine phosphate, exercise will be very hard.

Now you can see why it is so important to make sure that your homocysteine levels are optimal. Because optimal levels are a good indication that your body is methylating well. And good methylation is critical for optimal energy production.

Lipoprotein(a)

Elevated blood lipoprotein(a) has received less attention than homocysteine, and much less than cholesterol, but it is nevertheless a significant risk factor for atherosclerosis.

The best way to make sure that your lipoprotein(a) levels are low is to pick your parents well. That's because lipoprotein(a) levels are genetically determined.

This substance is an extremely sticky molecule. As it circulates in the blood, it has a marked tendency—greater than any other lipid—to adhere to sites of arterial wall damage and contribute to plaque buildup, arterial blockades, and atherosclerosis. You know that in some people high cholesterol levels increase the risk of atherosclerosis. But what you probably don't know is that 46 percent of cholesterol is made up of lipoprotein(a). And it is the lipoprotein(a) part of the cholesterol along with LDL cholesterol that is responsible for its damaging effects.

For the same reason that lipoprotein(a) causes heart disease, it is also associated with developing a condition called intermittent claudication.

People with intermittent claudication notice muscle cramps in their legs after walking only a hundred yards.

Lipoprotein(a) also interferes with the clotting mechanisms of blood, causing it to clot more easily. This creates an additional risk factor for heart attacks and strokes.

The acceptable statistical range for lipoprotein(a) is up to 80 mg/dL (some labs report as high as 130 mg/dL). But the optimal level is much lower. Most authorities state that the healthiest levels of lipoprotein(a) are below 20 mg/dL.

Linus Pauling, one of the greatest scientific geniuses of the twentieth century, argued over fifty years ago that an elevated lipoprotein(a) level was the single leading risk factor for heart disease.

You haven't heard more about this substance for a simple reason: Big Pharma hasn't been able to patent a drug to treat it. When this happens, as it no doubt will, you can expect a high-decibel campaign about a completely new discovery—a sad commentary on the way medicine is practiced in this country. Instead of being driven by physicians and their patients, who care the most, medicine today is driven by pharmaceutical corporations whose overriding interest is the bottom line. There's got to be a better way.

The good news is that you don't have to wait for the drug industry: there are already some excellent solutions. They're not patentable, but they work.

Years ago, Pauling discovered the way lipoprotein(a) damages the arteries and causes atherosclerosis. It does this by adhering to a part of the inner lining of the arteries called the lysyl residues. But lysyl residues are also present on a common amino acid called l-lysine. Pauling was able to show that taking l-lysine as a supplement diverts lipoprotein(a) from adhering to the lysyl residues in the arteries toward adhering to the lysyl residues contained in supplemental l-lysine. Taking l-lysine won't lower your lipoprotein(a) levels, but it will protect your arteries from it.

Another amino acid called n-acetyl cysteine can also help. One study showed that taking supplemental n-acetyl cysteine was able to lower lipoprotein(a) levels by as much as 70 percent. This is particularly effective when the n-acetyl cysteine is combined with vitamin C.

In men, one of the causes of increased lipoprotein(a) is a deficiency of the male hormone testosterone. If you are a man with elevated levels of lipoprotein(a), be sure to have your testosterone levels checked. If they are low, replacing your sagging levels with natural testosterone will help to lower lipoprotein(a). I will discuss this in much greater detail in chapter 15.

Coenzyme Q_{10} Deficiency

CoQ_{10} is a vitamin-like substance. It is a fundamental enzyme in the cellular conversion of oxygen to energy. Therefore, insufficient levels of it threaten energy production. Depletion is associated with aging, poor diet, the use of cholesterol-lowering drugs, diabetes, and heart disease.

Adequate CoQ_{10} is necessary for the integrity of all tissues—even more so for those tissues with a high metabolic need for energy, such as the brain, heart, and liver. Studies show that people with heart disease are deficient in CoQ_{10}, leading to decreased heart function. And according to Texas cardiologist Peter Langsjoen, MD, a CoQ_{10} deficiency can also lead to high blood pressure and congestive heart failure. Dr. Langsjoen has been using CoQ_{10} in his practice for more than forty years, and recently published his findings showing that by decreasing CoQ10 levels, statin drugs are the reason we are seeing an increase in congestive heart failure.

CoQ_{10} is made in the liver from the less complex forms found in foods such as CoQ_6 and CoQ_8. This is one more reason why optimal liver function is so important. The statistical range for levels of CoQ_{10} is between .75 mg/mL and 1.5 mg/mL, but most research indicates that levels above 1.5 mg/mL are required for optimal health. I strongly recommend supplementing with CoQ_{10} if your levels are lower than this. This is particularly important for anyone with atherosclerosis, congestive heart failure, or high blood pressure.

Anyone taking a cholesterol-lowering statin drug should definitely be on a CoQ_{10} supplement. Blood levels should be checked to be sure that the dose is adequate. The failure to do so means substituting one relatively minor risk factor (cholesterol) for a much more significant one (a CoQ_{10} deficiency).

Elevated Iron

The iron story is fascinating. Women have a much lower incidence of heart disease than men and also live an average of 10 to 15 percent longer. And this difference exists in every culture studied, regardless of diet, exercise, or stress. There is one exception, however—men who regularly donate blood. These men basically share the same desirable statistics as women.

Why is this so? Could it be that iron levels have something to do with longevity?

Inside the body, iron is a two-edged sword. On the one hand, it is critically important for the production of energy. Iron chemically binds to oxygen in hemoglobin molecules in the blood and carries the oxygen for delivery to the cells. Iron is also required for proper mitochondrial function. But it is also iron, in excess, that instigates damaging free-radical activity.

Because of their cyclic blood loss, menstruating women have less iron. But men, unless they regularly donate blood, have a tendency to develop higher iron levels. So do post-menopausal women who do not donate blood. Excessive iron consumption from supplements, or iron cookware, can also be a contributing factor.

Excessive iron levels can be discovered by examining the blood iron, iron saturation, and ferritin levels. With these blood tests, it will be easy for the doctor to diagnose an unacceptably high iron level.

I routinely check the iron levels of my patients and find that 10 to 15 percent of men and 3 to 5 percent of post-menopausal women have elevated levels. I make sure these patients are careful about their dietary intake of iron. I also recommend that they donate blood regularly, as this is the surest way to maintain optimal iron levels. In addition, natural substances, such as algae, colostrum, inositol hexaphosphate (IP6), and garlic, are able to lower iron levels.

In most labs, the reported range for serum ferritin levels is usually between 40 and 180 ng/mL. But in my opinion, and that of many experts in this field, any value over 70 ng/mL can indicate an excessive amount of iron in the body.

Antioxidant Deficiencies

I have already mentioned free radicals, the highly reactive molecules formed in the course of everyday energy production in the cells. In excess, they cause considerable damage to cells and tissues, and are major factors in disease processes and accelerated aging. Free radicals, for example, are always involved in the initial arterial damage that leads to atherosclerotic plaques.

The body has evolved an elaborate defense system of enzymes and other substances called antioxidants to prevent free-radical damage.

This system is stimulated by aerobic exercise and weakened by stress and infection. It is also undermined by exposure to pesticides, petrochemicals, and some other chemicals.

Certain nutrients are required to keep the antioxidant system running strong. Among these are vitamins, minerals, and amino acids. Fortunately, these substances are widely available in health-food and drug stores. Chief among them are vitamins C and E, CoQ_{10}, alpha-lipoic acid, the amino acid cysteine, and the minerals copper, manganese, selenium, and zinc. These supplements can help your body's fight against free radicals, and can also help prevent the development of atherosclerosis.

The secret to making sure your cells are protected from free-radical damage is to make sure that your E.Q. is optimal. It is only when the E.Q. is compromised that free-radical damage happens.

Elevated Blood Triglycerides

Triglycerides are fats produced in the liver from carbohydrates. The more carbohydrates you eat, the more triglycerides you will make. Other causes of high triglycerides are too much alcohol, low thyroid, certain drugs, overeating, and genetics. An elevated level increases your risk for cardiovascular disease, especially when combined with a low HDL, the so-called *good* form of cholesterol.

The influence of triglycerides on atherosclerosis seems in large part related to HDL. That's because high triglycerides cause a decrease in HDL. Harvard researcher Michael Gaziano, MD, pointed out the significance of this relationship in a 1997 article in the cardiology journal *Circulation*. He found that individuals with the highest ratio of triglycerides to HDL were sixteen times more likely to have a heart attack than those with the lowest ratio. Ideally, triglyceride levels should be below 120 mg/dl. An ideal HDL/triglyceride ratio is 1:2, and anything over 1:3 should be treated.

Improving this ratio can readily be achieved through weight loss, exercise, a low-carbohydrate diet, thyroid hormone replacement, and supplementation with fish oils, carnitine, and niacin.

Hypertension

The relationship between hypertension and atherosclerosis is well known. Simply put, elevated pressure in the arteries is a significant cause of atherosclerosis.

More than 50 million Americans have high blood pressure. Depending on your age, your blood pressure should ideally be between 120/80 and 140/80. If it is higher than this, the standard treatment is anti-hypertensive medication. However, strange as it may seem, many of the medications used to treat high blood pressure actually promote atherosclerosis—this is particularly true of beta-blocker and diuretic medications.

In most cases, hypertension responds well to a combination of treatments focusing on weight loss, exercise, a low-carbohydrate diet, and supplementation with CoQ_{10}, fish oil, and magnesium. Breath meditation (see chapter 14, Secret 7) is also beneficial because it helps relieve stress, a major contributor to hypertension.

Stress is often related to time urgency, the feeling that there just isn't enough time to accomplish what needs to be done. It will always be more attractive for the time-urgent individual to take a blood-pressure pill in three seconds than to alter thir diet, meditate, exercise, and take supplements. But for those who really want to live longer and better, the correct choice is clear.

For anyone with severe hypertension who has been on medication for many years, it may be difficult to eliminate the drugs. But adding in an alternative approach often allows a reduction in the medication.

The Great Cholesterol (Mis)Conception

Cholesterol is obviously involved in atherosclerosis, but not to the degree you have been led to believe. The whole issue of cholesterol has been overblown, oversold, and totally distorted as a public menace. It has become a fixation of the medical establishment and has spawned a huge industry. You have low-cholesterol foods. No-cholesterol foods. Cholesterol blood tests. And, most troubling of all, there is the increasing promotion of a very dangerous class of drugs called statins to lower cholesterol levels. The ads are everywhere. On TV. On the radio. In newspapers and magazines.

These drugs are even being promoted to healthy people with no evidence of any disease or condition as a smart prevention strategy. However, there are many good reasons why fixating on cholesterol—and, worse, trying to lower cholesterol with drugs—is a dangerous and medically unsound way to prevent heart disease. Here are five important reasons.

Reason 1

* Cholesterol is only one of many factors leading to heart disease. If all the risk factors aren't individually identified and treated, simply lowering cholesterol will not appreciably reduce your overall risk. In one newly published study, lowering cholesterol will prevent a heart attack in only 1 in 50 people with high cholesterol (and no heart disease).
* Studies repeatedly show that these medications demonstrate no beneficial effect at all for 70 percent of those who use them. The other 30 percent show a modest benefit at best.
* Many of the studies examining the effect of lowering cholesterol on the overall incidence of heart disease have been quite disappointing. One of the first and largest of such studies is the Helsinki and Oslo Heart Study. This study showed that there was a 34 percent decrease in coronary heart disease in patients taking the cholesterol-lowering drug. However, despite this, there was no reduction at all in deaths. Worse than that, the non-illness death rate (suicides and accidents) was more than twice as high in the drug group. Sure, they had less heart disease. That made their cardiologists happy. But they were pretty much dead anyway. Why? Because maintaining adequate cholesterol levels is critical to maintaining adequate brain function. Similar results were also seen in the Lipid Research Clinics Coronary Primary Prevention Trial, and many other studies.
* The usefulness of lowering cholesterol is related to age. A recent study in the publication *Cardiology* showed that in people over the age of sixty, the ones with the highest LDL cholesterol levels are the ones who live the longest. The authors of the paper concluded that lowering cholesterol levels in people over the age of sixty without evidence of existing heart disease was not warranted.

Reason 2

* It is not actually cholesterol per se that damages the arteries: it is oxidized LDL cholesterol. LDL cholesterol becomes oxidized when the body's antioxidant defenses become depleted. This occurs as a result of decreased mitochondrial function, excess stress, inadequate fitness, and deficient intake of antioxidant nutrients and other causes

of a decreased E.Q. It is very possible with the right treatment to have high LDL cholesterol with low oxidized LDL cholesterol. In that case, there would be no advantage to lowering LDL cholesterol.

* Following the steps in this book can help prevent cholesterol from becoming oxidized, thus preventing your high cholesterol levels from harming your arteries, no matter how elevated the levels are.

Reason 3

* The most common cholesterol medications are called statins. Statins are dangerous. They have a long list of serious side effects, some of which persist even after the drugs are withdrawn. Statin drugs inhibit the production of the vital co-enzyme CoQ_{10} that I discussed a few pages back.
* CoQ_{10} acts as a bodyguard for LDL cholesterol, accompanying the LDL in the bloodstream and protecting it from being oxidized. Remember that LDL only creates problems when it is oxidized. Recent research has found that the most susceptible LDL—LDL3—is equipped with CoQ_{10}.
* Research has proven that statin drugs deplete the CoQ_{10} that your body produces. The long-term effects of this depletion are potentially disastrous. This is what has motivated the International CoQ_{10} Association, a group of researchers and clinicians who study the uses of CoQ_{10}, to voice their concerns to the U.S. Food and Drug Administration. In 2001, these medical professionals urged that the FDA warn anyone taking statin drugs about the CoQ_{10} depletion that goes along with the drug.
* Studies have shown that heart failure is associated with a CoQ_{10} deficiency. Heart cells require a huge amount of energy, and are therefore the primary cellular consumers of CoQ_{10} in the body. As I mentioned before, it is probable that the resurgence of heart failure in the United States is because of the effects of statin medications.
* CoQ_{10} experts tell us that people taking these drugs do not develop symptoms of possible CoQ_{10} deficiency immediately. After a year or two, they say, people may complain of malaise and muscular aches and pains. It is interesting to note that recent medical reports have emerged about the side effects of statins, and particularly the

potential for muscle damage. In the summer of 2001, one major statin drug, Baychol®, was pulled off the market by the FDA. Nobody has yet connected the dots specifically, but this could be related to CoQ_{10} deficiency. Muscles need energy to work, and without enough CoQ_{10} nothing works well.

* Not just muscles, but all cells need CoQ_{10}, and any deficiency can have widespread medical implications.
* Common complications of statins also include paralysis and rheumatic joint disease. A report in the British medical journal *Lancet* pointed out that there is no overall decrease in the death rate from the use of cholesterol-lowering drugs. That's because any reduction in cardiac deaths is offset by an increase in non-cardiac deaths.
* In fact, the sobering truth is that lowering cholesterol with drugs can actually increase the death rate. Take, for example, a World Health Organization study that looked at the death rates of people with high cholesterol.

This study compared people taking a cholesterol drug called clofibrate to people that did not take any drugs at all, and just lived with their high cholesterol. Both groups were followed over an average period of 9.6 years. The results were startling, to say the least: there were 25 percent more deaths in the clofibrate-treated group than in the high-cholesterol group. The death rate *from all causes* was higher in the treated group than in the high-cholesterol controls during the trial. No particular disease accounted for the overall excess: the clofibrate group had more deaths from heart attacks, stroke, cancer, and other major diseases. The authors of the study offered two possible explanations for the increase in death rate: 1) a long-term toxic effect of clofibrate; and 2) the unhealthy consequences of reducing cholesterol.

Another article published in the *American Journal of Cardiology* further emphasizes the dangers of reducing cholesterol levels. This paper examined and analyzed the results of the Lipid Research Clinics Coronary Primary Prevention Trial. This trial studied the effects of lowering cholesterol levels in 3,806 normal, healthy middle-aged men with elevated cholesterol. They discovered that although these men had fewer deaths from heart disease, they had a significantly greater death rate from accidents and suicide.

Reason 4

* Common causes of high cholesterol include antioxidant deficiency, insulin resistance, low DHEA, low-fiber diets, low thyroid, low sex hormones, nutritional deficiencies, and stress. If you have elevated cholesterol, you may have any or all of these problems. Instead of introducing potentially harmful drugs into the system, it would be much better to correct the problems that cause high cholesterol in the first place. And drugs obviously don't do this. They just squelch the body's production of cholesterol, while the real causes are not addressed.

Reason 5

* The discussion on cholesterol requires a final touch to put it in full perspective. Cholesterol is in your body for a reason. It is the most abundant steroid in your body. It is needed. Less than 20 percent of the cholesterol in your body comes from your diet. Most of it is made in the liver. Cholesterol is much too important a molecule to be trusted to dietary intake alone. All your steroid hormones are made from cholesterol. All your cell membranes are made from cholesterol. Your brain and nervous system are almost entirely made of cholesterol.
* A low cholesterol level is associated with immune deficiency and with an increased risk of death from all causes, including cancer.

So, if It's Not Cholesterol, What Really Causes Heart Attacks?

I've explained the factors that cause the constriction, hardening, and narrowing of the arteries. A significant amount of blockage in the coronary arteries supplying the heart sets up the conditions for a myocardial infarction—a heart attack. But there are other factors than blocked arteries that are as much or even more responsible for heart attacks.

Increased clotting tendency

Many people with coronary-artery disease have an abnormal tendency to form clots. Excessive levels of lipoprotein(a) is often one of the main reasons, but there are also other causes. This increased tendency causes extensive clots at plaque sites.

It all starts when a plaque erodes, exposing its contents to the bloodstream. The clotting elements in the blood then adhere to it. When this happens, the plaque/clot combination is referred to as a "vulnerable plaque." Vulnerable plaques are dangerous. The clot part of the plaque may break off, be swept away by the blood, and cause a sudden and complete blockage of a coronary artery. The result is sudden death without any warning symptoms.

This clotting risk can be nearly reduced by taking the QuickStart and Super Fat nutritional formulas I developed (see chapter 12, Secret 5). This combination contains herbs, oils, and nutrients that effectively keep the blood thin. This often is the only remedy my at-risk patients have to take to correct this problem.

Infected plaques

One rather surprising cause of heart attacks involves the immune system. Researchers have discovered that common bacteria can grow on arterial plaques and infect them. As a result, the plaques may break off and cause a sudden heart attack in the same way that vulnerable plaques do. Furthermore, the infection can actually increase the plaquing.

The discovery was made when researchers found that people with coronary-artery disease who were regularly treated with antibiotics for other conditions were less likely to have heart attacks. Apparently, those who develop these infected plaques are unable to normally mount an effective immune response to prevent the infections. The immune-enhancing nutrients found in QuickStart, along with natural hormone replacement and stress reduction, can help your immune system prevent—and even eradicate—these infections.

Coronary-artery vasospasm

The coronary arteries are no different from any other artery. They are surrounded by smooth muscles that help to regulate the blood flow through them. When the smooth muscles constrict, they squeeze down the size of the artery and effectively decrease the blood flow. Likewise, when they relax, the blood flow is increased. Vasospasm refers to a condition in which these smooth muscles constrict and stay constricted, just like a muscle cramp. This causes a severe decrease in the blood flow to the heart muscle. If the vasospasm lasts longer than a few seconds, it may cause chest pain and sudden cardiac arrest. Up to 70 percent of all heart-attack deaths are preceded by a coronary-artery vasospasm.

Among its many important contributions to the body, the mineral magnesium helps to prevent vasospasm by keeping the smooth muscles around the arteries nice and relaxed. Most coronary-artery vasospasms are caused by a deficiency of magnesium, a deficiency that can be caused by diuretics, a poor diet, or an excessive intake of coffee, tea, or soft drinks. Magnesium supplementation (QuickStart is high in magnesium) can significantly reduce the risk of vasospasm.

Poor fat utilization

An overlooked—and extremely important—factor in the cause of heart attacks is the poor ability of those with coronary-artery disease to optimally metabolize fat for energy. *The heart, like all the other muscles in the body, prefers to burn fat as its primary energy source.* Anyone who suffers from impaired fat metabolism is at a significantly increased risk for the development of a heart attack, simply because the heart tissues are less metabolically adaptable, and that makes them more sensitive to fluctuations in oxygen. And, as I already pointed out, a decrease in fat metabolism is one of the hallmarks of a low E.Q.

The Facts on Bypass and Angioplasty

One of my major pet peeves is the escalating rise of various surgical plaque-removal procedures to treat coronary-artery disease such as bypass surgery and angioplasty. This is particularly bothersome because although these procedures can save lives, they entail a significant risk of death and neurological impairment, combined with a high degree of failure within five years. Furthermore, they do *nothing* to address the above-mentioned causes of heart disease.

Clinical studies show no significant difference in survival rates between those who opt for angioplasty or bypass surgery and those who choose to treat their disease medically. In 2020 the *New England Journal of Medicine* showcased a study demonstrating the ineffectiveness of either method to extend life following a heart attack.

In the study, researchers at the University of Toronto compared the death rate for four hundred Canadians with heart disease to a matched group of Americans. At the end of one year following a heart attack, the death rate was the same in both countries. However, the difference between how these patients were treated was illustrative:

* Three times as many Americans had angiographies.

* Three times as many Americans underwent angioplasty.
* Almost five times as many Americans underwent bypass surgery.

The Americans had three to five times as many dangerous procedures, and yet the death rate was the same. This and similar studies do not suggest there is no place at all for these procedures in the medical care of people with coronary-artery disease. But the results do strongly indicate that many angioplasties and bypasses performed in the United States are ineffective and unnecessary.

The main guiding diagnostic procedure used to determine whether or not a bypass or angioplasty should be performed is an angiography. An angiography is an invasive procedure that entails risk, albeit fairly low, of both stroke and death. It involves placing a catheter into the coronary arteries, and injecting a dye that can be seen on X-ray. Angiographies are supposed to be able to determine if the artery has a significant blockage or not. But there are substantial problems with angiographies.

Most studies show that there is very little agreement among cardiologists on exactly how to interpret the angiograms. For example, researchers at the St. Bartholomew's and the London Chest Hospitals in Great Britain randomly picked 209 angiograms that were performed in their hospitals. They then had two different cardiologists look at the angiogram results and interpret the amount of significant coronary-artery disease present in each case. The results? These cardiologists disagreed in 40 percent of the cases. It gets worse. There was a 30 percent disagreement between the two specialists on whether or not a given patient should go on to have an invasive procedure or should just be managed with medication. So, depending on which cardiologist looks at the angiogram, a patient has between a 30 and 40 percent chance of receiving an unnecessary procedure. Other studies, also published in leading journals, have concluded that angiogram interpretation is subject to error in as many as 70 percent of cases.

Adding up all these studies, you can't help but reach the rather shocking conclusion that when a physician tells his or her patient that an angiogram indicates the need for bypass surgery or angioplasty, there is perhaps a 70 percent chance that the interpretation is wrong. Moreover, if the interpretation is correct, the odds are only 10 percent that the bypass procedure or angioplasty will actually extend life.

How can this be? It seems so natural to conclude that if you remove the blockages, you eliminate the problem. But, as with many things in medicine, what seems rather obvious at first glance only turns out to be a small part of the whole picture.

The reason that angioplasty and bypass surgery are of such limited value is because these procedures don't treat the causes; they only treat the effect. The causes, meanwhile, are still at work, and the disease process is still advancing. *The most effective approach to the treatment and prevention of coronary-artery disease can occur only when all causal factors are considered.* The best therapeutic approach combines the timely and judicious application of drugs with remedies to correct and optimize E.Q.

The Value of Chelation Therapy

Chelation therapy is the safest and most effective form of treatment for most cases of coronary-artery disease. This method involves a series of intravenous infusions of minerals, vitamins, and a special amino acid called EDTA (ethylene diamine tetraacetic acid).

EDTA is an amino acid similar to those found in the proteins you eat. It has a strong attraction for toxic metals, such as arsenic, cadmium, lead, and nickel, which it binds up and escorts out of the body. It also has the ability to bind up and remove calcium deposits that are hardening into arterial plaques.

Chelation improves the function of individual cells and their enzyme systems, particularly the endothelial cells that line the arteries. And it also infuses the body with beneficial minerals, such as potassium and magnesium, which are typically deficient in people with heart conditions.

Arterial walls become softer and develop greater elasticity. This increases circulation, meaning more oxygen and nutrients get to the heart and all the other cells throughout the body. And with a huge amount of toxic material being removed, the grand effect is to significantly defuse the many risk factors that lead to heart attacks and strokes.

I offer chelation therapy to my patients in the context of a broad-based health-care approach, including the many steps outlined in this book. Along with other treatments, such as blood thinners, blood-pressure medication, and diuretics, chelation is successful at preventing cardiovascular deaths virtually 100 percent of the time. Blood pressure is reduced or normalized, and the need for medication can be reduced or even eliminated.

An added bonus is that it improves circulation *throughout* the body, not just to the heart. You can bet that if there is atherosclerosis in the coronary arteries, it is in all the other arteries as well. In fact, I recommend that everyone receive a course of chelation therapy when they hit their sixties, even if they are healthy and free of heart disease. My thinking is that there are very few of us who will reach that age without having gunked up our arteries to some extent.

Chelation therapy is effective, safe, and completely free of any significant side effects. Moreover, it is inexpensive. For those who would like to learn more about chelation therapy, not only in coronary-artery disease but in other diseases as well, there are several excellent books on the subject that can be found online or in the health section of any major bookstore. To find a doctor trained in chelation therapy, contact the American College for the Advancement of Medicine at 1-800-532-3688, or visit the organization's website at www.acam.org.

Now for the less encouraging news: unfortunately, the method is ignored by a majority of cardiologists. In its place are scare tactics, which seem to work pretty well. I can't tell you how many times a patient of mine had been previously told by a well-meaning cardiologist that an emergency procedure is needed to "save your life."

The reality is that studies have shown that over 90 percent of all cases of coronary-artery occlusion respond well to a combination of chelation therapy and medication: the only known emergency indication for surgical intervention is uncontrolled angina.

I know a number of cardiologists who are absolutely convinced that chelation therapy is not nearly as effective as angioplasty or bypass surgery. And when they see my patients, who tell them how much chelation has helped them, these doctors dismiss the improvement as a placebo effect. However, I have never met a single cardiologist who has called the method ineffective after giving it a decent chance. On the contrary, the few cardiologists I know who have been open to chelation and have given it a try have never gone back to the knee-jerk mentality of the necessity of surgery for each and every case of advanced arterial disease.

Cancer

Strictly speaking, cancer is not a disease of aging. It can strike at any age. But the incidence of the disease does rise sharply with age, which makes it reasonable to wonder what it is about the aging process that so greatly contributes to this problem.

The starting—and startling—point is this: if you are over fifty, it is very likely you already have cancer in your body. In fact, it's almost 100 percent likely. Autopsy studies of people who died in accidents, or from causes other than cancer, have confirmed that nearly every person older than fifty already has at least one cancerous tumor in the body. I am not talking about a few cancerous cells. I mean actual cancers. And, according to these studies, many of these people were found to have more than one cancer.

If this is true, why is it that only 25 to 30 percent of the population dies from cancer? And why is it that many individuals live well into their eighties and nineties without ever developing any problems from the cancers that must be present in their bodies?

The answer lies in the concept of "promotional factors."

Cancer Promotion

Cancer experts say that, on average, most of us have several cells a day that mutate into cancerous cells. This process is referred to as "initiation." Initiation is a normal occurrence at any age.

They also say that the immune system is equipped to quickly detect and destroy these cancerous cells before they can multiply and enlarge into a colony of cells large enough to form a tumor. Every now and then, however, a cancer cell develops the ability to elude detection, and a tumor is born. It is important for everyone to realize that, in these early stages of tumor development, the tumor is far too small to be identified by any sort of medical detection.

Often, this growth is snuffed out as it becomes visible on the radar screen of the immune system. But it also may just remain there in a state of limbo—contained, but not eliminated, by the body's defenses. It is this dormant stage of cancer that virtually everyone harbors, no matter what the age. These cancers are called "latent" cancers.

Because they are so small, latent cancers cannot be discovered except on an autopsy examination. You won't be aware of them. They produce no symptoms and they can't be detected by scans or X-rays. We only know they exist because of autopsy studies, which use microscopic examination to find them. As far as you or your doctor know, there is no cancer present at all. And as long as your immune system is operating effectively, and there are minimal promotional factors present, you will live a long, healthy life—free of any clinical cancer.

The term "promotional factors" refers to various influences and imbalances that favor the development of latent cancers into larger, clinically apparent cancers—the kind that can kill you. The precise ways these promotional factors influence cancer development are not clearly understood. But the primary central promotional factor was first proposed by Otto Warburg more than one hundred years ago.

Dr. Warburg, who received the Nobel Prize for medicine for his work with cancer cells, is considered to be one of the most influential physicians of the twentieth century. Dr. Warburg was able to prove that cancer cells primarily develop as a result of decreased energy production. More recent research has validated Dr. Warburg's conclusions by proving that increasing the energy production in cancer cells causes them to: (a) decrease their growth rate, (b) decrease their tendency to spread, and (c) revert to normal cellular metabolism. In addition, increasing a cancer cell's energy production also causes it to be less malignant.

In the aging process, the immune system steadily loses efficiency. This decline, along with the decline in energy production, permits the growth into full-blown clinical cancer of latent cancers that would otherwise be mired in the pre-clinical stage.

Let me share an example:

Ernest, sixty-three, came to my clinic with a problem of uncontrolled blood sugar. He had been diagnosed with diabetes several years before. It turned out that the diabetes was secondary to a very rare condition created by cancer of the pancreas. The pancreas is the organ that produces insulin, the hormone that controls blood sugar. Looking back on his medical history, it became apparent that he had had the cancer for at least eight years before its presence finally became apparent.

The case is typical of newly diagnosed cancers. By that, I mean the cancer is actually present and working in the body many years before any clinical indications appear. Many times, physicians see patients who only a few weeks before were feeling fine, but suddenly have health complaints and symptoms of disease. As they investigate, the doctors discover that their bodies are literally riddled with cancer. Such patients have often had annual physicals and blood tests that show nothing abnormal.

Experiences such as this indicate that, without symptoms, medicine is not yet sophisticated enough to recognize cancer in the latent preclinical stages. Once the diagnostic tools to do so have been developed, however, practitioners will be in a position to initiate therapy before the cancer reaches a symptomatic and more destructive stage.

The Promise of an Early Detection Method

Medical science is pursuing such technology. Researchers are striving to develop reliable methods to determine the presence of cancer markers, naturally occurring substances in the blood that represent pre-cancerous development. I have already seen some promising tests and methods that give an optimistic prospect for the future of cancer detection. But until then, here's the take-home message:

1. It is highly likely that you and I already have one or more latent cancers. And that under the influence of promotional factors that decrease energy production, such as decreased cardiovascular fitness, stress, poor nutrition, smoking, toxicity, etc., these otherwise harmless cancers may evolve into a clinically detectable and potentially life-threatening stage.
2. As the field of cancer-biomarker assessment further develops, we will have the capability to detect when a latent cancer is getting out of control, and treat them in their pre-clinical stage long before they reach the point of clinical detection. I strongly believe the coming years will bring major breakthroughs in combining blood-cancer markers with computer analysis to identify when a latent cancer is being promoted to a malignant stage.

Until that day, when cancer-biomarker assessments become refined and widely available to doctors, it behooves everyone to recognize that the body harbors latent cancers and to act accordingly. This means keeping our latent cancers in permanent confinement by making sure that our E.Q. remains optimal even as we get older. Otherwise, like giving a convicted criminal the keys to the jailhouse, you are giving them the power to break out. Following the recommendations in this book can help to keep cancer in check.

Osteoporosis

Osteoporosis is a disease in which bones become fragile and more likely to break. If not prevented, or if left untreated, the condition can progress until a bone breaks, typically in the hip, spine, or wrist. Women are affected four times more than men. Americans have been brainwashed into thinking that calcium deficiency is the cause of osteoporosis. This has now been proven to be untrue.

There are many factors in the onset of osteoporosis, but dietary calcium deficiency is not one of them. That's why taking calcium supplements does nothing to prevent the disease. The latest study that proves this point looked at 36,282 normal healthy women between the ages of 50 and 79. These women were randomly assigned to take either 1,000 milligrams of calcium with 400 international units of vitamin D a day, or a placebo. They were followed for seven years.

This extremely well-done and statistically significant study found *absolutely no benefit* from calcium and vitamin D supplements in preventing broken bones. What's more is that the study showed why: only a very insignificant amount of all that calcium was actually going to the bones. The bone densities of those on the supplements showed no improvement at all in the spine. The only "improvement" at all was in the hip area, and that was an insignificant one percent.

Osteoporosis is caused by excessive calcium loss, not by insufficient calcium intake. That's a very important distinction to make, so I will repeat it: the problem is excessive *loss*, not deficient *intake*. And what causes excessive loss?

It's a combination of hormone deficiencies combined with a lack of adequate diet, exercise, and sun exposure. All these factors are discussed in the chapters to follow.

Is It Safe to Take Calcium Supplements?

Calcium is the most abundant mineral in your body. Ninety-eight percent of it is used to build and maintain strong bones. Another 1 percent builds and maintains your teeth. The remaining 1 percent is spread throughout the body and serves essential chemical roles in muscle contraction, blood clotting, and the transmission of nerve impulses. Normal bone health doesn't rely just on calcium: vitamins C and K play a critical role, along with the minerals boron, magnesium, zinc, phosphorus, silicon, and strontium.

True calcium deficiency is essentially non-existent in this country. It doesn't even turn up in studies of inner-city children who are on calcium-deficient diets. The reason is that calcium is the only mineral with its own regulation system. When the level of dietary calcium falls, the body compensates for this through the action of vitamin D. Vitamin D increases calcium absorption from the intestines and decreases calcium loss from the kidneys. This system works so well that a normal calcium balance will be maintained even with low calcium intake.

The author of a definitive clinical review on calcium metabolism says it best: "Many official bodies give advice on desirable intakes of calcium but no clear evidence of a calcium deficiency disease in otherwise normal people has ever been given." In Western countries, the usual calcium intake is of the order of 800 to 1000 mg/day; in many developing countries, figures of 300 to 500 mg/day are found. There is no evidence that people with such a low intake have any problems with bones or teeth. It seems likely that normal people can adapt to have a normal calcium balance on calcium intakes as low as 150 to 200 mg/day. This adaptation is sufficient even in pregnancy and lactation.

I believe that the *indiscriminate* supplementation of calcium to strengthen bones is not only useless but also dangerous. Yes, you read that correctly. The food and supplement industries have achieved a major sales coup by convincing women that they will develop osteoporosis unless they take calcium supplements. Nothing could actually be further from the truth.

There is not a single well-controlled prospective study showing that calcium supplementation actually prevents osteoporosis. The term "prospective study" means the study followed the same group of people over many years. Statistical studies that are not prospective are often subject to error.

Preventing osteoporosis with calcium supplements is a nice theory, and it seems to make sense; but it just doesn't pan out, because osteoporosis is not caused by calcium deficiency. Instead of helping, supplementation can cause problems by putting an excess of calcium into the wrong parts of the body.

Can Calcium Supplements Cause Heart Disease?

What does the body do with all the excess calcium it doesn't need? It's certainly not reaching the bones. So where does it go? One common repository is the arteries. And yes, there's a connection here to arterial obstruction, calcified blood vessels, decreased circulation, and plaque.

Electron-beam tomography represents a state-of-the-art diagnostic technique for coronary-artery disease. Studies using this new technology demonstrate that the chances of dying of a heart attack go up in direct proportion to the calcium content of the coronary arteries. This fact raises serious concern for the cardiovascular health of people who consume large quantities of calcium supplements. Much of that calcium is just precipitating out on the arteries.

Can Calcium Supplements Cause Cancer?

What happens to someone taking supplementary calcium in spite of the fact that she or he does not have a deficiency? The first thing that happens is that vitamin D production is suppressed by the excessive calcium intake, which leads to a deficiency of this vitamin. Since vitamin D is critically involved in proper immune-system function, all this extra calcium results in an immune deficiency, which has been shown to lead to autoimmune diseases, inflammatory bowel disease, and cancer. The full magnitude of this problem remains unknown, but a glimpse into the many possibilities is provided by a paper published in 1998.

The paper, published in *Cancer Research* by the Department of Medicine at Harvard Medical School, found that the immune deficiency caused by elevated calcium intake resulted in an increased incidence of advanced prostate cancer. The authors state: "Our findings provide indirect evidence for a protective influence of high 1,25(OH)2D [vitamin D] levels on prostate cancer and support increased fruit consumption and avoidance of high calcium intake to reduce the risk of advanced prostate cancer."

Other studies show the same relationship with breast and colon cancer, and I'm sure that because vitamin D is so important for proper immune function, we will see the same problem with other cancers in the future.

Can Calcium Supplements Cause Deficiencies?

Another problem with calcium supplementation relates to the absorption of other important nutrients. Specifically, calcium blocks the intestinal absorption sites for magnesium and zinc. By loading up on calcium, you can create a deficiency of these other minerals. Many studies have confirmed that magnesium and zinc deficiencies are widespread.

What Else?

All this is bad enough, but it's not the end of the story. In the body's attempt to rid itself of excessive calcium intake, it channels the extra calcium to the kidneys for urinary excretion. And this, according to medical research, promotes kidney stones. You'll also find calcium deposits in joints and tendons, where they contribute to arthritis and tendinitis.

These facts certainly discourage me from recommending calcium supplements to my patients. With what we know about how the body deals with calcium, it seems like wishful thinking to expect that supplementation will somehow magically restore bones without creating any of these undesirable effects.

Depression

Depression often affects older people. Why? The problems of aging, lost vigor, and lost loved ones certainly provide ample reason to be depressed. But these are not the major reasons. Hormone deficiencies of estrogen, progesterone, thyroid, testosterone, and growth hormone are even more significant causes. And add to that the decline in neurotransmitters (brain chemicals) and methylation that happens to us as we get older.

As an example, take the case of George, sixty-four years old. He was reluctantly brought in to see me by his wife of thirty-six years. In front of him, she told me: "If you can't do something about him, I am going to lose my mind."

George had been a man of great passion and energy, but over the previous three years he had become grumpy and complaining. Six months prior to that, he had retired, and now he had no motivation and no interest in life.

"At least he was bearable when he was working," his wife said; "but now that he's home all day, he drives me crazy with his complaints and demands." George had tried counseling, to no avail. He had no idea why he was so negative. It was completely uncharacteristic of him. Three different antidepressant medications had been tried. Each one was stopped because of side effects, and the fact that they didn't work for him.

Ordinarily, George enjoyed sex, but he admitted, "If a naked supermodel walked into this room right now, I wouldn't even look at her! I have absolutely no interest." During that first visit, George began to cry, and I saw in front of me a man who had given up, who felt utterly helpless and hopeless.

Testing revealed an abnormally low level of testosterone, combined with an elevated level of estrogen, both common in men over sixty. Bio-Energy Testing revealed a thyroid deficiency as well, even though his blood thyroid tests had previously been found normal.

I prescribed natural thyroid and testosterone replacement, feeling that these would help elevate his depression and gusto. And, using the data from his Bio-Energy Testing, I established the right diet and exercise program for him. After three months, however, his condition had not improved, even though his testosterone level tested normal.

Growth-hormone replacement was an extremely expensive therapy at this time, and for that reason I wanted to try other things first, and did not initially test him. But now I did, and, not surprisingly, his growth hormone level was quite low. I then added growth hormone to his regimen.

After one month into this expanded program, George started to perk up. When I reevaluated him in three months, his wife told me he was "almost back to his usual ornery self." Ornery or not, George was thrilled. No counseling. No drugs. Not even exercise in his case (he was extremely resistant to that suggestion). It was just a matter of giving his body the hormones he so badly needed.

As an aside, George later admitted to me that he had contemplated killing himself because he loved his wife too much to put her through the agony of living with him. He never revealed his intention to me, or anyone, because he planned to stage the suicide as an accident so his wife would collect his life insurance.

George's case illustrates not only the powerful effect that hormones have on mood, but also the importance of prescribing *all* deficient hormones in orde to optimize the therapeutic effectiveness. Unfortunately, many physicians are unaware of the astounding impact that hormones can have on the function of the brain, and especially on mood.

The other major factor in age-related mood changes is neurotransmitter imbalances. Neurotransmitters are the brain chemical that determine not only how efficiently we think and remember but also our mood. And guess what happens to our neurotransmitter balance as we get older? It gets worse. The result is often insomnia, anxiety, and depression. That's the bad news.

The good news is that neurotransmitter imbalances can be treated without drugs simply by taking the right balance of free-form amino acids. Amino acids are parts of proteins. And certain amino acids are what the body uses to manufacture our neurotransmitters. By supplementing with these amino acids in the right doses, it is very possible to turn around all kinds of brain disorders, including mood changes. And one more thing.

In order for our neurotransmitters to be able to work, they require the methyl groups I talked about earlier. Those methyl groups are created in the mitochondria. It's one more reason why having a good E.Q. is so important as we get older—it helps to maintain youthful brain function.

Diabetes

The latest statistics from the Centers for Disease Control indicate that more than 100 million Americans are now living with either diabetes or pre-diabetes. As of 2015, 30.3 million Americans, 9.4 percent of the entire population, had diabetes.

Moreover, the disease is developing at the staggering rate of 798,000 new cases a year. That's equivalent to the population of Washington, DC, and about six times higher than the incidence in the early 1950s.

In my opinion, this development is a medical disgrace, a prime example of a distorted medical system that focuses almost entirely on the treatment of symptoms while basically ignoring prevention. Type 2 diabetes, a disease of contemporary living, is 100 percent preventable.

A recent survey revealed that only 8 percent of Americans regard diabetes as serious. Yet diabetes is deadly serious. It is the major cause of amputations, blindness, and kidney failure in adults, and a leading factor in disorders of the nervous system. People with diabetes are also two to four times more likely to develop stroke and heart disease. Diabetes doubles the risk of liver, pancreas, and endometrial cancer. And it increases the risk of colorectal, breast, and bladder cancer by 20 to 50 percent.

Diabetes is defined by high levels of blood glucose (sugar) resulting from flawed insulin secretion, insulin resistance, or both. Insulin is the hormone produced by the pancreas that controls blood-sugar levels. It causes blood sugar to move into the cells for use in energy production. In diabetes, insulin function is compromised.

Type 2 diabetes is the most common form of the disease. It develops slowly, usually among people over forty-five who are overweight. However, health officials have started to see a disturbing increase in type 2 diabetes among children. This is a development that parallels the soaring rise of juvenile obesity. Type 2 diabetes used to be known as adult-onset diabetes, but because kids are now getting it, this term has been dropped.

The guidelines in this book will prevent type 2 diabetes 100 percent of the time. That's because the primary cause of it is decreased energy production. In fact, type 2 diabetes is the poster child for diseases caused by low energy production. I wrote a book on this connection called *The Type 2 Diabetes Breakthrough*. Anyone with diabetes or a family history of diabetes should read and follow the advice in that book.

MY RECOMMENDATIONS TO YOU

Once you have read this book, start making my recommendations a part of your everyday life. Don't drive yourself nuts. Just start off easy, and then work into a mad frenzy later.

* In addition to all the important things you do for yourself to maintain optimum health, it's a good idea to enlist the help of a prevention-oriented, nutritionally aware practitioner. I have screwed up my plumbing and automobile several times by trying to fix problems myself. I learned the hard way that hiring someone who knows what they are doing is often essential to getting a good result.
* All of us over the age of fifty (that includes me) should have an annual checkup. Medicine is a rapidly changing field. Every year there are new discoveries, and it may be that your program can be improved or enhanced as a result of these developments.
* Nothing is more valuable a part of an annual checkup than Bio-Energy Testing. There are more and more doctors now using this test. You can find them at www.bioenergytesting.com. Preventing disease without Bio-Energy Testing is like treating high blood pressure without a blood pressure cuff. You have no idea if what you are doing is really working.
* Assume you have pre-clinical cancers and act accordingly. Promise to take better care of yourself and your immune system. Do this especially if you are going through a particularly stressful time.
* Think of your fortieth birthday as a good point in life to get your baseline studies. In fact, give yourself a birthday present in the form of a baseline evaluation. This evaluation should include Bio-Energy Testing and the other important tests mentioned throughout this book. The results of these studies on your health status at forty can be used as a base against which to compare in later years as you age and embark on an anti-aging program.

✳ 5 ✳

ENERGY AND WEIGHT

According to government statistics, more than 60 percent of American adults are overweight. One-quarter of American adults are more than just overweight—they are obese. This puts them at increased risk for every chronic disease there is, including diabetes, heart disease, high blood pressure, strokes, and cancer. And, very sad to say, our children are following suit. As I mentioned earlier, a weight problem among youngsters is now at an epidemic level and increasing. By all accounts, Americans appear to be the most obese people in the world, and they are growing more so every year.

Obesity is not just an appearance problem. It is a huge (pardon the pun) health problem—by far the single major risk factor for developing serious diseases. Medical experts say it is an aggravating, or independent, agent for more than thirty medical conditions.

If you are a man, you can't be healthy and overweight at the same time. If you are a woman, you can be healthy and overweight, but not healthy and obese. This difference between the sexes is because a woman's physiology normally allows her to put on excess weight (up to a certain extent) without its being a consequence of decreased energy production.

There are many reasons for obesity. These include bad eating habits, improper exercise, inadequate sleep, a stressful and sedentary lifestyle, and hormonal deficiencies. But the primary underlying cause is decreased energy production.

Maintaining a healthy level of energy production is critical for maintaining a healthy weight. But for many people, doing what it takes to keep energy levels high involves the challenge of replacing habits that don't work with new habits that do.

Habits are difficult to break, but it can be done if the will and the desire are strong enough. The good news is that once you develop new habits, they will be just as hard to break as the old ones. And the rewards are great. Healthy weight pays off in terms of a healthier life . . . and a longer life as well.

I would like to offer a different approach to weight loss here. It is an approach based on years of guiding my patients who were frustrated by resistant weight problems to a more normal, healthier weight. If this description fits you, the information here can help you reach this critical and elusive health goal.

Are You Too Heavy?

Most people determine if they are overweight by standing on a scale. But a more exact way of assessing obesity is often needed because your fat stores cannot be objectively measured simply by weighing yourself.

Your total weight, what you see on the scale, is a mixture of your muscle weight and your fat weight. This is important: *muscle weight cancels out the negative effects of fat weight*. Saying that someone has too much body fat is basically the same as saying she/he has too little muscle.

You might wonder how professional football players who have so much obvious fat can still be so quick and powerful. The answer is that underneath all that fat, there is a huge amount of muscle, which is not so obvious to the eye.

One of the best ways to determine how much fat and muscle weight you have is by using an electronic technique called bio-impedance measurement. Bio-impedance testing is quick, safe, easy, and readily available in fitness centers and from anti-aging physicians. It involves passing a small level of electrical current through the body. Since muscle and fat conduct current in different ways, it is possible to determine how much of each is present.

Ideal body-fat measurements are 12 to 18 percent for men and 18 to 22 percent for women. Without pulling any punches, let me say that, to the degree your body-fat measurement is greater than this, you are unhealthy and are at risk for diseases that are otherwise completely preventable. This is especially true for men. As I mentioned earlier, some women (about 30 percent) can even have a body-fat percentage as great as 30 percent and still be healthy, but this can only be determined by Bio-Energy Testing. Unless you have a Bio-Energy Test that proves otherwise, if you are a woman with a fat percentage over 22 percent, assume you have a health problem.

Heaviness Officially Defined

The National Institute of Diabetes and Digestive and Kidney Diseases of the National Institutes of Health is the lead federal agency responsible for biomedical research on obesity.

From this resource, we have the following official definitions.

Overweight. An excess amount of body weight that includes muscle, bone, fat, and water.

Obesity. Most people think the term "obesity" simply means being very overweight. But obesity specifically refers to an excess amount of body fat. Some people, such as bodybuilders or other athletes with a lot of muscle, can be overweight without being obese. Everyone needs a certain amount of body fat for stored energy, heat insulation, shock absorption, and other functions. As a rule, women have more body fat than men. Most health-care providers agree that men with more than 25 percent body fat and women with more than 30 percent body fat are obese.

Obesity = Energy Deficit

There is no more obvious disorder of energy balance than obesity. And perhaps the most important point regarding obesity and energy production relates to fat metabolism. Let me explain.

To repeat, every time anyone eats a meal, the energy from that meal is stored as fat. It doesn't make any difference whether the meal is carbohydrates or fat. Practically speaking, *it all gets stored as fat.* This is how we are designed.

The fat stored from your last meal is meant to meet your energy requirements until the next one. But what if your body's ability to produce energy from this stored fat is impaired? What if your body can store up fat easily, but does not break it down for energy production as well as it puts it on? *In this case, you will not only gain weight because you can't break down your fat stores, but you will also produce less energy as well.* The two go hand in hand. Gaining weight and having low cellular energy are two sides of the same coin: an inability to burn or metabolize fat. This is a very common scenario as people get older, and is also why they are often unable to lose weight.

Except for those individuals who are fat simply from chronic super-sizing, all obese individuals have a serious flaw in the ability to produce energy efficiently. Without measuring energy production and correcting the underlying disorders of energy production, it becomes almost impossible to permanently correct obesity.

Here are the facts. Without correcting the underlying energy disorder:

* 75 percent of all those who lose weight regain it within three years.
* 95 percent regain it within ten years.

Why were the 5 percent who initially lost weight able to keep it off? No doubt because somehow they managed to correct the energy-production deficit that caused their obesity in the first place.

Low energy production causes obesity. And obesity causes low energy production.

Many people fall into such a deep hole from this vicious cycle that it appears impossible for them to escape. What initiates this vicious cycle in the first place?

Too Much Insulin

The answer, and the first step toward obesity, involves a loss in energy production resulting from insulin resistance. Before explaining what this means, let me take a moment to give you a brief background.

Our bodies are made of fats and amino acids. You consume these raw materials in your food. Your body extracts them from food in the digestive process and, after they are processed in the liver, uses them as needed.

Carbohydrates are also consumed. But the only use for carbohydrates is as an energy source. Nothing in your body is made of carbohydrates. Nothing at all! This is why nutritionists will tell you that there are *no essential carbohydrates*. When a nutritional item is termed "essential," it means that it must be present in the diet in order to maintain health. There are essential fats and amino acids, but there are no essential carbohydrates.

Think of carbohydrate foods as treats. Put them in the same general category as chocolate cake. You don't need to eat chocolate cake to be healthy, but it is nice to have some every now and then.

Carbohydrate foods aren't totally useless. Your body extracts vitamins and minerals from many of these foods. And assuming it has not been processed out (as in refined flours and grains), the fiber contained in the carbohydrates is used by the body as roughage to promote elimination of waste products and a healthy microbiome. But the truth is that the major ingredients in many carbohydrate foods are sugars. And sugars are not essential to anything.

The absorbed sugars extracted from the carbohydrates represent a raw material for energy production. That's all. And the reality is that the body can make all the energy it needs from fat and amino acids alone. It doesn't need any dietary sugar. Sugar is not essential to your health.

When carbohydrates are consumed, the body does one of two things with the extracted sugars: it burns them for energy, or it stores them as fat. The decision whether to burn or store is primarily determined by hormones. And the most important hormone in this scenario is insulin. Insulin is secreted by the pancreas according to how much carbohydrate is in your diet.

The connection between carbohydrate consumption and obesity is this: *The more carbohydrates you eat, the more insulin the pancreas makes. And the presence of too much insulin is a primary cause of obesity because insulin diverts ingested carbohydrates to fat storage while at the same time blocking the breakdown of fat stores.* It makes you fatter because it not only increases your fat stores, it also blocks your body from burning fat for energy.

But there's even more to this story. Outside of exercise, a hormonally balanced individual produces his or her energy almost completely from stored fat. However, as energy expenditure is increased during activity, the body begins to shift from mainly using fat stores to using carbohydrates stored in the body as glycogen. That's because carbohydrates offer 7 percent more energy per molecule of oxygen consumed than does fat. But remember that the body can only store a very small amount of glycogen, only enough to provide energy for one or two hours. By comparison, fat stores can provide energy for days and even weeks.

Because insulin prevents the breakdown and metabolism of our stored fat, in a state of insulin excess your body will have to get a majority of your energy from your glycogen stores.

This means two things.

1. Only a few hours after eating, your glycogen stores will become depleted and you will begin to run out of energy. This is a state known as hypoglycemia, or low blood sugar.

2. You will have a persistent craving for carbohydrates to replenish the exhausted glycogen stores.

The Insulin/Carbohydrate Vicious Cycle

Too many carbohydrates in your diet sets up a vicious cycle. The carbs stimulate your body to make more insulin. The more insulin you make, the more difficult it is for your body to access fat for energy, and so the more your body will rely on your glycogen stores. The more you use up your glycogen stores, the more carbohydrates you need to eat to replenish them. Ad infinitum.

The nasty effects of this cycle stem from the resulting hypoglycemia and decreased energy production. They include fatigue, lack of endurance, anxiety, depression, headaches, and insomnia. Another very common effect is a persistent weight gain. Weight that you are absolutely not able to lose, even when you exercise and limit caloric intake. Let me repeat. In a state of insulin excess, *you will not be able to lose weight, even if you exercise and limit calories until you are blue in the face.*

The end result of this insulin/carbohydrate vicious cycle is a condition called insulin resistance. Insulin resistance refers to the decreased ability of the body's cells to respond to insulin. Hence, they are described as being resistant to the hormone. Insulin resistance occurs when there is a decrease in energy production combined with excessive carbohydrate intake, genetics, hormonal deficiencies, insomnia, various nutrient deficiencies, stress, and lack of exercise.

How do you know if you are eating too many carbohydrates? Well, one sign is weight gain. But the best way to find out is through Bio-Energy Testing. If you are over-indulging in carbs, the test will show this as an abnormally low C-Factor (Carbohydrate Factor—see chapter 7).

The Enlarged Fat Cells/Insulin Resistance Vicious Cycle

When the body's cells become resistant to insulin, the pancreas responds by making more insulin, which of course only makes the situation worse. Ultimately, a state of chronic insulin excess develops, which continuously blocks the utilization of fat stores for energy production. This, in turn, results in the low energy production and excessive fat stores that cause obesity.

As this situation continues, the fat cells themselves become progressively larger (the fat cells become fatter). They expand to such an extent that the insulin receptor sites on the membranes become stretched and distorted and are then unable to properly respond to insulin. In other words, these engorged fat cells become resistant to insulin, which, in turn, acts to further increase the already-elevated insulin levels.

How Weight Gain Causes Low Energy

There's still more to this drama of vicious cycles. We've seen how low energy production causes weight gain. Now let's look at how weight gain, in turn, causes low energy. I personally believe that the low-energy state comes first, but this is pretty much a moot point. The reality is, when most people become concerned about their weight, both factors are in full force—low energy production and obesity.

Obesity results in low energy production in several known ways. First, it leads to decreased muscle mass. This is primarily a result of the decreased levels of activity and exercise commonly seen in overweight people. But it is also a side effect of the hormonal deficiencies that helped to cause the obesity in the first place. Since muscle mass is metabolically active tissue, the decrease in muscle mass serves to further lower energy production. This is measured by Bio-Energy Testing as an abnormally low M-Factor (Metabolic Factor—see chapter 7).

Second, weight gain causes a variety of sleep disturbances. These disturbances are often manifested by snoring and daytime sleepiness, but they are frequently present without symptoms and often can only be detected in a sleep lab. A very common problem with weight gain is that it interferes with the body's ability to enter into what is known as the *slow-wave* stage of sleep. Since the majority of growth-hormone production occurs during slow-wave sleep, this leads to a deficiency of growth hormone. The most common consequence of growth hormone deficiency is a decrease in muscle mass and an increase in fat mass. Additionally, sleep disturbances are known to decrease energy production.

Third, the sleep disturbances associated with weight gain create more insulin resistance. How this occurs is still unknown, but the fact that it happens is well documented.

> ***Note to obese men:*** Excess estrogen levels can happen in two ways. One, the fat cells will cause increased estrogen production. And two, as men age, a greater proportion of our testosterone gets converted to estrogen. This not only causes fat gain but can also contribute to sexual dysfunction, prostate enlargement, and prostate cancer.

Next, weight gain causes an excess of estrogens. This is because fat cells metabolically increase estrogens in the body, independent of ovarian and adrenal-gland production. In excess, estrogens suppress the mitochondria, resulting in a significant reduction in energy production. Estrogens also cause the body to retain and increase fat stores.

Finally, overweight people quite naturally engage in less physical activity, which means they will burn fewer calories. How much do you think you would like to go jogging or play basketball if you were twenty or thirty pounds overweight? Often, overweight individuals are exercise-intolerant—they all too easily slip into anaerobic energy production, which makes exercising very difficult. This is where Bio-Energy Testing can be so helpful. It can pinpoint the exact exercise zones for maximum fat burning and metabolism, even in obese people.

Other Weight-Control Aggravators

The factors already discussed form the basis for most of the weight-control problems for overweight individuals. But there are still several others that can confound a weight-loss effort.

One is sunlight deficiency. Several studies examining the effects of sunlight deficiency have demonstrated a significant association with low energy production in both animals and humans. This occurs as a result of hormonal deficiencies associated with a lack of sunlight, plus other as-yet-unidentified effects of sunlight on the metabolism.

Stress is another cause of decreased energy production. In many individuals, prolonged stress decreases the metabolic rate through its negative impact on the output of the adrenal glands. This leads to low blood sugar, low energy production, and weight gain.

Inadequate water intake also depresses energy production. And dehydration can lead to overeating because it can mimic the feeling of hunger.

Insomnia and lack of adequate rest can lower energy production as well. And then there is the issue of emotional eating. In our overfed society, much of what we consider hunger can have more to do with emotions than with real physical need. I believe that everyone, skinny and fat alike, has an eating disorder to some extent. Periodic fasting (see chapter 11, Secret 4) can help you identify how much of a reality this might be for you.

Training yourself to be comfortable and relaxed when you are hungry is a major step toward solving the problem of emotional eating. An invaluable technique to help you develop this strength is to fast once a week and use the breath-meditation exercise when you feel hungry. This won't lessen your feeling of hunger, but it will help you control all the emotions that hunger stirs up.

Metabolic Weight Loss

If you have a serious weight problem, you now know the possible reasons for it. What's next is to lose the weight. Anybody can lose weight. There are hundreds of books that will tell you how to do this. That part is easy. What's hard is keeping the weight off. And to do that, you must normalize your energy production. You must make that the primary goal.

How Much Fat Do You Lose While You're Sleeping?

Your energy production when you are resting quietly is referred to as your resting metabolism. A tenet of the energy-deficit theory of aging is that no matter what age you are, or what genetics you've been dealt, your resting metabolism should ideally be at youthful levels. From the perspective of weight gain, resting metabolism can best be described as that measurement which determines how much fat you burn while you are sleeping.

It has often been said that the only way to really become rich is to make money while you are sleeping. I can promise you it is also true that the only way you can control your weight is to lose fat while you are sleeping. And the only way to do this is to optimize your resting metabolism.

The process of optimizing your resting metabolism literally involves each and every one of the secrets I've developed in this book. Often the most critical aspect of optimizing resting metabolism is a reduction in dietary carbohydrates to what is right for your genetics, combined with weight-lifting, exercising at your fat-burning rate, adequate sleep, and natural hormone replacement. Having an optimal resting metabolism forms the basis of what I refer to as permanent metabolic weight loss.

You're Not Too Fat—You're Too Weak

The more I have researched the dynamics of what makes some people thin and others fat, the more I have begun to appreciate the importance of muscle mass. I am convinced that the low resting metabolism consistently seen in almost every overweight person is to a large extent due to decreased muscle mass.

I am so convinced of this that I tell my patients that for permanent weight control, it is much more important to gain muscle than to lose fat. Their decrease in muscle mass is the result of frequent dieting, genetics, hormonal imbalances, aging, and lack of proper exercise. Careful attention to all these factors is critical to success. Any weight-loss program that doesn't seriously focus on increasing muscle mass is doomed to failure.

How to Increase Your Energy and Lose Your Fat Permanently

Step 1—Diagnosing Insulin Resistance

Do you have insulin resistance going on that is contributing to excess weight in your body? The most reliable way I have found to assess the presence and degree of insulin resistance is with Bio-Energy Testing.

Another easy way to determine insulin resistance is simply to check a fasting insulin blood level. The normal range for fasting insulin in the United States is 5 to 25 micro units per milliliter (μiu/mL), but any value greater than 10 μiu/mL means that insulin resistance is present. This so-called normal range for fasting insulin levels in the United States only serves to demonstrate how common insulin resistance is, since it means, statistically speaking, that more than half the *healthy* people in the United States have a degree of insulin resistance.

Is it just coincidental that half the population of the United States is insulin-resistant and half the population is overweight? I don't think so. I believe it just indicates that insulin resistance is the cause of weight gain in an overwhelming number of people. Insulin levels need to be brought down below a minimum of 10 μiu/mL before successful weight loss can occur.

An additional, sensitive way to make the diagnosis is with a fasting blood-lipid test. Since insulin acts to divert foods to fat, it causes an elevation of fats in the blood. An elevation in cholesterol and triglycerides alerts me to the possibility of excess insulin. An elevation of a fraction of triglycerides known as VLDL (very-low-density lipoprotein) is a particularly strong indicator.

Step 2—Addressing Insulin Resistance

Dietary carbohydrates stimulate the production and release of insulin. So it would seem that the most immediate and effective way to reduce the tide of insulin in the body is to reduce carbohydrate consumption. And indeed, that is key.

One of the most important things that Bio-Energy Testing can tell me about my patient is whether or not he is carbohydrate-sensitive. Carbohydrates stimulate the release of insulin in everyone. However, some people release much more insulin than normal after a carbohydrate meal. This condition is referred to as a carbohydrate sensitivity. If you are carbohydrate-sensitive, you should be very careful not to eat more carbohydrates than you actually need.

How much should you cut back? That varies greatly from person to person. A useful guide is to keep cutting carbohydrates back until the C-Factor measurement on Bio-Energy Testing is over 90 (more about this in chapter 7), and the fasting insulin is less than 10 μiu/mL. In some cases, almost all dietary carbohydrate must be eliminated in order to achieve these goals.

Using the Glycemic Index

Researchers have discovered that certain carbohydrates stimulate the release of more insulin than others. This observation has led to a ranking of carbohydrates according to their insulin effect. This list is known as the glycemic index, and here is how it works.

When carbohydrates are designated with a high-glycemic rating, this means they cause the release of elevated levels of insulin. Middle- and low-glycemic carbohydrates release progressively less insulin.

Carbohydrate-sensitive individuals should decrease the consumption of carbohydrates in general, but should particularly avoid foods that have a high-glycemic rating. Limited amounts of low- or middle-glycemic carbohydrates may be permitted, depending on the testing results.

Step 3—Diet Concerns

Besides monitoring your intake of carbohydrates, there are three other dietary considerations that must be addressed.

* The first relates to total calories. In order to lose weight, total calories must be carefully restricted. That means restricted enough to result in fat loss, but not enough to cause muscle loss. The correct caloric intake is extremely important and very individual, and another reason why Bio-Energy Testing is so helpful. Through it, you can determine your resting metabolic rate. Increase this number by 10 percent and that's the number of calories you should eat per day to lose weight. Be

The Glycemic Index

High-Glycemic

- Bread (white), cookies, crackers, pancakes, pastry, pretzels. Most flour products, with the exception of pasta.
- Barley, cold breakfast cereals (including muesli), chips, cooked cereals (except slow-cooked oatmeal), corn, millet, rice (white).
- Bananas, mango, melons, papaya, pineapple, pumpkin, raisins.
- All sweets. This means anything that tastes sweet, including barley malt, corn syrup, fruit juices, high-fructose corn syrup, honey, maltodextrin, maltose, maple syrup, molasses, and sugar. Always check ingredient labels for sugars. Anything that ends in the suffix *-ose* is a sugar. The exceptions in the sweet category are pure fructose and the herb stevia.
- All root vegetables, with the exception of yams. This includes beets, carrots, potatoes, and sweet potatoes.
- Beer and wine (even low-alcohol). All liquor other than vodka and gin.

Middle-Glycemic

- Apples, oranges, peaches, pears, and plums.
- Ezekiel brand bread.
- High-protein pasta, and yams.
- Garbanzo beans, kidney beans (canned), navy beans, peas, and pinto beans.
- Gin and vodka.

Low-Glycemic

- Black-eyed peas, chickpeas, kidney beans, lentils, and lima beans.
- Soybeans and soy products, such as miso, soy protein, tempeh, and tofu. Be aware that soy products will often contain sugar.
- Apricots, berries, cherries, grapefruit, grapes, milk, and nuts.
- Slow-cooked oatmeal and 100 percent wholegrain rye bread.
- Fructose. This is the only low-glycemic sugar. It is quite sweet.

very careful about using charts, formulas, or calculations to determine your resting metabolic rate. These are virtually always off by as much as 400 to 800 calories.

* The second key consideration is to avoid hydrogenated oils, also known as trans fats. I discussed these before. Hydrogenated oils are commonly found in baked goods, margarine, mayonnaise, and almost any packaged convenience food. The health warnings on hydrogenated oils/trans fats have now been sounded far and wide, and they have been replaced in many products, but they are still out there and are still dangerous.
* The third consideration is to learn to be comfortable with hunger. When you are hungry, it indicates that your glycogen stores are exhausted and that you are meeting your energy requirements from your fat reserves, which is exactly what you are trying to achieve. If you feel hungry between meals, just relax. It's absolutely okay to be hungry. In many cases it is even necessary in order to be successful. Don't immediately run to the cookie jar or pull out a 40–30–30 bar from your desk drawer. Drink a glass of water and get on with your day. You will often find that hunger lessens as you get over the hump and begin to access your fat stores better. Please don't yield to hunger. The majority of the time that people feel hunger, it's for emotional reasons, anyway.

Step 4—Supplements

Nutritional deficiencies are often lurking behind insulin resistance. For people who are genetically susceptible to insulin resistance, missing or deficient nutrients cannot be adequately supplied by diet alone. They must be provided through supplements that, in order to be effective, must be taken in the correct form and dosage. That is why I developed QuickStart, a powerful nutritional formula in powder form that contains the necessary nutrients in their proper potency (see appendix A for the ingredients list). QuickStart is a key element for my patients with stubborn weight problems.

In addition to this formula, I also recommend flax oil—or, better yet, Super Fats—and the amino acid L-carnitine to help bring down elevated insulin levels. One scoop of QuickStart is blended with one tablespoon of flax oil or Super Fat, and this smoothie is taken in the morning and often again in the afternoon.

Patients with mild insulin resistance are usually able to resolve the problem by avoiding the high-glycemic carbohydrates, taking the supplements, and exercising regularly. Obese individuals may require the additional help of the following specialized supplements.

CoQ_{10}. I discussed this critical enzyme earlier. Not surprisingly, it is often deficient in overweight people. If your fasting blood CoQ_{10} level is below 1.5 mg/L, you should supplement with enough of this enzyme to reach this minimum level. Typical doses are in the range of 100 to 300 milligrams per day.

Alpha-lipoic acid. Alpha-lipoic acid is an essential nutrient for fat metabolism. It is made by the body; but, as with everything else, it also becomes depleted as we age. The decline is even more marked in individuals with insulin resistance. The recommended dose is 200 to 600 milligrams daily.

Conjugated linoleic acid (CLA). There are several studies in both humans and animals verifying the fat-metabolizing effect of conjugated linoleic acid (CLA), a naturally occurring oil amply contained in animal fats. Strict vegetarians tend to be particularly low in this oil. CLA, at doses ranging from 1000 to 2000 milligrams three times a day, helps lower the insulin level.

Growth-hormone stimulators. The amino acids L-lysine and L-glutamine and several peptides (anamorellin, ipamorelin, MK677) stimulate the body to produce extra growth hormone. This is especially useful in a weight-management program because overweight people are often deficient in growth hormone. Growth hormone is the key hormone in maintaining an optimal fat-to-muscle ratio, so you can see how important it is for weight control.

Take 3000 mg of L-lysine on an empty stomach when you first wake up in the morning, and then take 2000 mg of L-glutamine on an empty stomach at bedtime. The peptides should be taken according to your doctor's advice.

Step 5—Natural Hormone Replacement

The hormone deficiencies most often responsible for low energy production and weight gain are progesterone (in women), testosterone (in women and men), the adrenal and thyroid hormones, and growth hormone.

Successful long-term weight control very often requires replacement of these hormones on an individually tailored basis. Since I believe a weight-loss program may not succeed without such replacement, I suggest consulting a physician specializing in anti-aging medicine who is experienced in working with natural hormones.

Step 6—Correct Exercise

Understand this—you cannot lose weight by simply exercising. Exercising is critical for a successful program, but it must be accompanied with the other measures I have mentioned. The reason it is critical has to do with "set point." Here's how this works.

Your brain is constantly monitoring what is going on in your body. It wants to maintain the status quo. This is true for your weight. Your set point refers to your current weight. Your brain does not want your weight to go below your set point. It wants to keep your weight the same.

When you start losing weight, your brain takes that to mean that you are either starving or are very sick. So in order to prevent you wasting away, it acts to decrease your metabolism so that your body is burning fewer calories. This is why after you have lost a little weight, you find that the weight loss starts to decrease, and eventually you reach a plateau. And that is where exercise becomes critical.

Exercise sends a message to your brain basically saying, "I guess you must not be sick or starving to death because if you were, you would not be exercising like this." It lets your brain know that the weight loss you are experiencing is okay, and it stops your brain from decreasing your metabolism. So, make sure that you are regularly exercising during your entire time of weight loss as well as at least six months after you have reached your desired weight.

The other significant benefit of exercising along with changing the way you eat is that it ensures that the weight you lose is only fat and not muscle. Without exercise, you will lose muscle in addition to fat. And that will cause you to regain the weight.

FBR training. When you exercise at a heart rate equal to your fat-burning rate (FBR), your body is burning fat as fast as it can. As the exertion level increases beyond this point, the proportion of energy produced from fat metabolism actually decreases until you reach a point at which you don't burn any fat at all. Unfortunately, due to their energy-production deficit and insulin irregularity, overweight people usually spend all their exercise time at this latter level. Instead of burning fat, they are only burning their limited supply of glycogen. I call that exercising too hard to lose weight. It's counterintuitive, but it happens.

Proper exercise for fat loss means spending more time at a lower level of exertion. This means a minimum of thirty to forty-five minutes a day exercising at the FBR. For individuals with an aversion to exercise, this is good news indeed. Exercising at this level is very comfortable. So comfortable, in fact, that you could be exercising at this rate while talking on the phone, and the person you are talking to would never guess you were exercising at all.

Exercising at your FBR—for example, on a walk, bike ride, treadmill, or stationary bicycle—is the perfect kind of exercise for people who want to lose weight. Your FBR can only be determined with Bio-Energy Testing. You can fairly accurately guess it by noting what your heart rate is at an exercise level in which you are just starting to feel slightly out of breath.

Circuit training. Circuit training consists of a particular kind of weight training, also known as resistance training. If you are not familiar with weight training, you will definitely need to work with someone with experience, such as a personal trainer, to get you started and periodically check up on how you're doing. The circuit training I have found most useful is performed within the following specific parameters.

1. The resistance training must exercise the muscles of the arms, chest, back, abdomen, and, most importantly, the legs. This would include arm curls, military presses, bench presses, pullups, abdominal crunches, and squats or lunges.
2. The exercises are performed in 3 or 4 sets of 25 repetitions.
3. The sets are repeated continuously for 35 to 40 minutes.
4. At the end of each set, wait until your heart rate has dropped to your FBR before starting the next set.

Additional pointers. Rome wasn't built in a day. Neither will you get in shape the first day, or maybe even the first month. In fact, when you first start exercising, you probably will not be able to do half as much as you would like. Just be patient. It will all come around as you continue forward and get in progressively better shape. Just remember this: you have the rest of your life to get this together.

Perform the FBR training three days a week, and the circuit training a different three days a week. Take one day a week off to rest and be lazy. A successful program will usually result in losing anywhere from ten to fifteen pounds the first few weeks. Most of this is water loss, so don't get too excited. After this period, expect to lose about one to two pounds of weight per week. When you have lost the weight, you will only need to exercise for thirty minutes three times a week to maintain your health, your optimum energy production, and your new weight.

Step 7—Sleep, Sunlight, and Water

I can't emphasize strongly enough the importance of adequate rest in order for your body to generate good energy. Be sure to get in seven or eight hours of quality sleep on most nights—*this often means disciplining yourself to go to bed earlier.*

And while I am in emphasis mode, I should also remind you about getting enough sunlight and drinking enough water.

Getting enough sleep, sunlight, and water is free, at least so far. But even though they cost you nothing, please don't think they are any less important than the other things we have been discussing. It may not be obvious, but sleep, sunlight, and water are all important for helping you with your weight problem and putting you on the fast track to be permanently bursting with energy.

The Shallenberger Blue Plate Special

FOOD, SUPPLEMENTS, AND LIQUID FOR A MORE STREAMLINED YOU

Carefully follow the instructions below. They work. In almost all cases, this approach will lead to one to two pounds of fat loss per week.

FOOD

Breakfast: One scoop of QuickStart blended with one teaspoon of flax oil or Super Fats.

Eggs, meats (meats include fish, poultry, and red meat), cheese, oils, coffee with heavy cream, and regular, unsweetened yogurt are optional.

Lunch: Salad with dressing, cheese, and meats, or stir-fried vegetables with meat.

Dinner: Meats, vegetables, salad, beans.

Snacks: A little of what you had at the last meal.

Desserts: One piece of whole, fresh fruit from the middle- or low-glycemic list, eaten right after dinner.

Exceptions: Two meals per week with rice, bread, or pasta.

GENERAL EATING GUIDELINES

Eat slowly and be relaxed. Chew your food well. Enjoy your meals. Eat only what you need. Feel free to not clean your plate and put some of the meal away for next time. Salt and spices are unlimited. Cream may be used in moderation. You may use one tablespoon of fructose or xylitol a day as a sweetener. Do not eat anything for at least three hours before bedtime.

INTERMITTENT FASTING

Intermittent fasting is one of the easiest and healthiest ways to lose weight. Not only will it cut down calories without all that counting, but is also stimulates the production of very important hormones and enzymes. In fact, it is a healthy thing to do even if you don't need to lose weight. Here's what I recommend:

Pick one day a week, and on that day eat a large high-protein, high-fat, low-carbohydrate breakfast. Eat a similar smaller lunch, and skip dinner. Make sure that you drink at least one quart of water during the day. You may squeeze the juice of a lemon in the water if you want to. You may have coffee or tea, but nothing added that contains calories. The next week, on the same day skip both lunch and dinner. After one week of doing this, add in a second day in which you also skip lunch and dinner. Don't do more than two days per week. That will be too much for your body, and will not result in any more weight loss.

DRINKS

Water is your preferred beverage. (See chapter 8, Secret 1, for how much to drink.)

Definitely limit your diet sodas. One per day, if at all.

Coffee or tea can be taken, up to 16 ounces a day.

Herbal tea is unlimited.

No fruit juice.

SUPPLEMENTS

Immediately after you wake up, take 2 grams of L-lysine with a glass of water. Wait at least forty-five minutes before eating.

As noted above, take QuickStart in the morning.

Take 2000 milligrams of conjugated linoleic acid (CLA) three times per day.

Take 100 milligrams of CoQ_{10}, 1000 milligrams of L-carnitine, and 100 milligrams of alpha-lipoic acid two times per day.

Take another scoop of QuickStart blended with one teaspoon of flax oil around 3 or 4 p.m.

Take 2 grams of L-glutamine at bedtime.

Laurie's Journey to Looking and Feeling Great

When I first saw Laurie, she was forty-three years old and weighed 220 pounds. Most of her weight gain had occurred during the previous nine years, a prolonged period of marital and job stress. During this time, she exercised only sporadically. She had gone on several diets, lost twenty or thirty pounds on them, but soon put the weight back on. Now, she complained, "I can't seem to lose weight no matter what I do."

Sound familiar?

Before her weight explosion, Laurie had weighed 150 pounds and had felt and looked great at that weight. But now, at 220, her body-fat percentage was almost 50 percent—half of her, 110 pounds, was fat. The other 110 pounds reflected her lean body mass, which essentially equates to her muscle mass. Assuming she had a healthy body-fat percentage of 22 percent before she gained all that weight, her fat would have been 30 pounds, and her muscle mass 120 pounds.

So what was her problem? Was it that she gained eighty pounds of fat, or that she lost ten pounds of muscle mass? The answer is that the ten pounds of lost muscle is actually more of a contributing factor to her obesity than the gained eighty pounds of fat. This is because muscle tissue is extremely active metabolically and burns a significant amount of fat calories even while sleeping. The more muscle mass you have, reflected by a greater lean-body-mass percentage, the greater your daily fat-calorie expenditure will be. Laurie's ten-pound decrease in muscle mass was easily enough of a loss to prevent her from successfully burning her fat stores.

Every time Laurie embarked on a weight-loss plan, she lost much more than she'd bargained for. Each time, she indeed did lose weight, but the lost weight included muscle loss. This is because weight-loss plans do not focus on the real problem with weight gain, a decrease in energy production. In fact, weight-loss programs only aggravate the situation, because in the absence of proper metabolic management, calorie restriction causes the body to lower its energy production even more.

The only way to lose just fat and no muscle is by combining calorie restriction with proper exercise, sleep, sunlight, supplementation, and hormonal replacement if it is needed.

Laurie's muscle loss also increased her insulin resistance. This is because muscle cells have an enormous number of insulin receptors.

Loss of muscle mass, therefore, results in a loss of total body-insulin receptors, in turn causing elevated insulin levels.

Because her muscle loss caused her metabolism to decrease and her insulin resistance to increase, Laurie ultimately regained all the fat she had lost—and then some. She gained back the fat, but unfortunately not the muscle. Over the years, this yo-yo effect caused her to lose enough muscle to put her in a hole she couldn't climb out of.

But it wasn't just a lack of exercise and repeated dieting that caused her problems. It was also the fact that she had gone from being thirty-four to forty-three years old and had developed the hormonal deficiencies that come with getting older. Since hormones play such an important role in maintaining muscles, a common side effect with deficiencies is a loss of muscle mass. All these elements fit into the equation of solving Laurie's weight problem.

Hormone replacement and correct exercise

The first thing we did was to look at Laurie's Bio-Energy Testing results. Chapter 7 will tell you all you need to know about this important advancement in weight management. The results provided the necessary information to customize a personal and effective program for this unhappy woman.

Bio-Energy Testing indicated that Laurie had low thyroid activity, known as hypothyroidism. Like so many cases of hypothyroidism, her blood testing was in range. Only her Bio-Energy Testing was sensitive enough to diagnose the problem. The primary effect of her low thyroid function was to lower the resting metabolic rate. The resting metabolic rate refers to how many calories your body burns in a day. It's close to impossible to lose weight with a low resting metabolic rate. Her Bio-Energy Testing revealed that her resting metabolic rate was only 76 percent of optimal. Based on this reading, I prescribed enough thyroid hormones to return her metabolic rate to normal.

Laurie's Bio-Energy Testing also determined her FBR. I explained to Laurie that she needed to begin exercising three times a week for thirty minutes at her FBR. Another three days a week, I had her performing circuit training. She hired a personal trainer to teach her how to do this. Then, every six to eight weeks she would meet with the trainer to update her progress and alter her exercise protocol as needed.

Next, her Bio-Energy Testing revealed a C-Factor of 50. As you will see in chapter 7, this meant that her consumption of carbohydrates was completely suppressing her fat metabolism. Instead of burning fat for energy, her body was living off carbohydrates. Clearly, she was eating way too many carbohydrates, and was already insulin-resistant. I told her that if she wanted to permanently cure her weight problem, the carbs were going to have to go.

Finally, hormone testing revealed that she was in a state of relative estrogen excess, and that her DHEA was depleted. This did not surprise me. As an anabolic hormone, DHEA is very much involved in the production of muscle tissue, and it is also extremely valuable in correcting insulin resistance. You will learn all about these hormones and others in chapter 15.

To overcome these imbalances, I prescribed a DHEA supplement and a topical progesterone cream for her estrogen excess. All her hormone levels were regularly rechecked to ensure that she was being administered the correct doses for her individual needs.

Laurie was determined to beat her weight problem. So, armed with new information and several natural prescriptions, she set off to remake herself. And she succeeded. Within a year she had lost fifty-five pounds of fat. More importantly, through her exercise program, she had gained five pounds of muscle.

As an additional reward for her tenacity, Laurie no longer needed to adhere so strictly to carbohydrate avoidance, because her fat loss, muscle gain, and hormonal replacement had completely eliminated her insulin resistance. She had literally made her body over. Additionally, Laurie was like so many of my patients who are addicted to carbohydrates. Once she had experienced what these non-essential treat foods were doing to her, she no longer considered them a treat. She had completely lost her desire for them.

Now, more than eleven years later, she still has her former figure back and continues to maintain her desired weight simply by following the guidelines I recommend in this book.

Laurie's case is not exceptional. In fact, it's typical. When energy production is normalized, it is possible for any overweight person to achieve—and maintain—a permanent and healthy weight level.

MY RECOMMENDATIONS TO YOU

* Carefully follow the food and supplement instructions above.
* Obtain a weight-composition analysis using bio-impedance testing, available at most health spas. The ideal body-fat percentages are 18 to 22 percent for women and 12 to 18 percent for men. If your measurements are in line, follow my recommendations to avoid developing a weight problem.
* If your body-fat percentage is above these levels, you have a weight problem that needs to be resolved. The most efficient way to do that is to obtain Bio-Energy Testing. (See chapter 7 for the details.) The test will provide you with your particular exercise zones, and accurately measure your resting metabolism and fat-burning capacity. You can find a clinic offering Bio-Energy Testing at www.bioenergytesting.com. You will probably have to travel to get this test done, but the incredible information you will get is well worth it.
* Regardless of what blood tests show, if your metabolism is below normal you may very likely need thyroid hormone replacement in order to be successful. If your physician isn't familiar with physiological hormone replacement and won't prescribe thyroid replacement unless the blood tests are out of the normal range, I suggest finding another doctor who can help you. For a referral, contact either the American College for the Advancement of Medicine at 1-800-532-3688 or www.acam.org, or the American Academy of Anti-Aging Medicine at 1-561-997-0112 or www.a4m.com.
* Exercise three days a week for thirty to forty-five minutes at your FBR. Spend another three days with thirty-five to forty minutes of circuit training. I very strongly recommend that you work with a personal trainer to help you achieve your goals.
* Obtain a Bio-Energy Testing recheck after every twenty-five to thirty pounds of fat loss. The reason is that energy measurements will improve as weight comes off, and the program will have to be adjusted accordingly.
* As you lose weight, you can also monitor progress from time to time with additional bio-impedance analysis. A correct exercise program will result in putting on muscle weight even as you lose fat weight,

so your overall weight may not reflect your net fat loss, and the best way to follow your results is by bio-impedance analysis. You can also measure your waist, thighs, and hips, and take a good look in the mirror as you take off the weight and tone yourself up.

* The hormones intimately involved with weight management are DHEA, estrogen, growth hormone, progesterone, testosterone, and the thyroid hormones. Unless your physician has been trained in natural hormone replacement, you will need a specialist in this field. Contact the organizations listed for a referral.
* This is important! Animal studies clearly show that when the animal has lost weight, the brain, thinking that the weight loss indicates that something is wrong, will work to get the animal to regain the weight. This will go on for about six months after the weight is lost. The same thing happens with people. So, once you have lost the weight, you are only halfway home. You still have to stay on your game and not regain the weight for at least six months before you can relax even a little bit.
* Practice regular breath meditation, and be sure to get plenty of water and a full night's sleep. Oh, and don't forget about sunlight.

* 6 *

ENERGY AND DETOXIFICATION

As you've watched friends and relatives over the years, you've no doubt wondered why some people age so much more rapidly than others. The basic reason is that those who age faster are the ones with low E.Q.s. Their cells do not have enough energy to maintain a youthful functioning body. And that's sad, because it is only going to get worse over time.

Genetics aside, toxicity is one of the greatest factors influencing the age-related decrease in energy production. By toxicity, I mean the progressive accumulation of harmful substances, referred to as toxins, in the cells and tissues of the body.

Toxins can obviously come from the environment in the form of chemicals, cigarettes, food additives, heavy metals, and pharmaceutical drugs. But surprisingly, the overwhelming source of toxicity is the body itself. Each and every cell in the body takes in oxygen and nutrients, and from these substances produces energy *and* waste products. The wastes materialize in the form of organic acids. They are very toxic and must be eliminated from the body in order to maintain youthful energy production. Other sources of toxicity in the body include infections in the bowels, the mouth, and the sinuses.

Regardless of the source, the important thing to know is that toxins decrease cellular energy production. Since the very tissues and organs that are responsible for eliminating toxins require substantial energy production themselves, a vicious cycle is created, resulting in a persistent decline in energy production and increase in toxicity as people become older.

All the secrets I'll be sharing with you in Part Two relate to detoxification and improving your energy level. But before I begin giving you practical how-to information, I want to give you a good understanding of toxicity and detoxification (toxin removal).

Your Internal Sewer

It's not a very pleasant scene in our intestines. Basically, you're looking at an internal sewer, teeming with bacterial and fungal life, putrefied matter, incompletely digested foods, dyes, pesticides, preservatives, and probably a fair share of parasites.

Your body deals with this mess in a number of ways. First and foremost, more than 90 percent of your immune-system activity occurs in the intestinal tract where the immune cells are constantly working to prevent any of the toxic soup from entering the bloodstream. As you would imagine, a job like that requires a huge amount of energy. But, even as good as a highly energetic immune system is, it still can't prevent all the bowel's toxins from finding their way into the bloodstream.

Fortunately, before it enters the general circulation, the blood that circulates in the intestines and picks up all the nutrients and toxins then passes through the liver, where the toxins are filtered out. I say "fortunately" because, if the liver was not there to do this job, you would die within a matter of hours from your own internal toxins—that's how important the liver is to your health.

The liver also requires an enormous amount of energy production to accomplish its critical janitorial services. As long as it functions optimally, it can effectively protect the rest of the body from toxicity; but as illness and the aging process erode this energy production, liver function diminishes. As a result, more toxic materials, many of them carcinogenic, are able to get through the liver and into the general circulation. This can turn into another vicious cycle in which the liver cells cannot effectively detoxify because they themselves are toxic and can't produce enough energy to do the job well.

Oral Toxins

These days, more and more doctors and dentists are becoming aware of how important dental health is to overall health. Poor dental health can cause cancers, heart disease, autoimmune conditions, abscesses, diabetes, and a host of difficult-to-treat symptoms. But poor dental health is not the only way your mouth could be making you toxic. The other way is the dentists themselves!

One of the very real problems that still plagues modern dentistry is the routine use of silver amalgam fillings. Since the late 1800s, dentists have been using silver amalgam fillings as a preferred treatment for cavities. Many years ago, I was shocked to learn that 50 percent of these amalgams are composed of mercury, an extremely toxic heavy metal. An average amalgam filling contains about 780 milligrams of mercury, enough to exceed the U.S. Environmental Protection Agency's non-dietary mercury intake standard for a hundred years.

Dentists have always thought that once amalgam fillings were mixed and put in place, the mercury was somehow locked in. Some years ago, however, researchers learned that this is *not* the case. They revealed that mercury vapor is *continuously* released in the mouth by the activity of brushing, chewing, and drinking hot liquids, making people with silver amalgams constantly exposed to mercury every day.

Mercury is more toxic than arsenic, cadmium, or lead. Other than fluoride, it is the most toxic of all naturally occurring substances. Organic mercury, called methyl mercury, and the inorganic form found in the vapor from amalgams are the most toxic forms. There is no known non-toxic level for mercury vapor.

The vapor easily enters the body, where levels of mercury build up with time. *Mercury is a potent suppressor of mitochondrial activity*, and it damages brain and nerve tissue; the adrenal, pituitary, and thyroid glands; the heart and lungs; and hormones and enzymes.

Additional research indicates that as mercury collects in the body's tissues, it suppresses the immune system, forms mutated strains of fungi and bacteria, and contributes to allergies and autoimmune disorders, such as lupus, multiple sclerosis, and rheumatoid arthritis.

Mercury penetrates the placental membrane easily and has been found to damage the brain and nervous system of unborn babies. For that reason, the American Dental Association has recommended that silver amalgam fillings not be placed in the mouths of pregnant women. What is ignored is the effect of the mercury fillings already in place in these women.

Mercury depletes the immune system. In one study, immune helper cells, which regulate immune-system operations, were significantly suppressed in every person tested until their silver amalgams were removed. Furthermore, these same immune cells were determined to be almost immediately suppressed when silver amalgams were placed in the mouths of those previously without them.

Other studies have revealed that the ingested mercury released from silver amalgam fillings causes the yeast organisms commonly found in the intestines to become resistant to the normal function of the immune system.

The federal Occupational Safety and Health Administration (OSHA) and the Environmental Protection Agency (EPA) have declared that left-over scrap dental amalgam is a toxic hazard to dental personnel, to the dental office, and to the environment. Ironically, these agencies require very rigid legal protocols for the handling and disposal of the exact same dental material that is placed in our mouths.

Chronic mercury poisoning can affect all the body tissues and can mimic many common diseases. Many people recover from diseases after the fillings are removed, and the residual mercury is chelated (chemically removed) from the body.

Please remember that because of genetic susceptibility, some individuals are very sensitive to certain toxins, whereas others are much less sensitive. This is why the various side effects from medications only happen to certain people, not to everyone. And it is also why mercury is so much more of a problem with children and certain genetically susceptible adults.

Modern medicine tends to downplay the effects of environmental toxicity, because it often only affects those individuals who are sensitive and leaves the rest of us alone. Many people who are suffering from chronic environmental poisoning such as that stemming from mercury dental fillings are told that it is all in their head because they are the only ones affected. Perhaps in some cases this is true, but I have seen many patients over the past fifty years get much better when those fillings are removed and they are placed on an aggressive detoxification program. The following are the most prevalent signs and symptoms of chronic mercury poisoning.

- Cardiovascular effects—Alterations in blood pressure, feeble and irregular pulse, irregular heartbeat, pain and pressure in the chest.
- Neurological effects—Coordination difficulties, chronic or frequent headaches, dizziness, speech difficulties, tremors.
- Psychological effects—Anxiety, depression, fits of anger, irritability, loss of self-confidence, loss of self-control, memory loss, nervousness, shyness, timidity.
- Respiratory effects—Emphysema, persistent cough, shallow and irregular respiration.

* Other effects—Abdominal cramps, allergies, anemia, bleeding gums, bone loss, cold and clammy skin, colitis, diarrhea, edema, excessive perspiration, excessive salivation, fatigue, foul breath, joint pains, loosening of teeth, metallic taste in mouth, muscle weakness, sub-normal temperature.

But dental fillings containing mercury are not the only problem that a dentist can give you. Another is root canals. Here's the potential problem with root canals.

To perform a root canal, the dentist removes both the nerve and the blood supply of an infected or cracked tooth. This makes the tooth a dead piece of bone in the middle of living tissue. This leads to a chronic state of infection and inflammation. Even if the root canal seems successful in that it does not hurt, it is still a source of infection and inflammation. And that's the problem.

In susceptible people, the infection, inflammation, and toxicity associated with a root canal can easily trigger the immune system to be chronically activated, causing cancer, allergies, autoimmune disorders, and chronic pain. As long as you are young and strong and your energy production is optimal, it is unlikely that a root canal will cause one of these diseases. But it is likely that eventually, over time, it will create enough toxicity that the E.Q. drops and things start falling apart.

There is so much to say about the potential dangers of root canals in susceptible people that it is impossible to completely cover the controversy in this book. So, for those of you who are anticipating a root canal, let me recommend that you read *The Root Canal Cover-Up* by dentist George Meinig. Dr. Meinig does a great job laying out the facts about root canals, facts that have been vigorously suppressed for the last fifty years.

Before I finish this section, let me just emphasize how important I think it is for all of us to only consult with a biological dentist who is familiar with ozone therapy when it comes to procedures. Biological dentists have received important training that strictly mainstream dentists have not received. They know all kinds of healthy, safe, natural ways to treat dental problems that are not taught in dental school. I have to drive three and a half hours to see a biological dentist, and I consider myself lucky for that.

One last piece of advice about this very important topic. Never, ever have a dentist not fully trained in biological dentistry remove a root canal or remove mercury-containing amalgams. It is not safe. There are special measures that should be taken to protect the patient from the toxicity that happens with these procedures. You can find biological dentists at: www.iaomt.org, www.holisticdental.org, and www.iabdm.org.

Chronic Sinus Infections—Just Watch TV

The inflammation stemming from allergies and chronic sinus infections is a very common source of toxicity. All you have to do is watch TV and count the advertisements for sinus medications to know this is a big problem.

Allergies to foods and inhalants are one cause. Interestingly enough, as people age, allergies tend to disappear. This is because allergies are an overreaction of the immune system. The immune system requires a huge amount of energy to operate, and as people grow older and energy production declines, immunity declines as well, resulting in a decreased incidence of allergies. Nevertheless, long before the allergies have gone away, chronic sinus infections have often taken root, and a depressed immune system only makes them harder to eliminate.

The persistent use of antibiotics, steroid nasal medications, and antihistamines has the end result of creating chronic fungal infections that are resistant to therapy. Doctors trained in ozone therapy can often eliminate these infections, but that is the only therapy that I have found to be successful.

So, what's a chronic fungal infection of the sinuses do? It's not good. The immunologically reactive materials—such as free radicals, immune complexes, immunoglobulins, and peroxides—that our immune system uses to fight these chronic infections are highly toxic and must be cleared by the liver.

As one of the body's most metabolically active organs, the liver is unable to clear these toxic reactive materials without solid energy production. No surprise there. Furthermore, these toxins can react with the mitochondria in the liver cells and elsewhere to decrease energy production even more.

Detoxification to the Rescue

The process of eliminating toxins is referred to as detoxification. Without adequate detoxification, toxins can accumulate in the tissues and gradually, over many years, turn the body into a veritable toxic waste dump.

Imagine how much efficiency is lost by organs trying to carry out their functions under the burden of a half-century's buildup of pollution and poison. It's easy to understand why their function deteriorates at an accelerated rate. And by understanding how your body eliminates these toxins, you will be able to assist it and prevent toxin accumulation and the inevitable decrease in energy production that comes from it.

The Lymph System

The first step in the detoxification process occurs when the cells excrete their waste products into the lymph fluid. Imagine the cells of your body aligned like a brick wall, but instead of cement, they are separated by fluid, called the lymph fluid. The lymph fluid meanders through a network of lymph ducts, and eventually dumps its cargo of wastes into the bloodstream just above the heart.

Two factors are required to assist this flow into the bloodstream. One is movement, meaning activity that moves the muscles of the arms and particularly the legs. I don't mean exercise, just the routine walking and arm movements that occur in everyday life. People who especially need to be aware of this are those with disabilities or sedentary jobs where they sit for long periods of time—office workers, truck drivers, or writers, for example. If you work at such a job, be sure to get up every thirty minutes or so and walk around, madly waving your arms. (I'm kidding, of course, but you get the idea.)

The second factor is lying down. No problem there, huh? I'll bet you didn't realize that lying down was so vital to your health. Here we finally have a health concept that pretty much everyone can handle. Lying down allows the lymph fluid to gravity-drain. So when you sleep, the body is busy cleaning up the mess that was made during the day. Detoxification and repair are actually the primary activities of the body during sleep.

The Kidneys

After the lymph fluid is dumped into the bloodstream, the circulation carries the toxins to the kidneys and the liver. Certain toxins are selectively removed in the kidneys and dispatched to the bladder, where they are eliminated through the urine.

In order to do their jobs, the kidneys require water—pure water, and plenty of it. Not coffee, not juice, not alcohol, not milk, not soda—all these are liquids that may, in fact, actually impede kidney function—just water. And water is one of my secrets for better health and energy.

The Liver and Intestines

The toxins that aren't eliminated by the kidneys are processed in the liver and channeled out into the intestinal tract. Here, dietary fiber acts like a sponge and absorbs the toxins, escorting them out of the body through the feces.

This is why fiber is so important. Fiber, I should point out, is the roughage in vegetables, fruits, and whole grains. Your body doesn't absorb fiber. Instead, this material acts as a broom, keeping the intestines clean. Fiber absorbs the waste products removed by the liver and carries them out in the stool.

People who eat diets high in processed, refined carbohydrates, such as white bread and pasta, often don't have adequate fiber. Among other harmful effects, they run the risk of having toxins reabsorbed back into the body, which just makes the liver have to work harder.

Fiber also enhances regular bowel movements and helps prevent constipation. Chronic constipation is a major cause of toxin accumulation in the tissues.

Why Your Liver Is the Most Important Organ in the Body

The body is a dynamic, interacting organism. It is affected by even the slightest alterations in the environment, as well as by diet, emotion, and thought. These influences are continually changing, of course, and the changes can easily throw the body out of balance. Not to worry, however. The body has an almost miraculous ability to diagnose and correct these imbalances as they occur.

This ability is handled by the body's homeostatic regulation (body-balancing) systems. And nothing is more important to a healthy body than the optimal functioning of these systems, which are controlled by interactions between the brain and the liver.

These two organs, the brain and the liver, are not only designed to correct homeostatic disturbances but in fact actually require the disturbances. That's right, in order for your body to be fully healthy, it needs to be constantly challenged.

Most people would think the most important organ in this activity is the brain. And it's true that the brain has the most direct incoming and outgoing connection with all the cells and organs in the body. But it's not the most important simply because it is, for the most part, invulnerable.

The brain sits in its ivory tower like a general, separated and protected from most toxins and infections by what is known as the blood-brain barrier. This barrier allows only a very select group of molecules to come into actual contact with the brain.

Contrast this with the liver. Unlike the brain, the liver is on the front line, where all toxins are directed. From bacteria to viruses and pesticides, every toxin in the body must be cleared by the liver. Not only that, but it is also responsible for processing every nutrient you eat. Not a single molecule you ingest, no matter whether it's a vitamin, a mineral, fat, amino acid, or carbohydrate, can be used by the cells of the body until it is first processed by the liver.

Additionally, the liver regulates the balance of all the protein, fat, and carbohydrate in the blood. In combination with the spleen and intestines, the liver is the center of regulation and maintenance for the immune system. And it also regulates the balance of the entire hormonal system.

Nothing that occurs in the body is not in some major way regulated by the liver.

In contrast with the brain, moreover, the liver is not separated by a protective wall. It is right smack in the middle of all the dirty action. It is, therefore, a vulnerable organ, and it needs all the help and care it can get.

The fact that the liver is so vital to the maintenance of homeostasis, while at the same time so vulnerable to damage and dysfunction, is why I regard it as the most important organ in the body.

Let me put it another way. If you want to be healthy, do everything you can to help and protect your liver. Going forward in this book, you will see that a huge part of my program involves therapies and lifestyle habits geared toward helping the liver. I have often thought it's not accidental that the word *liver* starts with the word *live*.

Just to review, the following basic ingredients prevent the accumulation of toxins, increase energy production, and, hence, slow down the aging process: water, fiber, sleep, movement, exercise, and nutrients that assist the liver and intestines. Along with these, it is important to try to limit exposure to toxic conditions and substances that can interfere with the elimination process by adding to the overall toxic burden. These substances include pharmaceutical drugs, cigarette smoke, GMO foods, processed foods, inhaled or ingested environmental chemicals, silver dental fillings, and root canals.

✳ 7 ✳

BIO-ENERGY TESTING

Breakthrough Technology That Tells You If You Have an Energy Crisis

Okay, so you have decided that you want to optimize your energy production and extend the length and quality of your life. Now what? Before you can effectively start improving your energy production, the first step is to learn exactly how good (or bad) it is, and where any potential problems may lie.

Additionally, once you get started on your re-energizing program, you will want to be able to test how effective it is. Why wait until something goes wrong to learn that what you had been doing was missing a few crucial steps? You will want to make sure that your personalized program is really helping you to realize your energy potential.

The most reliable way to determine your needs and test how well your wellness program is working for you is through Bio-Energy Testing. I would have a tough time treating patients if I did not have access to Bio-Energy Testing. Thanks to Bio-Energy Testing, I can now measure every aspect of my patients' energy production easily, accurately, safely, and non-invasively. Furthermore, this technology has enabled me to discover and verify the efficacy of all the secrets presented in this book.

Each one of the secrets has been found to improve E.Q. That literally means slowing down and even reversing the aging process. I don't know this because I read about it somewhere, or because it sounds like a really good theory. I know the secrets work because I have proved it, using Bio-Energy Testing with thousands of my patients.

In the world of anti-aging medicine, your chronological age is unimportant. It's how efficiently your body produces energy, not how old it is, that counts. That's what indicates how healthy you are, how well you will feel and function as you age, and how long you will likely live.

Bio-Energy Testing

Bio-Energy Testing involves the use of a scuba-like mask, coupled with a computerized analyzer. The analyzer is able to measure how much oxygen the body is using and how much carbon dioxide the body is producing at any given time. These measurements are taken for about ten minutes with the patient resting quietly in a chair, and also while exercising for about fifteen minutes on a special computerized bicycle called an ergometer.

Additional measurements are determined using digital blood-pressure readings, body-composition analysis, lung capacity, and heart-rate readings.

To obtain the name of a health-care practitioner in your area trained in the use of Bio-Energy Testing, please go to www.bioenergytesting.com.

The cost for Bio-Energy Testing will vary depending on where you have it performed, but it typically runs in the area of $250 to $350. If you have a Bio-Energy test, it will be the best money you ever spent on yourself. When the test is performed by a physician, it is often reimbursable by insurance, although this will vary with the policies of each insurance company.

Before I discovered all the advantages of Bio-Energy Testing, I was the same as most anti-aging physicians. I just had to assume that the programs I put my patients on were actually working to slow down the aging process. Now, using Bio-Energy Testing, I can measure the E.Q. of every patient before and after treatment. And with this information I can verify whether or not my recommendations are effective. Quite simply, if it is increasing the E.Q., the program is working, and if it isn't, something is missing, and it isn't working. In that case, back to the drawing board.

Preliminaries to Bio-Energy Testing

Here are some insights and tips you should have prior to testing.

The test is usually performed in the morning, before noon. You should not eat or drink anything other than water. And be extremely lazy before the test—both physical and mental exertion should be kept to a minimum. Avoid any strenuous exercise for five days and any exercise at all for forty-eight hours prior to the test.

Record your resting heart rate for several days prior to the test. This is done by wearing a heart rate monitor to bed. Heart rate monitors can be purchased at bicycle shops and sporting-good stores, and typically cost around $50 to $80. They come equipped with a strap outfitted with an electrode that goes over the heart. You read your heart rate on a little monitor that looks like a watch. Just before bedtime, attach the electrode. Place the monitor on a bedside stand so you can read it in the morning without having to sit up or reach over. In other words, with very little effort.

When you wake up, gently roll over and read your heart rate.

Record your wake-up heart rate in this manner for several mornings. The readings should be very similar to each other. For most people, the readings will be between 55 and 70 beats per minute. People in better condition will have lower readings. Some athletes may have a resting heart rate of less than 40.

Average out your readings when you go for your Bio-Energy Test.

Resting Testing—The First Test

After you arrive at the testing center, the technician will record your age, sex, height, and weight. She will also determine your body composition (your body's percentages of fat and muscle) using an electronic device called a bio-impedance analyzer. Your blood pressure will be taken sitting down and, right after that, standing up. All these measurements will be entered into the computer.

After the technician applies a heart rate monitor strap to your chest, you will be placed in a comfortable chair. You should be relaxed, mentally and physically, and not be concerned about the outcome of the test. Failure to adequately relax can influence the resting measurements.

Within a few minutes of your settling down in the chair, the technician will place a special face mask similar to an oxygen mask over your mouth and nose. There is no discomfort, so relaxing shouldn't be a problem. As you just lie back and relax, the analyzer will determine how much oxygen your body is taking in, and how much carbon dioxide it is putting out.

Exercise Testing

After the resting measurements are taken, the fun really begins. You are placed on an ergometer, a fancy name for an exercise bicycle that uses a computer to measure how hard you are working. The seat of the cycle is adjusted so your leg is straight when the heel of your foot is on the pedal in the most extended position.

The technician will help you to put on what can best be described as a scuba mask that covers your nose and mouth. Now you will begin to cycle. For the first several minutes, very little effort will be required of you. Then the workload on the ergometer will gradually increase, so you will have to work harder to turn the pedals. As the level of exertion increases, your heart rate will also increase. The test continues until the technician notifies you that you have entered into anaerobic energy production. At this point, the test is concluded.

If you are a person who exercises regularly and is in good shape, then you will find that the exercise testing will work you pretty hard. If you are not in good shape, you will find that the exercise testing seems easy. Why? Because someone in good shape is going to be able to work much harder before becoming anaerobic than someone who is not fit.

Oxygen Consumed = Life

Oxygen is an extremely high-energy molecule. Animals, including humans, convert oxygen, nature's highest-energy molecule, to water, nature's lowest-energy molecule. In this process, energy is released. *It is this precious energy that powers every aspect of your life.*

This process also generates carbon dioxide as a waste product. The amount of carbon dioxide produced is in direct proportion to the amount of energy being generated from fat, as opposed to the amount being generated from glucose. Fat metabolism produces less carbon dioxide than glucose metabolism.

Fortunately, all the oxygen enters the body through the lungs, and all the carbon dioxide is eliminated from the lungs. Thus, the energy-conversion process can be gauged by measuring how much oxygen and carbon dioxide are coming in and going out with each breath you take. That's precisely what the Bio-Energy Testing analyzer is busy measuring.

The total amount of oxygen taken in is used to determine the total amount of energy being produced. The ratio of oxygen going in to carbon dioxide coming out is used to determine whether your body is producing energy from fat or glucose. It is also used to determine when your body starts to become anaerobic.

What Bio-Energy Testing Can Tell You

When I evaluate a patient with Bio-Energy Testing, besides measuring that person's E.Q., I can also determine the following critical metabolic measurements:

- The M-Factor (resting metabolism)
- The C-Factor (carbohydrate factor)
- The Fat-Burning Factor (fat metabolism)
- The optimum exercise zone for that person, centered around the FBR and the ATR
- The Fitness Factor (strength and fitness factor)
- The Lung Factor (lung capacity)
- The Biological Index (overall score)
- The optimum caloric intake for weight loss
- The optimum caloric intake for longevity

I will show you how these measurements are used to increase your energy levels, fine-tune your disease-prevention and anti-aging program, and improve your overall health.

Bio-Energy Testing lets me offer my patients the most efficient and accurate health, aging, and fitness assessment available. It can diagnose a decrease or increase in E.Q., as well as pinpoint what factors may be working to suppress energy production. This makes Bio-Energy Testing the ultimate tool for anti-aging medicine, medical diagnostics, personal fitness training, and weight management.

Who Can Benefit from This Test?

- Anyone wanting to verify that the anti-aging program is working
- Anyone, even an older person, who wants to feel and function like a younger person
- Anyone interested in preventing the diseases of aging
- Anyone needing help with weight control
- Anyone wanting to maximize workout efficiency
- Anyone who is interested in slowing down the aging process
- Anyone with arthritis, diabetes, heart disease, or high cholesterol
- Chronically fatigued individuals
- Anyone who has a disease they can't cure

How the Bio-Energy Testing Analyzer *Knows*

Imagine a salesperson trying to persuade a prospective buyer to buy a thermos.

"If you put something cold into it," he says, "it will stay cold. If you put in something hot, it will stay hot."

The man buys the thermos and then comes back a few weeks later.

"There's no problem at all with the thermos," he says happily. "It works great. It keeps hot things hot and cold things cold. But what I don't understand is: how does it *know*?"

In order for you to understand how the Bio-Energy Testing analyzer *knows*, take a short tour through some of the measurements used in Bio-Energy Testing, and see how they relate to the process of energy production in the body. This information can get incredibly complex, but I've attempted to keep it as simple as possible.

The Man Behind the Curtain

The Bio-Energy-Testing analyzer measures the real-time breath-by-breath intake of oxygen and the production of carbon dioxide. The computer then records all the readings.

Due to the effects of coughing, sighing, and other forms of irregular breathing, there are often artifacts in the recorded readings that do not accurately reflect true oxygen and carbon dioxide levels. The computer program identifies these artifacts and eliminates them. It then takes the remaining readings, averages them, and uses them to make its calculations.

Calculating Energy

All the oxygen that we depend so much on only has one destination. It eventually ends up in the mitochondria in the cells and is used to produce energy. Thus, the amount of oxygen that is consumed directly correlates with the number and function of the body's mitochondria. To the degree that we have optimal amounts of mitochondria and to the degree that our mitochondria are functioning effectively, we will consume larger amounts of oxygen. Oxygen uptake gives us a direct look at our mitochondrial function.

When the mitochondria use oxygen to produce energy, about 60 percent of the energy gets released as heat. That's how we keep warm.

The remaining 40 percent gets harnessed in the form of a molecule called adenosine triphosphate (ATP). It is ATP that every one of your cells uses to carry on its various functions. Put another way, the amount of energy your body has to perform all its functions is directly dependent on how much ATP it can produce. So, when I say that Bio-Energy Testing is measuring your body's ability to produce energy, I mean that it is measuring your body's ability to produce ATP. This is how *it knows*.

Look at the following equations, which show how oxygen is used in the mitochondria to produce ATP.

Fat + 23 molecules of oxygen →
16 molecules of carbon dioxide + 130ATP

This equation shows that when only fat is being metabolized by oxygen to produce ATP, there is a ratio of 5.6 (130:23) molecules of ATP produced per 1 molecule of oxygen consumed. Thus, by measuring how much oxygen is consumed, the amount of ATP being produced from fat can be easily determined by multiplying this amount by 5.6.

Glucose + 6 molecules of oxygen →
6 molecules of carbon dioxide + 36ATP

In the case of glucose (the sugar that carbohydrates break down to), there is a ratio of six (36:6) molecules of ATP being produced per 1 molecule of oxygen being consumed. Again, when only glucose is being metabolized, we can simply measure oxygen consumption and quickly determine ATP production by multiplying this amount by 6. Note also that glucose results in 7 percent more ATP production per molecule of oxygen than fat. This is why glucose metabolism is said to be a more efficient form of energy production than fat metabolism.

Fat or Glucose?

The only problem with this particular scenario so far is that during the Bio-Energy Testing procedure, the body is producing ATP from both fat and glucose. Therefore, in order to determine total ATP production with accuracy, it is necessary to know at all times what percentage of the oxygen being consumed is metabolizing glucose and what percentage is metabolizing fat.

For example, when oxygen is metabolizing glucose, the ratio of carbon dioxide produced to oxygen consumed is 1 (6:6). So, when the Bio-Energy Testing analyzer determines that the ratio of carbon dioxide to oxygen is 1.0, it knows that oxygen is metabolizing glucose exclusively

When fat is being metabolized, there is a ratio of .7 (16:23) molecules of carbon dioxide produced for every 1 molecule of oxygen being consumed. Thus, the analyzer will determine that oxygen is metabolizing fat exclusively when the ratio of carbon dioxide to oxygen is .7.

For the mathematicians in the crowd, it is important to note that this relationship of carbon dioxide produced to oxygen consumed from fat and glucose is linear. This means that it is possible to know exactly how much fat or glucose is being metabolized at all times simply by measuring the ratio of carbon dioxide to oxygen.

By constantly measuring both total oxygen being consumed and the ratio of oxygen consumed to carbon dioxide produced, the Bio-Energy Testing analyzer is able to accurately determine two things: 1) how much ATP is being produced; and 2) what percentage of the ATP is being produced from fat and what percentage from glucose. These two things may not sound like much information, but they are critical to mitochondrial function. And they can be used to calculate your entire energy-producing capability.

Bio-Energy Testing at a Glance

Using the information provided by the analyzer during both rest and exertion, the Bio-Energy Testing computer program then calculates the following:

1. How much ATP your body produces at rest.
2. How much ATP is produced from fat at rest.
3. The maximum ATP you can produce aerobically under exertion.
4. The maximum ATP you can produce from fat under exertion.
5. The maximum amount of aerobic work your body can perform.

These calculations are then compared to what would be predicted for each individual according to sex, height, and weight, using standard ATP-prediction databases. The results are used to determine your M-Factor, your C-Factor, your Fat-Burning Factor, your FBR (fat-burning heart rate), your ATR (anaerobic threshold heart rate), your Fitness Factor, and, of course, your E.Q.

Healthy—Not Healthy for Your Age

Two additional factors need to be addressed regarding these calculations. They both have to do with how the determinations of predicted ATP production are arrived at. The first is age.

Keep the goal in mind. From the anti-aging perspective, what you want to do is to maintain youthful levels of ATP production even as you get older: you want to be healthy for a young person, not healthy for your age. Therefore, it does not make sense for older people to compare their ATP production to what is typical for their age bracket.

There is general agreement in the anti-aging, exercise physiology, and in longevity literature, that, for all practical purposes, the effects of aging do not begin to become measurable to anyone but world-class athletes until after the age of forty. Therefore, when looking to maintain youthful levels, a reasonable benchmark for ATP production would be those levels that are typical of a forty-year-old.

So, for anyone over the age of forty, all their ATP-production measurements are compared to a database with a default age of forty. Take the case of a sixty-two-year-old woman. Her Bio-Energy Testing results will not be comparing her to what would be considered normal and expected for the average sixty-two-year-old. Instead, the computer will compare her readings to those expected of the average forty-year-old woman with the same weight and height.

On the other hand, since those under forty are too young to have experienced the effects of the aging process, they are compared to their own age group.

Correcting for Fat

The second factor that has to be taken into consideration for the calculation of predicted ATP production is percentage of body fat.

All the formulas used to predict ATP production use weight as part of the input to the equation. This makes a lot of sense, because it stands to reason that the more someone weighs, the bigger they are, and the more ATP they should be expected to produce. However, this expectation is true for every tissue but fat.

Because fat is metabolically inert tissue, it makes very little ATP. In this case, using the predictive formulas as they are classically used would result in unreasonably high predicted levels of ATP production in anyone who has an excess of body fat. This would cause them to have a falsely depressed expectation for ATP production secondary to their excessive body fat. A man who weighs 200 pounds, 75 pounds of which is fat, should not be compared to a man who weighs 200 pounds but only has 30 pounds of fat. The second man will obviously produce more ATP, simply because he has more metabolically active tissue.

To account for this potential inaccuracy, the weight used in determining predicted resting ATP production is corrected, using this body-fat analysis: the weight of overweight men is corrected to a weight based upon an ideal body fat of 18 percent. The weight of overweight women is corrected to an ideal body fat of 22 percent.

Your M-Factor (Metabolic Factor)— How Much ATP Your Body Produces at Rest

Now that the right adjustments to accurately predict ATP production have been made, take a look at what Bio-Energy Testing is going to tell about how much ATP you make.

By measuring how much ATP your body produces at rest, the Bio-Energy Testing analyzer can determine your resting metabolic rate. Your resting metabolic rate (RMR) reflects your overall metabolic rate. Those with high RMR's have high metabolic rates, and those with low RMR's have low metabolic rates.

Your RMR is especially valuable for weight control because it is used to compute how many calories your body will burn in a day. It is also a much more accurate way to diagnose low-thyroid states than blood testing.

Dietitians have used many formulas to estimate RMR; but for most people, especially those for whom it is the most important, these estimates are almost always inaccurate. Bio-Energy Testing is unique in that it precisely measures your exact RMR. Once your RMR is measured, your M-Factor can be determined.

For people younger than forty, the M-Factor is equal to the ratio of their measured RMR as determined by Bio-Energy Testing compared to the average RMR of a healthy person of the same age, weight, height, and gender.

For those over forty, the M-Factor equals the ratio of the measured RMR compared to the average RMR of a healthy forty-year-old of the same weight, height, and gender. The optimal M-Factor is 100 percent. This would indicate that the person being tested is producing the entire amount of ATP that is predicted.

Since the M-Factor declines with aging, it is an excellent yardstick of your rate of aging. But it is not only an excellent way to determine how well your anti-aging program is working; it also supplies the critical information needed to establish the correct therapeutic program for optimum energy production and weight control.

Remember that 2004 study where the researchers looked at how long individual mice lived based upon their RMRs? They found that the mice with the highest RMR's lived a whopping 36 percent longer than the mice with the lowest readings—an astounding testimony to the effect of resting ATP production.

Low M-Factors aren't just a result of getting older. They also decline from disease. And they vary considerably depending on muscle mass, sleep quality, diet, genetics, fitness, and hormone levels (particularly thyroid and adrenal hormones). Nutrient deficiencies, especially the B vitamins, coenzyme Q_{10}, fatty acids, and magnesium, can also play a significant role in determining the M-Factor.

In particular, your M-Factor can signal significant decreases in thyroid function (hypothyroidism) that often go undiagnosed. A low M-Factor is the most sensitive indicator of low-thyroid states, even when thyroid blood tests show normal values (see chapter 15, Secret 8).

Your C-Factor—How Much ATP is Produced from Fat at Rest

As stated above, when glucose is being metabolized, there is a one-to-one ratio of carbon dioxide produced to oxygen consumed. When fat is being metabolized, the ratio is .7. Since the Bio-Energy Testing analyzer measures carbon dioxide production as well as oxygen consumption, the percentage of fat being metabolized can be determined by examining this ratio.

Based on my own measurements and those published, when an optimally healthy person is resting, he/she should be able to produce at least 75 percent of his/her total ATP production from fat. I have measured some competitive athletes who made almost 90 percent of their resting ATP from fat. But this is a superhuman level. Seventy-five percent is more than enough. But less than that indicates decreased fat metabolism. And since fat provides most of our overall energy, decreased fat metabolism causes major decreases in total energy production.

The reason the body can't produce 100 percent of its resting energy from fat has to do with the brain. Unlike every other organ in the body, the brain can utilize only carbohydrates for energy. Since the brain is active even in a resting state, there is always going to be some carbohydrate metabolism going on in the brain.

Once the percentage of resting ATP production from fat is measured by the analyzer, the computer presents it as the C-Factor. The C-Factor is formulated on a scale of 50 to 100, as shown below.

* A C-Factor greater than 100 indicates that 75 percent of the resting ATP is from fat. This points to optimal resting fat metabolism.
* A C-Factor between 90 to 100 is also acceptable because, even though it indicates that less than 75 percent of the resting ATP is from fat, the fat metabolism is still good.
* A C-Factor less than 90 is starting to indicate a problem with resting fat metabolism. For example, a C-Factor of 80 indicates that only 50 percent of the resting ATP production is from fat.
* A C-Factor of 50 indicates that none of the resting ATP is coming from fat; it is all coming from glucose. This points to a severe impairment of resting fat metabolism.

Why Is It Called C-Factor?

It turns out that when you are at rest, and not exercising, the amount of carbohydrate in your diet determines how much fat your body is burning more than any other single factor. The more carbohydrates you eat, the less fat you will burn. The reason is actually quite simple.

When you feed your body carbohydrates, it will take the most energy-efficient path it can. Rather than store the carbohydrates for later use and in the meantime rely on fat metabolism, it will just take the easy way out and burn the carbohydrates for energy. And that means it will burn less fat.

The more carbohydrates you eat, the less fat your body will need to burn. If you eat too many carbohydrates, your body will not need to burn any fat at all. Given this, the effect of dietary carbohydrate on fat metabolism is one of the major factors in premature aging, low energy production, obesity, and many other diseases and health problems.

This suppressive effect of carbohydrates on fat burning is quite individual. There are some people who can have a relatively high intake of carbohydrates and still maintain an optimal C-Factor. Most people, however, need to maintain a very modest intake of carbohydrates in order to avoid suppressing fat metabolism.

Let me offer a very graphic example to make my point.

A forty-two-year-old movie actor came to my clinic to have his energy production analyzed with Bio-Energy Testing. He was an avid exerciser, and took an array of supplements as part of an anti-aging/preventive medicine program.

He had no complaints, and his physical and routine laboratory examination was almost completely normal. The only problem he had was a modest elevation of a blood fat called triglyceride. When I first saw him, I thought this young man looked like the epitome of health. Looks can be deceiving, however, especially in health.

When tested, this man had a greater than 40 percent reduction in his total aerobic ATP production. That means a 40 percent reduction in his E.Q., which placed him in the category of a severe energy deficit.

Additionally, his C-Factor was 50. This meant his resting energy production from fat was zero. Essentially, he had no fat metabolism. He was spending his days living strictly off his carbohydrate stores.

I have learned not to be too surprised by such findings, and I immediately asked him about his diet. That's when he confessed that every day for the previous two months, he had been consuming two milkshakes blended with cookies at a popular fast-food restaurant. It was his only bad habit. But it was one that was going to make him age faster and impair his health in the years to come.

I asked him to continue everything he was currently doing except drinking the milkshakes. I also asked him to avoid all other carbohydrates, including fruit, grains, legumes, sugars, and tubers.

He repeated his Bio-Energy Testing only three weeks later and was much happier the second time around. In only three weeks, his E.Q. had doubled. It had increased to 130 percent—that of the average man two years younger. From energetic rags to riches in only three weeks simply from dramatically decreasing dietary carbohydrate!

Not surprisingly, this second test revealed that his C-Factor was now maximal at 101. Cases such as this form the majority of what I see on a daily basis in my clinic. So if you haven't already figured it out by now, that's why resting fat metabolism is presented as "C-Factor": the C stands for carbohydrate.

* A C-Factor greater than 90 indicates that you are eating an optimal amount of carbohydrate for your genetics and lifestyle.

* A C-Factor less than 90 indicates that for your genetics and lifestyle, your intake of carbohydrates is excessive and is impairing your fat metabolism.
* A C-Factor of 50 indicates that your intake of carbohydrates is so excessive that it is completely suppressing all fat metabolism.

It is important to note here that resting fat metabolism can be impaired by factors other than carbohydrates. Every now and then, I see a person who is on a very low-carbohydrate diet, but who still has a low C-Factor. This is fairly unusual, but it can happen because, again, resting fat metabolism is also influenced by other factors.

Deficiencies of the adrenal hormones cortisol and DHEA, the anabolic hormones HGH, progesterone, and testosterone, and the thyroid hormones T_4 and T_3 also play a significant role, along with deficiencies of amino acids, B vitamins, chromium, coenzyme Q_{10}, essential fats, L-carnitine, lipoic acid, and magnesium; excessive dietary intake of trans-fatty acids; insulin resistance; and sleep disturbances.

Any one or any combination of these factors can result in a low C-Factor even in the presence of a low-carbohydrate diet. However, in a resting state the demand for ATP is pretty minimal, so these factors usually have only a small effect on the C-Factor score compared to the carbohydrate effect.

If your C-Factor is less than 90, you are eating too many carbohydrates for optimal energy production. Sometimes the amount of dietary carbohydrate that will suppress fat metabolism is quite small. In fact, after observing the C-Factors of hundreds of my patients, I can report that there are a great many people out there who seem to be genetically programmed so that, in order to optimally burn fat, they must eat almost no carbohydrates at all. But this is not always the case.

About 15 percent of people have bodies that need carbohydrate. In these people, I see a pattern in which the E.Q. is optimal and the C-Factor is low. What is happening in these people is that their particular mitochondria prefer to burn glucose to fat. This metabolic type is caused by a combination of mitochondrial genetics and lifestyle. In this group, it is actually important to make sure that they eat enough complex carbohydrates, because if they don't, they will feel tired and lack stamina.

Why Is the C-Factor Important?

The C-Factor is important because it specifically looks at resting fat metabolism.

A hundred years ago, before cars, central heating, washing machines, and other conveniences people now take for granted, the everyday lifestyle involved much more exertion. In fact, people probably spent most of their waking hours in activities that involved exertion.

But today, most people are like me. I drive to work. My work consists of sitting down all day and walking from one room to another. When I get home, I exercise for thirty minutes, then I rest from my hard day of mental activity. And finally, I go to sleep for eight hours, and then start all over again.

On the weekends, I might work in the garden, ride my horse, sail my boat, or set out on a bike ride. The point I am making is, except for my daily thirty minutes of exercise, I am in a resting state for twenty-three and a half hours every day. So, for me, and for every one of you who has a similar contemporary lifestyle, resting fat metabolism is critically important—because that's the state people are in 98 percent of the time.

The three most important considerations for your overall health are your resting metabolism (M-Factor), your resting fat metabolism (C-Factor), and your mitochondrial function (E.Q.). Two of these three measurements are resting measurements. And the reason they are so important is because 98 percent of the time, the majority of people in today's modern society are in a resting state.

The fact that you can burn fat well while exercising is relatively unimportant. What you do in your resting state is really what it is all about. And that's why your C-Factor measurement is so critical to your health.

Fat-Burning Factor—Maximal ATP Production from Fat

Once the resting energy-production readings have been determined, Bio-Energy Testing then determines how well your mitochondria function under an exertional stress. It does this by examining how well you can make ATP while exercising.

Once you start the exercise phase of the test, the computer will steadily increase the resistance every fifteen seconds. This will cause you to progressively work harder and harder.

As your exertion increases, your rising energy demands will cause your body to metabolize increasing amounts of fat into ATP. And so, as the resistance becomes harder and harder, your body will be burning more and more fat.

This increase in fat burning can only go on for a limited amount of time, however, because as I mentioned before, fat metabolism is not as energy-efficient as glucose metabolism. Remember that you get 7 percent more ATP from glucose than from fat. Therefore, as the resistance becomes harder and your energy demands increase, at some point your body will start to shift from burning fat to burning glucose.

It is at that point that you will have reached a level of exertion where you are burning the maximum amount of fat your body is able to metabolize. As you continue to increase your exertion level beyond this point and your need for ATP steadily increases, you will be metabolizing progressively more glucose and less fat. This point of maximum fat burning can be determined by the Bio-Energy Testing analyzer. It is used to determine your Fat-Burning Factor.

As exercise intensity continues to increase, and you are are progressively burning more glucose and less fat, you will eventually get to a point where you are metabolizing no fat at all. At this second point, all ATP production will be coming entirely from glucose. Called the anaerobic threshold, this marks the point where you have reached your maximal aerobic ATP production.

Your Fat-Burning Factor refers to the maximal amount of ATP you can produce from fat. Like the other Bio-Energy Testing factors, it is a percentage calculation, which compares your measurement to one expected from a healthy person of your sex, height, and weight. Based on my own clinical measurements and those published, a healthy person should be able to produce at least 60 percent of his/her maximal aerobic ATP production from fat. Less than that indicates impaired fat metabolism.

The computer determines your Fat-Burning Factor and presents it in the following way:

* A Fat-Burning Factor greater than 100 indicates that your body is able to produce at least 60 percent of your maximal aerobic ATP production from fat. This points to optimal fat metabolism.

* A Fat-Burning Factor less than 100 indicates that you are producing less than 60 percent of your maximal aerobic ATP production from fat. This points to less-than-optimal fat metabolism.

* A Fat-Burning Factor less than 70 indicates you are producing less than 30 percent of your maximal aerobic ATP production from fat. This points to a severe impairment of fat metabolism.

I want you to be healthy, not just healthy for your age. Therefore, for anyone younger than forty, the Fat-Burning Factor compares them to healthy people of the same age, weight, height, and gender. But for those over forty, the Fat-Burning Factor compares them to healthy people of the same weight, height, and gender who are forty years old.

The Difference Between C-Factor and Fat-Burning Factor

The difference between C-Factor and Fat-Burning Factor is as follows: The C-Factor is a measurement of resting fat metabolism. Resting fat metabolism is almost always a function of carbohydrate intake. So, if your C-Factor is decreased, you can bet that you are eating too many carbohydrates. The exception would be if your C-Factor is low but your E.Q. is greater than 100. In that case, the low C-Factor indicates that your body does well with carbs.

The Fat-Burning Factor is not as influenced by carbohydrate intake as the C-Factor. It is more affected by other determinants of fat metabolism. These other determinants include dietary deficiencies of essential fats, excessive dietary intake of trans-fatty acids, insulin resistance, low thyroid function, adrenal exhaustion, and sleep deprivation. They also include deficiencies of B vitamins, chromium, coenzyme Q_{10}, L-carnitine, lipoic acid, and magnesium; hormone deficiencies; and toxicity.

Additionally, the C-Factor and Fat-Burning Factor measurements are very important for people who find it hard to maintain a healthy weight. They often have a low C-Factor along with a low Fat-Burning Factor. Functionally speaking, that means the majority of their daily energy needs are being met by carbohydrate metabolism. No wonder they can't lose weight. They're burning carbohydrate instead of fat.

Fat—Your Primary Energy Source

Fat has received an enormous amount of negative press over the years. Yet fat is absolutely central to energy production. Many nutritionists still profess that carbohydrate is the body's primary energy source. But they are wrong.

My use of Bio-Energy Testing has taught me an amazing fact: *a decline in fat metabolism is more responsible for the effects of aging and degenerative disease than any other single factor.* This is because fat is the body's ideal energy raw material. We were designed that way. The body has the capability to store huge amounts of fat. But it can only store a tiny amount of carbohydrates. Add these two facts up. If carbohydrates were the main energy provider for cells, then we are all designed wrong.

I discovered the amazing value of fat quite by accident. It happened as I was analyzing the Bio-Energy Testing results of several hundred people. As I studied the data, I gradually became aware of a certain pattern. The younger, healthier, and more athletic a person was, the more efficiently he/she burned fat. However, the older or sicker people were, the less energy they produced from fat metabolism, and the more they began to obtain their energy needs from carbohydrates.

The average healthy twenty-two-year-old man or woman obtains close to 80 percent of their daily energy needs from fat. But by the time they reach fifty-five years old, she or he would be lucky to be producing half the needed energy from fat. As people aged or developed illnesses, I saw this consistent shift from fat metabolism to carbohydrate metabolism over and over again.

A decrease in energy production from fat results in a corresponding decrease in *total* energy production. This is because, outside of an occasional brief period of exertion, fat is the major source of energy in the healthy body.

The fact that fat metabolism plays the key role in energy production is emphasized in many research papers. In a 2002 paper, the researchers were able to restore youthful levels of fat metabolism to a group of old rats. When they did this, they were able to restore the aging rats' energy production to that typical of younger rats, "thus delaying mitochondrial decay and aging." They proved that better fat metabolism equals better energy production.

Are You Burning Fat Efficiently?

Is it any wonder that obesity is now epidemic in the United States? We have these bodies that are designed to go long times without eating. But instead of going without food, three squares a day has become the reality. We truly have caveman bodies living in a supermarket world.

The constant eating, combined with high carbohydrate intake and low fat intake, has just about completely shut down the nation's fat metabolism. But the evolutionary process of storing meals as fat has not changed. We can store the fat, but we can't burn it. The result? The perfect recipe for weight gain.

Aging, gaining weight, low energy, and disease all go hand in hand. They're just different sides of the same problem—an inability to burn or metabolize fat. There are two proofs of this.

One is the fact that an increase in body fat is one of the most consistent hallmarks of the aging process. The other is that the risk for developing every disease from cancer to diabetes is increased in those who are fat.

And, despite what you may hear from many so-called experts in the diet industry, excessive carbohydrate consumption—not fat—is the major dietary cause of weight gain. It is also the leading cause of diabetes and high cholesterol.

It seems like a reasonable-enough assumption that eating fat causes fat gain, but the science doesn't support it.

Determining Your E.Q.

Your E.Q., or Energy Quotient, is a measurement of your maximal aerobic energy production. It tells you how well your body is able to produce energy from oxygen. To the degree that your E.Q. is over 100, you are highly efficient at producing energy from oxygen. To the degree that it is below 100, the opposite is the case.

A high E.Q. means you are in an optimum state of health. A low E.Q. doesn't mean you have a disease or are even sick. But it does indicate that your health is in jeopardy. You are aging faster than you should, as well as increasing your risk for every disease, from cancer to arthritis.

During the exercise part of Bio-Energy Testing, your exertion level is steadily increased until you get to your anaerobic threshold. This is your point of maximal aerobic energy production. At this point, your body is producing ATP from oxygen as efficiently as it can.

The Bio-Energy Testing analyzer measures how much ATP you are producing at this point. Then the computer program compares your ATP production to that expected for the average healthy person. Just as with the other measurements, for anyone younger than forty the computer compares them to healthy persons of their age, weight, height, and gender. But for those over forty, it compares them to forty-year-old healthy people of the same weight, height, and gender.

The computer determines your E.Q. and presents the results in this way.

* An E.Q. greater than 100 indicates that your body is able to produce ATP from oxygen at a very healthy level. This points to optimal health.
* An E.Q. less than 100 indicates that your body is not able to produce adequate levels of ATP from oxygen. This points to less-than-optimal health, accelerated aging, and increased risk of disease.
* An E.Q. less than 66 indicates that your body is only able to produce less than 66 percent of the amount of ATP it needs to be healthy. This points to a severe impairment of ATP production. It means your mitochondria are in a true state of emergency. Your body is aging much too rapidly and is on the fast track toward disease.

Your E.Q. at Work

Take a look at what this means in principle. It's time to brag now.

Suppose you are, like me, an over-fifty man who does all kinds of things to be healthy. You have a special diet you stick to. You have a regular exercise program. You work on not getting overly stressed. You take nutritional supplements and, just as I do, you also take supplementary hormones to boost your sagging levels.

Then suppose you have your energy-production efficiency determined using Bio-Energy Testing. Your E.Q. turns out to be 130 (as mine was recently). What does this mean? Well, it's really good news.

An E.Q. of 130 means your body is producing energy 30 percent more efficiently than a man twenty-plus years younger. It means you are aging at a snail's pace. It also means your risk of developing disease is at an all-time low. It is basically the same risk that the average thirty-year-old has. What risk is that? Essentially no risk at all.

But there's even more good news. Such a wonderful E.Q. reading confirms in your mind that all the measures you are taking to slow aging and stay healthy are working for your particular genetics. In other words, you are not wasting your time, energy, and money on a program that will not deliver.

But what if you don't come out with an E.Q. as good as mine? What if, like many of my patients, your E.Q. is less than 100 the first time I measure it? What does that mean?

Well, first of all, it is good news. It tells you in no uncertain terms that your health program is not working with your particular genetics. So, rather than continuing an ineffective regimen, you and your health-care practitioner can use the information from your Bio-Energy Testing to come up with a program that *will* work.

There is no one health program that will work for everyone—this is just common sense. For some people, a vegetarian diet is just what they need. For others, such a diet spells disaster. The same is true for supplements, hormones, exercise programs, etc. Bio-Energy Testing is essential if we want to know if all those things you do to stay healthy are in fact really working.

The Ferrari and the Clunker

I'll turn to the automotive world for a moment and put you behind the wheel of a brand-new Ferrari to illustrate my point.

The tank is filled with the highest-octane gasoline available, to accommodate the Ferrari's high-performance engine. The fuel pump and the carburetor are delivering the gas to the cylinders. The spark plugs are new. The battery has plenty of juice.

This is analogous to your having good lungs, a good heart, and good circulation. Everything is set for a great ride.

But what if the engine is out of tune? That new Ferrari will run no better than an old clunker. In fact, a well-tuned old clunker will most surely outperform a poorly tuned new Ferrari.

When your body is highly tuned, your E.Q. will be 100 or higher.

Nothing is more tied to mental and physical functioning and disease prevention than optimum energy production through an optimum E.Q.

Your FBR—Fat-Burning Heart Rate

Are you keeping up so far? Here's a quick review.

Your M-Factor directly correlates with aging, health, and weight management. It can signal significant decreases in thyroid function (hypothyroidism) that might otherwise go undiagnosed. It should be greater than 90.

Your C-Factor should be greater than 90. If it isn't, and if your E.Q. is less than 100, it means you're probably eating too many carbohydrates, and your energy production from fat is being suppressed as a result.

Your Fat-Burning Factor should be greater than 100. If it's not, then you are not burning fat efficiently. This could happen from eating too many carbohydrates, but it could also indicate various nutritional or hormonal deficiencies.

Your E.Q. should be greater than 100. That way, you can be assured that your health and anti-aging program is really living up to your expectations.

Now look at how Bio-Energy Testing can help you dial in your exercise program.

During the exercise part of the test, as you continue to work harder and harder, your body will burn more and more fat to meet your increased energy needs. But as I mentioned above, there will be a point at which your body has reached its maximum level of fat burning. I refer to the heart rate at this point as the fat-burning heart rate, or FBR.

Your FBR defines your point of recovery during your exercise period. By "point of recovery," I mean the point at which your cells have recovered from the stress and strain of hard exercise. It is important for your exercise period to include some time at this point of recovery.

Why? Because the body always responds best to a stimulus when it is repetitive and not continuous. Your brain, for example, will learn best if you alternate periods of learning with periods of mental rest. Your muscles will also respond better if you work them and then rest them, rather than continually stressing them and not allowing for a recovery period. In order to be really effective, therefore, all exercise programs must have hard, challenging periods of time alternating with periods during which the body can recover.

This is one reason why knowing your FBR is so valuable. It tells you when your particular body has recovered from your exertion.

The other way that knowing your FBR can be helpful has to do with exercising for fat loss. When you are exercising at your FBR, your body is burning fat as fast as it can. You are training your body to burn fat more efficiently when you are exercising at your FBR. But when your exercise intensity drives your heart rate beyond your FBR, the proportion of energy produced from fat metabolism declines, and your body begins to burn glucose instead. So, always exercising above your FBR is actually counterproductive for fat loss.

Time and time again, I see frustrated patients who are overweight in spite of the fact that they are exercising harder and harder. The problem? They are exercising too hard. They are spending no time at all at their FBR, and their entire exercise period is only training their body to burn glucose, not fat. No wonder it doesn't work.

A few years ago, I published an article: "Is Your Patient Exercising Too Hard to Lose Weight?" which stressed this fact. It can be found in appendix C, and I highly recommend you read it if weight control is an issue for you. But whether you want to lose weight or not, it is always better to spend a portion of your exercise at your FBR.

Your ATR—Anaerobic Threshold Heart Rate

As you keep on exercising harder and harder and your heart rate escalates beyond your FBR, you will eventually reach a point of exercise called your anaerobic threshold. At this point, your cells have completely maxed out their production of ATP from oxygen. I refer to your heart rate when you reach your anaerobic threshold as your ATR, or anaerobic threshold heart rate (not to be confused with an ATM). As you exercise harder and go above your ATR, you are entering into anaerobic metabolism.

Exercising above your ATR is forcing your cells to come up with energy that they cannot easily come up with. It is stressing the heck out of them. If you were to do that for long periods of time, you would actually hurt them by increasing free-radical production. So, why would you want to do that?

It's because when you spend small increments of time above your ATR, it forces your cells to adapt to the stress, and the result is that over time they will become much better at utilizing oxygen and increasing energy production more efficiently. And that is exactly what we want out of our exercise time. It also maximizes your circulation, stimulates your detoxification systems, and strengthens your heart and lungs more than any other point of exercise.

But exercising above your ATR hurts! It is not fun. You will be way out of breath. Your heart will be pounding, and your muscles will be crying for you to stop. That is why it is only done for very short periods of time.

Now imagine someone who has a low E.Q. and can't produce ATP well from oxygen. That person's body will be forced into anaerobic metabolism with very little effort—almost as soon as any kind of exertion begins. He/she will easily go into anaerobic metabolism, and will experience many of the above symptoms, even at very low levels of exertion.

Over the years, I have been astounded to see many people with E.Q.s so low that they go into anaerobic metabolism simply by walking across the room. These people are commonly labeled with chronic fatigue syndrome or fibromyalgia. They inevitably complain of all the symptoms associated with anaerobic metabolism, including anxiety and panic states, breathlessness, mental confusion, muscle aches and pains, a profound lack of endurance, and severe fatigue. Unless the causes of their decreased E.Q. are successfully addressed, their lives are quite limited.

In chapter 13, you will learn how to use all three of these exercise zones—FBR, ATR, and anaerobic—to get the most out of your exercise regime. And this is important. If you do it right, you only have to spend twenty to thirty minutes, three times a week, exercising.

Your Biological Index—How Old Are You Really?

Alas, all things remaining the same, your E.Q. will steadily decrease with every birthday you have. And other factors, such as decreased fitness, excessive carbohydrates, illness, nutrient and hormonal deficiencies, stress, drugs, and toxicity can compound the problem.

This decline results in a diminished function in every single cell, organ, and tissue in the body, and is behind all the symptoms and diseases of aging. Since the brain, the heart, and the liver are the largest consumers of energy in the body, these organs are the most affected. But the bad news is—no part of your body is spared.

Your age only reflects how long you have been alive; and other than spending more for life insurance, or getting into the movies for less, your age turns out to be relatively unimportant. What is important is not your age, it's how efficiently your body is able to produce energy. That's what determines your health, your rate of aging, and your resistance to disease—*and that's what your Biological Index is all about.*

In determining your Biological Index, the computer analyzes all the factors mentioned above and then presents you with an overall energy score. If your Biological Index is greater than 100, you are well on your way to cheating Mother Nature out of the aging process. You can rest assured that all the time, energy, and money you spend to keep healthy is really doing what it's supposed to do.

If your Biological Index is less than 100, it gives you a goal to strive for over the years. Any increase is solid evidence that what you are doing is working.

Now that you are familiar with the importance of these vital Bio-Energy Testing measurements, it's time to move on and introduce you to the practical steps you can take to improve each and every reading.

PART TWO

EIGHT SECRETS FOR IMPROVING YOUR ENERGY PRODUCTION

✳ 8 ✳

SECRET ONE—WATER

Water has absolutely no nutritional value. Your body cannot produce energy from water. Nevertheless, all energy production, and indeed life itself, would very quickly come to a halt without water.

You can go without eating for weeks, but you cannot go without water for more than several days. The reason: 75 percent of your body is composed of water, and every single aspect of your biological functioning will quickly break down without enough water in your system.

A very simple home experiment can demonstrate this. Put a bit of baking soda and vitamin-C powder into a glass. What happens? Absolutely nothing! Now add a little water and watch the powerful reaction that develops. In your body, the same effect is at work.

Without adequate amounts of water, every biochemical reaction, including those essential for the proper generation of energy, is compromised. Take the brain. It is an organ with highly complex biochemical reactivity. The speed at which these reactions occur is critical: your information processing and thinking activity depend on it. While most other organs in the body are made up of 75 percent water, the brain consists of 85 percent. When it becomes even slightly dehydrated, your mental speed declines markedly, and greater levels of dehydration result in delirium and seizures.

Another critical aspect of water relates to detoxification. *Water is the only solvent the body can use to rid itself of toxins.* When water leaves the body, whether it's through your kidneys, skin, stool, or breath, it takes toxins with it. So, the more water that leaves your body, the more toxins it is eliminating. And the less water that leaves your body, the fewer toxins it is eliminating.

Some toxins are environmental and enter the body, but the majority are formed inside the body as the waste products of normal metabolic function. Without any water intake, these toxins would accumulate so rapidly that, in most cases, you would be seriously ill within four or five days. With a less-than-optimal intake you wouldn't die, but you wouldn't be able to flush out the toxins fast enough, and this would lead to toxin accumulation, decreased energy production, decreased organ function, and ultimately disease.

Yet another vital function of water is the maintenance of body temperature. Your body's ability to cool itself depends on adequate water intake. High fevers associated with acute illnesses, such as the flu, are often the result of dehydration. And if you are intolerant of hot weather, chances are you are significantly dehydrated. Think of water as the coolant you put in your car. If the level goes down too far, the engine overheats. It's the same with your body.

Few People Drink Enough

Despite its fundamental importance, it is amazing how few people actually drink enough water. In my clinic, I find that many of my healthy preventive medicine patients are somewhat dehydrated. They all state that they feel great, and have no symptoms; yet when I check their body's water level, they are clearly deficient.

And when asked if they are thirsty, none of them ever respond positively. Although thirst is a pretty good indicator of *acute* dehydration, in chronic states of dehydration the body adjusts by retaining fluids, so thirst doesn't occur.

Thirst turns out to be a poor indicator of whether or not you have an adequate level of water in your body. A 1998 article in the *American Journal of Hospital Palliative Care* dramatically points this out. The researchers reported that fluid depletion, even in severely dehydrated, dying people, resulted "in relatively benign symptoms," of which thirst was not a common one. The bottom line is just because you're not thirsty, it doesn't mean you are not dehydrated. The only way to be sure you have adequate water levels in your body is to drink plenty of water.

Fereydoon Batmanghelidj, MD, an expert on water and author of an excellent book, *Your Body's Many Cries for Water,* points out that, unlike a camel, the human body has no water-storage system to draw on in times of need. And those parts of the body most acutely affected by a water shortage are the areas without a direct blood supply, particularly cartilage in the joints. Painful joints, including those with arthritis in them, can be a result of inadequate water intake.

This overlooked issue was singled out in *Preventing Arthritis,* a book by Ronald M. Lawrence, MD, PhD, a pain specialist. "I have indeed found that joint and pain problems are helped by water, and made worse when a patient is dehydrated or hardly drinks water at all," he says.

Cured with Water

Years ago, Sarah, a seventy-two-year-old woman, made an appointment to see me and reported the following medical history: Eight months earlier, she had started to experience nausea. Her appetite had gradually diminished, and she had begun to lose weight. Her physician had prescribed various medications, including ulcer drugs, but nothing improved her condition. Two months went by, and Sarah began to develop a severe pain in her right hip. Her doctor knew she had arthritis damage in this hip, and concluded that the increase in pain meant it was finally time for a hip replacement.

After several weeks of continued pain, she was admitted to the hospital and had the surgery. Following the procedure, her nausea worsened to the point that she vomited almost everything she ate. She was prescribed more pain medication and was ultimately placed on significantly high doses of strong narcotics. She was then discharged from the hospital but returned with continued nausea, weight loss, and vomiting (no complaint about thirst).

Scans, X-rays, and blood tests failed to reveal any abnormality; but since she was obviously dehydrated, she was treated for fluid replacement with intravenous salt water. Miraculously, her symptoms improved, and after the third day she was allowed to return home.

Two months later, Sarah came to my clinic complaining of persistent joint pain, continued dependence on narcotic medication, and relentless nausea and vomiting. The case stumped me. I tried a homeopathic approach, but was unable to make any inroads. It was not until I recommended that she drink six ounces of water every hour that the situation changed.

Within several days, she had completely turned around. The stomach symptoms disappeared. The pain went away. It turned out that Sarah's entire range of symptoms was due to dehydration. Had she been adequately hydrated from the beginning, she might have been able to avoid the surgery, and all the misery she experienced during those many months. Remarkably, during the entire time, Sarah never once complained of thirst.

Water Purity

When I talk to my patients about water, I emphasize the importance of *pure* water. Regular tap water is often contaminated by chlorine, fluoride, hard minerals, heavy metals, or pesticide and drug residuals. This means that the water not only carries toxins with it into your body, but these toxins actually reduce its important solvent duties once inside.

Don't assume your water source is clean. According to a 1993 statement from the Environmental Protection Agency, 819 cities across the United States served up unacceptably elevated levels of lead to some 30,000,000 customers. Additionally, one fourth of all the public water systems in the United States had been found in violation of federal standards for water purity. Several epidemics of infectious diseases had been traced to contaminated public and ground water, and had led to recalls of meats and vegetables. And this was almost thirty years ago. Do you suppose things have gotten any better since then?

I have been testing water for many years, and rarely do I find any well or city water pure enough to generate optimum detoxifying effects in the body. To counter this, I recommend that my patients install a home purification unit. The key word here is *purified*. Water labeled as drinking water, mineral water, or spring water is often just not pure enough. Ideally, water should be labeled "purified." The two best ways to have purified water in your home are by using either a reverse osmosis or distillation method. My favorite is reverse osmosis, because distillation units are complex and expensive and don't remove as many potentially harmful materials. If you buy bottled water, be sure it says "purified" on the label.

MY RECOMMENDATIONS TO YOU

* One easy way to check if you are dehydrated is to look at your urine specific gravity during the day. This can be easily done with an inexpensive urine dipstick. Readings between 1.005 and 1.020 indicate a state of good hydration. Readings between 1.020 and 1.030 indicate moderate dehydration. And readings between 1.030 and 1.040 indicate severe dehydration.
* Drink at least a quarter to a half of your weight in ounces of water per day. If you have joint or muscle aches, try drinking the maximum for a few weeks to see if it makes a difference. For example, if you weigh 180 pounds, drink a minimum of 90 ounces daily (that's approximately eleven eight-ounce glasses of water).
* On hot days or when exercising, twice that amount may be needed.
* Once your body is used to drinking this amount of water, you will begin to feel thirsty if you aren't getting enough. But as a rule, don't rely on thirst to remind you to drink water.
* Since your lymphatic system has been collecting toxins and dumping them into your bloodstream during the night, it's good to get into the habit of helping the kidneys by drinking sixteen to thirty-two ounces of water when you get up in the morning. This may take some getting used to, but it's worth it.
* Alcoholic drinks, coffee, juice, sodas, and tea are not water. Nor are they substitutes for water. In fact, through their diuretic action, they can actually intensify dehydration.

* 9 *

SECRET TWO—REST

Get plenty of rest. That's the age-old physician's prescription for sickness. It's also an age-old prescription for staying healthy. And today, even in this time of medical marvels, it still holds true. As you will soon see, nothing is more critical to optimal energy production than sleep.

I find that the issue of adequate rest and sleep appears to be a major challenge for my patients. I am constantly reminding them that rest is really important. Not getting enough of it can be a major barrier to all their health and anti-aging goals. Yet it often doesn't really sink in. Perhaps it's just too simple a concept.

And the attitude of catching up on lost sleep "when I have the time" just doesn't cut it. Without adequate sleep, your resting metabolic rate and your E.Q. will decrease. Sleep deprivation shortens your life and increases the likelihood of a variety of diseases, including cancer, diabetes, and obesity.

My observation over the years has been that those people who sleep the best usually feel the best, and tend to be the healthiest ones.

According to a 1997 article in the *New York Times Magazine,* many sleep researchers believe that sleep deprivation is reaching "crisis proportions." This is not just a problem for serious insomniacs but for the populace at large, the article said, and added, "People don't merely believe they're sleeping less, they are *in fact* sleeping less—perhaps as much as one and a half hours less each night than humans did at the beginning of the 20th century—often because they choose to do so."

In an October 2000 report published in the British journal *Occupational and Environmental Medicine,* researchers in Australia and New Zealand found that sleep deprivation can have some of the same hazardous effects as being drunk. Getting less than six hours a night can affect coordination, reaction time, and judgment, they said, posing "a very serious risk."

In 1999, Eve Van Cauter, a sleep researcher at the University of Chicago, reported in *Lancet* that lack of adequate sleep can create a pre-diabetes state in the body, which can, in turn, contribute to obesity. Van Cauter's suggestion came after a study in which six young healthy men were allowed only four hours of sleep each night for a week. During the week, the subjects were tested and found to have impaired glucose tolerance, essentially a pre-diabetes state. The sleep-obesity connection is troubling from all angles. Obesity itself impairs sleep, thus setting the stage for a vicious cycle.

Van Cauter also points out that two very important hormones, growth hormone and leptin, are secreted primarily during the sleep hours. Leptin is a critical hormone with respect to eating and weight management. It signals the body to stop eating carbohydrates. "With the low-leptin levels of sleep debt, your body will crave carbohydrate even though you've had enough calories," says Van Cauter. And we've already seen the damage that too many carbs can do.

Your Two-Phase Body

The body's physiology basically runs on two twelve-hour phases. The time between 6 a.m. and 6 p.m. is called the *catabolic* phase. During this phase, your body is willing to do pretty much anything to keep you up and running, meaning it is going to continually sacrifice Peter to pay Paul. Simply stated, if your left leg needs something your right leg has, your body will borrow it from the right leg and give it to the left. If your heart needs a certain raw material more urgently than your adrenal gland, the body will make sure your heart gets it, and your adrenal glands will have to make do. This process, called catabolism, permits damage to certain tissues in order to keep others with a higher priority running efficiently. But don't worry: your body is quite smart.

Enter phase two, the *anabolic* cycle, from 6 p.m. to 6 a.m. This is when the body repairs all the damage and borrowing that went on during the catabolic phase. The process, called anabolism, transpires primarily when we are sleeping (or should be). This is a key point. The body repairs damage through the medium of subtle energy fields that cannot be effective during the active part of the day. These fields organize the repair effort and reach their maximum potential during sleep, particularly the deeper levels of sleep.

This is precisely why sleep is so important. *Without an adequate sleep period, we are unable to fully repair the damage we create during the day.* A chronic lack of adequate sleep results in accelerated deterioration of the body, leading to premature aging. Sleep is even more important for those who exercise and/or lead very active or stressful lives.

If You Don't Snooze, You Lose

The current stress-oriented 24/7 culture isn't doing much to help people stay healthy. I love capitalism, but the daily decisions people make often reflect a greater desire to make sacrifices for money than for health, and getting enough sleep is a good example of this. In fact, for too many, the prevailing attitude has become: *if you snooze, you lose.*

You will often meet people who actually brag about how little sleep they need, saying "I can get by on only four to five hours of sleep and still exercise and have a fully productive day." While this macho attitude may be impressive, I'm sure these people have no idea how negatively it is impacting their health.

Many won't go to sleep early enough because they want to watch TV. Having been convinced by the news industry that news actually changes from day to day, they can't see going to sleep until they have been brought up to date. Better to get your news in the morning, right after exercising.

Mr. Sandman Says . . .

- Take your sleep time seriously. The body is designed to go to sleep when the sun is down and to wake up with the sunrise. So, adjust your sleeping schedule accordingly.
- Work toward getting eight hours of good, uninterrupted sleep in a fully darkened room, ideally before the sun comes up. If you can't do this, blacken your room or use eyeshades so it is still dark after the sun has risen.
- Avoid food or alcohol for three hours before bedtime.
- Lights left on in the room interfere with sleep. The production of melatonin, perhaps the single most important hormone for the immune system, occurs during sleep. It is immediately cut off by exposure to light (except red light). Decreased melatonin production is thought to be one of the factors leading to breast cancer.

* If you have to get up in the night for a trip to the bathroom, don't turn on the lights. If you need light, use a red-colored night light—red light does not seem to curtail melatonin production.
* If you routinely get up to urinate, restrict your fluids before bedtime so you don't have as many trips.
* Chronic insomnia is a serious health problem. If you have this problem, don't think you're solving it by taking drugs. You're not. Studies show that sleeping medications interfere with the development of the deeper levels of sleep. So instead treat the problem by following my other secrets in this book—exercise, adequate water intake, breath meditation, sunlight, and supplements can go a long way toward relieving insomnia. Also limit or eliminate your intake of all caffeinated drinks. Certain herbs, particularly chamomile and valerian, are especially helpful to induce sleep. If you are over forty-five, take melatonin before bedtime. Melatonin, even in very high doses, has no negative effects. I take 180 mg every night, and I sleep like a teenager.
* Don't use anything electric on your bed, such as electric blankets or heating pads. These devices create an electrical field that significantly interferes with the anabolic repair process. Even when they are turned off, electric heating systems still maintain an electric field because they have transformers. That's right. Even when they're off, they're on. Just get rid of them, and get a good comforter. You'll like it better anyway.
* Keep your cell phone either more than four feet away from you at night or put it in airplane mode. The electromagnetic fields generated by it can interfere with sleep.

10

SECRET THREE—SUNLIGHT

Sunlight is absolutely essential to health. Sunlight deficiency will not only seriously limit energy production; it will seriously compromise your health in other ways as well. Despite the fact that people couldn't possibly survive without it—and despite the fact that humans were created without the benefit of sunscreen or sunglasses—the sun has become something of a medical scapegoat, so much so that for many it is virtually synonymous with the deadly skin cancer called melanoma. This hysteria is unfounded.

It makes no sense at all to indict the sun for the rise in melanoma. Or, as some experts have done, blamed it on the hole in the ozone layer that lets in more of the sun's ultraviolet (UV) rays. The hole is restricted to the area over Australia, Argentina, Chile, South Africa, and New Zealand, and so offers no explanation for the dramatic increase in melanoma *all over the world.* We have always been exposed to the sun. One hundred years ago, the average exposure was much more than it is today. And yet the incidence of melanoma has dramatically increased, even as our average sun exposure has decreased. Clearly, the increase cannot be caused by the sun.

I believe we can attribute a good deal of the increase in melanoma to the very same factors that have brought about an increase in every other type of cancer: decreased energy production, poor food choices, stress, and toxicity.

In 1982, a comprehensive report by the National Research Council on Diet, Nutrition, and Cancer concluded that much of the rising cancer rate in the US was due to the typical American diet. And, according to the National Academy of Sciences, 60 percent of all cancers in women, and 40 percent of all cancers in men, may be due to diet alone.

Smoking and passive exposure to cigarette smoke have also been linked to the increased incidence of all cancers, including melanoma.

Although there is no doubt that overexposure to the sun—and the resulting sunburn—definitely increases the incidence of a type of common, normally benign skin cancers called basal cell carcinoma and squamous cell carcinoma, it plays no role at all in melanoma.

What is known is this, and sun worshipers should pay heed: sunburn, even a slight sunburn, does cause premature aging of the skin, including wrinkles and pigmentation. So it is advisable during the summer to limit exposure between 10 a.m. and 3 p.m. These are the hours during the day when the sun's rays are most intense and more likely to cause skin damage.

Am I telling you to stay out of the sun? No, far from it. Just be cautious. There's no big secret about that. It's common sense.

My anti-aging and energy secret involves the flip side of all this: that is, the essential and positive aspects of sunlight, and just how valuable it is to your health. I am more concerned about people not getting enough sunlight. And I consider sunlight deficiency a mostly overlooked issue.

According to the late Dr. John Ott, an expert in the biological effects of light therapy, there is no doubt that too much UV is harmful. "But the fear of ultraviolet is causing people to overprotect themselves from sunlight to the point that they are creating a deficiency of a very essential life-supporting energy."

Don't Become Eclipsed

Shut-ins, sun-shunners, and office workers run the risk of sunlight deficiency. Your doctor may not tell you this, but sunlight deficiency results in biological imbalances that will lower your energy production. It also causes myriad clinical problems including anxiety, depression, hypothyroidism, insomnia, osteoporosis, and a suppression of the immune system, leading to both breast and prostate cancer.

Sunlight Deficiency = Energy Deficiency

Are you getting enough sunlight? The fact that sunlight is an important factor in energy production is well established. Many studies have shown a decrease in the resting metabolism of both animals and people when they do not receive enough sunlight. The decline in resting metabolic rate commonly seen in everyone during the winter is a direct result of decreased exposure to sunlight. Sunlight deficiency is not usually an issue for those who live in the middle latitudes, because sunlight is readily available there all year long. But for the rest of us, it can be a big issue.

For those in colder climates, the shorter days of winter and late fall can be problematic. Bundled up from head to toe, millions leave for work and return from work in the dark. And the weather keeps them inside during the day, for weeks and even months, without exposure to sunlight. This single factor is undoubtedly what triggers flu epidemics and explains why they tend to occur primarily during the cold months.

Well, you may be thinking, I work in a glass-encased office building and the light comes streaming through the glass. Sorry, that's not much help. Glass interferes with the absorption of certain spectra of UV light that are critical to the functioning of the immune system. Exposure to sunlight through windows is better than none at all, but it is of limited usefulness and will not completely provide for your biological needs. You need the real thing—sunlight sans glass.

Sunlight exposure is also important for those who work under conventional fluorescent lights. These lights are unable to produce many of the important wavelengths that our bodies need. And the imbalance of the spectrum from fluorescent lights creates a relative deficiency of the wavelengths that are not present in fluorescent light. If possible, try to have *full-spectrum* fluorescent lighting installed. It's no substitute for the sun, but it's less harmful than regular-spectrum fluorescent lights.

Sun Healing

Here's how important sunlight is to our health. In the late 1800s and early 1900s, tuberculosis was a serious and widespread problem without an effective treatment. During this time, a Danish medical researcher named Niels Finsen developed an ultraviolet (UV) light treatment to treat an infectious skin disease called lupus vulgaris, for which there had previously been no cure. Finsen and his successors were able to demonstrate a remarkable 98 percent success rate simply by exposing affected areas of the body to UV light. UV refers to the radiation that comes naturally from the sun. Some man-made lamps can also produce UV, but for most people, the sun is the primary source of UV.

Finsen subsequently discovered something even more exciting. He had wondered whether the success of the treatment was due to a direct anti-microbial effect of the light on the skin, or whether the results could be explained by the effect of the light on the immune system. To determine this, he treated a number of people with lupus vulgaris by exposing only the unaffected parts of their skin to the light. He discovered that even when infected skin was not directly treated, the infection cleared up just as rapidly as it did for those whose infected areas he treated directly. Which is to say, the light itself was not killing the infection, but instead it was stimulating the immune system to do its job better.

For his breakthrough in demonstrating the healing power of light, Finsen was awarded the Nobel Prize in physiology and medicine in 1903. The award was given "in recognition of his contribution to the treatment of diseases, especially lupus vulgaris, with concentrated light radiation, whereby he has opened a new avenue for medical science."

What Finsen didn't know, but is known today, more than a century later, is that he was stimulating Langerhans cells in the skin. These cells are vital to immune-system function. They are important antigen-presenting cells, meaning they communicate (that is, present) the infection to other immune cells. This, in turn, initiates a proper immune response. Certainly, it is the effect of sunlight on the Langerhans cells that at least partially accounts for the most amazing of all stories regarding the use of sunlight to treat disease.

Following Finsen's breakthrough research, a medical doctor named Auguste Rollier opened a sun clinic in the Swiss Alps, high above the cloud layer. Here, at Le Chalet, as he called his clinic, he developed the therapeutic use of sunlight, along with a balanced diet, exercise, fresh air, and rest, into a powerful healing art form. This was in an era before antibiotics, and Rollier documented many impressive cures for tuberculosis and other incurable diseases.

His patients resided in hospital rooms, which had huge glass windows oriented to the sun. In addition, each room had a balcony large enough to accommodate a bed. And, whether in beds or chairs, his patients exposed themselves to the sun for about two or three hours a day in the summer, and three or four hours a day in the winter.

Rollier was convinced that sunlight combined with excessive heat had negative effects on his patients, so he did not allow them out in the middle of the day during the warm summer months. He treated his patients with this controlled exposure to sunlight during periods lasting as long as eighteen months. The results? Deformed, sick children with spinal tuberculosis were literally transformed into healthy, energetic, fully functional youngsters with straight backs, completely free of disease. You would be absolutely amazed at the before-and-after pictures. Sunlight is a powerful healing agent!

Rollier's success with tuberculosis and other infectious diseases was so significant that he established some thirty-five sun clinics from 1903 to 1940. At the height of his Alpine healing enterprise, he was able to treat more than a thousand people a day. Rollier published extensively on the curative power of the sun, reporting not only miraculous cures of tuberculosis but also success against abscesses and bone infections. His treatments were also effective for rickets, various anemias, and a variety of non-healing wounds.

For the record, there were no cases of basal cell or squamous cell carcinoma or melanoma observed in any of his patients *after* he treated them in these clinics. This is undoubtedly because he made sure that his patients became gradually accustomed to the sun without getting sunburned.

In recent times, the prevailing sunlight-causes-cancer bias has motivated researchers to focus on proving that doses of UV light high enough to cause sunburn can damage the Langerhans cells. In these studies, researchers invariably exposed various human cells in a test tube to extremely high doses of an unnatural spectrum of artificial light. I have not seen one study that actually used sunlight. The other problem with the studies is that they were done in a test tube, not a live animal. Test tube studies always have to be viewed with some skepticism, especially when there is no clinical proof to back them up.

These experimental conditions represent exposures to light spectrums that don't exist in nature and are known to cause skin damage. It is therefore not surprising that the exposed cells became damaged and exhibited changes consistent with cancer and impaired immune activity. Had the researchers paid attention to the work of Finsen and Rollier, they would have learned that both doctors achieved their healing results without ever inducing skin damage or sunburn.

Finsen and Rollier are classic examples of why you can't always translate isolated laboratory test-tube findings to real life. Many times, the results bear little resemblance to what happens in vivo—that is, inside the body.

To further make my point, I'll cite a study conducted by dermatologists at the University of Turku in Finland, published in the journal *Experimental Dermatology*. The researchers found that high doses of UV light could indeed damage Langerhans cells in a test tube. But when real skin is exposed to UV, even high doses of it, they found that the Langerhans cells are actually up-regulated, meaning they are stimulated. This study suggests that, in reasonable doses, sunlight actually stimulates and enhances immune-system function and efficiency, and helps to explain why Finsen and Rollier were able to cure the incurable.

I am convinced that correct sunlight exposure and a healthy diet will prevent the very same skin cancers that some say are caused by the sun. And who knows if the inadequate level of sunlight exposure that so many sun-fearing people get these days might be responsible for many of our immune-related diseases.

The Sunshine Vitamin

Sunlight is the *rate-limiting* factor in the production of a very overlooked vitamin—vitamin D. The term rate-limiting means that if a necessary substance in a particular chemical reaction—in this case, sunlight—is not present, then the reaction simply will not take place. Your skin tissue makes vitamin D, the amount of which depends on your exposure to sunlight. Insufficient sunlight results in a deficiency of vitamin D. It's why vitamin D is known as the sunshine vitamin. Some people think that the diet can supply enough vitamin D, but this is wrong. Even a diet extremely high in Vitamin D cannot raise vitamin D blood levels as high as five minutes of exposure to the sun.

The implications are immense. For one thing, as discussed in chapter 4, vitamin D promotes the body's absorption of calcium, essential for the normal development of healthy teeth and bones. Without adequate exposure to the sun, vitamin D levels fall to a dangerously low level, a level so low that osteoporosis can result.

In 1979, the *British Journal of Medicine* published a study on the vitamin D levels of twenty-three older people followed for sixteen months. In July, they had normal vitamin D levels; but by November, the levels had dropped an average of 19 percent—and by the following February, 65 percent. At this point, almost half of the group had levels consistent with the development of osteoporosis. This is a startling demonstration of the powerful results of sunlight deficiency.

Another common disorder associated with aging is gradual hearing loss due to otosclerosis, an abnormal growth of bone tissue in the inner ear. The growth prevents the ear from working properly. The hearing loss is sometimes accompanied by chronic ringing in the ears (tinnitus). Otosclerosis is a multifactorial disease (caused by a variety of factors), among them, a deficiency of vitamin D.

A 1985 study published in *Otolaryngology and Head and Neck Surgery* indicated for the first time that supplementation could help some people, as a low level of the vitamin may contribute to demineralization of bone tissue in the ear. Today, vitamin D is part of the medical treatment for otosclerosis. But it's my guess that if people got an adequate amount of sunlight during their lives, there would be much less otosclerosis in the first place.

The Penetrating Power of Sunlight

Most people think sunlight affects only the very outermost skin, but this is far from reality—several inches far.

To see how deeply light penetrates, William Campbell Douglas, MD, a pioneer in the use of ultra-violet light therapy, offers a simple experiment in his fascinating book *Into the Light.* Simply darken the room you're in and hold a flashlight under your hand. The light actually shines through the entire thickness of your hand.

How much stronger is sunlight?

Try the same experiment with some cloth between your hand and the light, and you will find the results are not all that different. The light still comes right through. To quote Dr. Douglas, "It doesn't take a rocket scientist to figure out that if you can see the light illuminating the top of your hand, then, obviously, the light has penetrated through your hand."

And that's just a flashlight—sunlight is much more powerful. It can indeed penetrate into the body, even through clothing, where it can be very beneficial, causing an increase in energy production, increased vitamin D synthesis, and a markedly improved immune system.

Sunlight and Your Immune System

A commonly overlooked fact is that vitamin D is deeply involved in the proper functioning of the immune system. Although the full mechanisms of this connection are unknown, a glimpse into the possibilities is provided by a paper published in 1999 in *Cancer Research* by the Department of Medicine at Harvard Medical School. These researchers found that the vitamin D deficiency caused by elevated calcium intake resulted in an increased incidence of advanced prostate cancer. The authors state: "Our findings support increased fruit intake and avoidance of high calcium intake to reduce the risk of advanced prostate cancer." Other studies show the same relationship with breast cancer.

Breast and prostate cancer aren't the only cancers associated with low vitamin D production. In an amazing nineteen-year study, published in *Lancet* in 1985, researchers found that men with the lowest levels of vitamin D (even though the levels were still within the normal range) were more than twice as likely to develop colon cancer as individuals with the highest levels. Although the so-called normal range of vitamin D in the blood is 20 to 100 ng/mL, the studies show that having vitamin D levels between 50 and 70 ng/mL reduces the overall chance of getting *any* kind of cancer by 30 percent!

MY RECOMMENDATIONS TO YOU

* Remember that too much of anything, including sunlight, can be harmful.
* The best time of day for sunbathing is during the morning hours.
* Start off your exposure to the sun gradually, and cover your face. Sunbathing should not include the face, because it already gets plenty of exposure and excessive sun will cause wrinkles and pigmentation on the face and neck.
* Never expose your skin to an amount of sunlight that will create more than a barely perceptible reddening of the skin twenty-four hours later. If you are fair-skinned, this may be no more than ten minutes at first.
* Don't use sunscreens when you sunbathe. They interfere with the full spectrum of the light. Use them only in situations, such as in certain athletic activities, where cover protection is impractical, and without sunscreen you will become burned.
* Wear a hat so the thin, ultra-sensitive skin of your face, head, and neck is protected. The skin in these areas receives much more exposure to sunshine than other parts of the body. Protecting these areas can minimize wrinkles, age spots, and blemishes that will make you look older than you really are.
* If you live in the northern or southern latitudes, take two or three capsules of cod liver oil per day in wintertime, just to ensure an adequate dietary intake of vitamin D. If possible, during this period of the year try to get outside in the middle of each day for at least twenty minutes.

✳ 11 ✳

SECRET FOUR—SUPPLEMENTS

For many people, one sure way to amplify energy production is to take the right nutritional supplements. This is very individual, because the need to supplement your diet is determined by your lifestyle and your genetics. Some people will need much more of a given vitamin or mineral than will others. There are even a few of us who can get all they nutritionally need from a healthy diet alone. I know: I have seen them. They come into the clinic and test out beautifully on Bio-Energy Testing, despite the fact that they take no supplements at all. It can happen, but for most of us this would just be a pipe dream.

It may seem like a fairy tale in this day and age, but once upon a time (not so very long ago) taking vitamin and mineral supplements was a controversial issue for doctors. The American Medical Association and many physicians emphasized that a *balanced diet* was enough to provide all the nutritional requirements for the average Joe or Jane. Many physicians even maintained that supplements could be dangerous, although there was no evidence of medical injury from their proper use.

In recent years, the tide of opinion has turned significantly. The 1990s witnessed a huge worldwide wave of scientific validation for the use of supplements, ranging from vitamins and minerals to the most esoteric rainforest herbs. Moreover, mounting consumer and patient interest has forced many doctors to rethink their attitude and modify any anti-supplement bias.

In addition, it is now widely recognized that large numbers of people don't eat a healthy balanced diet. Instead, they eat unbalanced diets heavy in processed convenience foods, thereby guaranteeing themselves nutrient deficiencies that can only lead to health problems.

Today, physicians are routinely exposed to positive articles on the beneficial aspects of proper nutritional supplementation in the *Journal of the American Medical Association* (*JAMA*) and other leading medical publications. This represents a 180-degree turnaround from the past. We now see a plethora of articles citing all the many benefits of supplements, including the following:

* How B_6, B_{12}, and folic acid help prevent heart disease
* How chromium supplementation aids diabetes
* How coenzyme Q_{10} rescues ailing hearts and also protects against the dangerous side effects of cholesterol-lowering medication
* How oral magnesium tablets prevent fatal cardiac arrhythmias
* How a simple extract of rice bran can cause cancer cells to revert back into normal cells
* How vitamins A, C, E, and the mineral selenium combat the development of cancer

Keeping up with the nutritional research is almost a full time job. The information is torrential. The question is no longer "Should I be taking supplements?" The question now is "Which are the most important supplements for me, and at what dosage?"

Proper, effective supplementation is really an individual matter, and not a matter of RDA—recommended daily allowance. The RDA refers to the minimal amount of a nutrient that is required to stave off a deficiency disease. It has nothing to do with what is required for optimal health. RDA's don't take into consideration an individual's unique physiology, physical condition, size, sex, degree of exercise and activity, or environment. As such, in a well-fed country, they are completely useless.

Precise nutritional needs can only be determined using some fairly sophisticated testing, along with a detailed history and physical examination. Even after all that, it still often boils down to trial and error.

My central criterion on whether or not someone needs a nutritional supplement is simple. It is based entirely on how well a person produces energy. That's because virtually any nutrient deficiency will result in a decrease in energy production. Therefore, if my patient tests out well on his/her Bio-Energy Test, I can be assured that all their nutritional needs are being met. Conversely, if the test results indicate poor energy production, then I know that something is missing. And sometimes that something is a nutrient. What nutrient? That is best determined by what nutrient or nutrients improve energy production.

Principles of Supplementation

I have been testing the biochemical and nutritional patterns of my patients for over forty years. This experience has taught me some important general principles regarding nutritional supplementation.

First Principle

Vitamins and minerals don't work unless they supplement a good diet. *Taking supplements while on a fast-food, high-sugar, low-fiber diet is a complete waste of time and money*. Sorry, it just doesn't work that way.

Surprised? You shouldn't be. Taking supplements and eating a poor diet is like building a house on quicksand. Even if you took a hundred supplements three times a day, it would be impossible for you to get all the nutrition you need. Every nutrient requires numerous other nutrients to be present in order for it to exert its own particular effect. Only a non-toxic, nutrient-dense, high-fiber, high-protein diet, such as I will discuss in the next chapter, can guarantee this.

Second Principle

Supplements should be taken in a balanced way. Typically, people read a magazine article extolling the virtues of a new super-nutrient, then rush out, buy the supplement, and start taking it.

Forgotten in this approach is that additional supplementation of other nutrients is often required to preserve the balance needed to support and bring out the effect of the super-nutrient.

Always remember that vitamins and minerals work together as a team. For example, vitamin E, the amino acid cysteine, and selenium work together to form glutathione peroxidase, a star antioxidant enzyme produced in the body. Taking one without also taking the others may not make sense.

Your supplementation program should always reflect respect for balance and synergism. A broad range of nutrients, not just popping the supplement of the month, will serve you best.

Third Principle

The issue of dosage is often abused. When you increase the amount of one nutrient, you may need to increase the amounts of some or all of the others if you don't want to invite an imbalance.

The principle is this: it is best to use relatively small doses of many nutrients rather than large doses of any one nutrient. This is extremely important.

This approach is particularly valuable when it involves antioxidant nutrients, such as vitamin C. Back in the 1970s, some medical and nutritional experts declared it unproven, but today almost everybody is aware that a reduction in antioxidant defense systems leads to cancer, heart disease, chronic infections, and many other degenerative diseases. So, the search is on to find ways to keep these systems functioning optimally.

This has led to the thinking that the more antioxidant nutrients you take, the more likely it is that the antioxidant defense systems will be enhanced. But is this true? Is it possible to take too much of an antioxidant and minimize its effect? Greater minds than mine have advocated routine mega-doses of antioxidants, especially vitamin C, as a way to improve antioxidant defense mechanisms. But are they right?

I first started to consider this question in earnest after reading an article published in the *International Journal of Biochemical Cell Biology* in 1995. The article compared mega-doses, typical supplemental doses, and RDA doses of vitamin E. The researchers reached the following conclusion: "Further increases in vitamin E to megadose levels did not provide additional protection from oxidative stress." This means that the large doses did nothing to improve anti-oxidant defenses, any more than the standard doses.

In another study on vitamin C, the results were the same. The mega-doses were no more effective at immune stimulation than more conservative doses.

In these two studies, mega-doses were not helpful, but neither did they produce any negative effects. However, the results of a 1983 article in *Acta Vitaminol Enzymol* are a little troubling. These researchers concluded that mega-doses of vitamins C and A both caused an increased destruction of red blood cells secondary to oxidative damage. Oxidative damage is precisely the same thing that increasing anti-oxidant defenses is supposed to stop.

In yet another study, the author asserted that "ascorbic acid (in large doses) decreases the detoxification of cyanide derived . . . through diminishing the availability of cysteine," and thus renders the liver more susceptible to oxidative damage. Cysteine, an amino acid, is a precursor to glutathione, a primary antioxidant and detoxifying protein in the liver. So, taking too much of one anti-oxidant, in this case vitamin C, ironically resulted in the depletion of another anti-oxidant, in this case cysteine.

These reports prompted me to conduct a small experiment in my clinic. I divided a group of volunteer patients in half, according to whether they took mega-doses of vitamin C or more moderate amounts. I then infused a solution of hydrogen peroxide into their bloodstreams. I used hydrogen peroxide because it is safe, and because it is known to tax the anti-oxidant defenses. Blood samples were taken immediately after the infusion and analyzed for how much oxidation was present. The analysis showed that the antioxidant defenses of those on moderate doses of vitamin C was significantly greater than those taking the mega-doses. I also discovered that the strongest antioxidant responses appeared to be in those who took moderate doses of vitamin C *and* regularly engaged in aerobic exercise.

This study, and the others I have cited here, have convinced me that mega anti-oxidant supplementation is neither necessary nor even desirable as a routine preventive measure. Moreover, such mega-dosing may, in fact, decrease the body's ability to defend against oxidative stress. The point I want to leave you with here is this: avoid mega-dosing on your own. It is a therapeutic concept that is often very useful in acute clinical situations, but the chronic use of these high doses should only be done with the guidance of a nutritionally savvy physician.

My Super Immune QuickStart With Super Fats

QuickStart in combination with Super Fats is the complete nutritional supplement I developed way back in 1992, and vigorously recommend to my patients. I'll tell you why.

I have put a lot of thought and twenty-five years of experience into the formulation of this unique blend of nutrients, herbs, oils, fiber, and amino acids. While it was never meant to be a substitute for a healthy diet, I believe the spectrum and doses of QuickStart/Super Fats reflect the current state of the art in medical and nutritional science.

I first began to make QuickStart for my own patients long before it was ever commercially available. The feedback I got from my patients was so gratifying that in 2000, I decided to make it available to everyone.

But here's the point. I did not write this book to sell QuickStart and Super Fats. I created QuickStart long before I wrote this book, simply because there just wasn't anything comparable to it on the market. And also because I wanted to save my patients the money and time required to take all the ingredients separately.

I don't really care if you use QuickStart and Super Fats or simply take all the ingredients they contain in a separate form. In fact, in case you want to do that, I have included all the ingredients along with their doses in the Appendix. The ingredients in QuickStart and Super Fats represent my idea of a complete supplement program for everyone. Nothing has been left out. If you decide to make your own substitute, that's fine. As long as you're happy, I'm happy.

That said, here's what it's all about. QuickStart comes in powder form. I tell my patients to use it as part of a power-breakfast smoothie that will literally give them a rocket-launch boost-off each morning.

It makes a one-stop therapeutic formula that provides all the supplementary nutrition and immune enhancement most people will need. It is also designed to improve the immune system and to assist the detoxifying activity of the liver.

I haven't yet performed any double-blind clinical studies to demonstrate that QuickStart is better than any other herbal/nutrient mixtures. I just know it gets the results my patients and I are looking for.

The reason for this gratifying effect is that the formula works on so many basic levels. It is formulated to alkalinize tissues, enhance immunity, improve brain function and circulation, increase energy production, and stabilize the appetite. *More importantly, it is specifically designed to provide all the various nutrients your liver needs to keep your body maximally detoxified.*

It is important to mention that QuickStart does not contain meaningless amounts of many nutrients just to make the label look good. Every ingredient is tried and true, and is added in its *full therapeutic dose.*

And I not only recommend QuickStart to my patients—my whole family takes it every day. It's a fabulous way to start the day.

THIRTEEN REASONS TO TAKE THE QUICKSTART FORMULA

1. It provides both preventive and therapeutic benefits.

2. It comes as a fine powder that ensures maximum absorption, even for individuals with less-than-perfect digestive systems.

   Because of the complex nature of the digestive tract, capsules and tablets are not the best way to deliver nutrients. Much of the vitamin content of pills can be ruined in the manufacturing process.

Moreover, tablets and capsules often do not adequately break down, which means that much of their content may not be fully absorbed.

It would require over forty large-sized capsules to pack the same amount of nutrients found in a routine dose of QuickStart. Few people will take that many pills for very long. The formula has been carefully formulated and scientifically manufactured so that each vitamin, mineral, and herb present is delivered in the most effective form. If needed for a specific therapeutic reason, other supplements can easily be added to the mix.

3. The formula mixes quickly and easily with water as a breakfast drink. Compared to pills, this is a much more natural and less complicated way to take nutrients.

4. It's more affordable than all the bottles of pills that would be required to get similar protection. Back in 1999, I used the catalog of a major supplement retailer to determine what the total cost of all the ingredients in a one-month supply of QuickStart would be if they were purchased separately. The results came to a tally of $163. Since QuickStart sells for $65 a container, that represents a difference of almost $100 per month. It's probably even more economical now.

5. It satisfies the appetite and is thus beneficial as an aid for weight control. The contents are low in carbohydrates and high in energy-boosting ingredients. It is suitable for all diets, including strictly vegan diets.

6. QuickStart detoxifies the liver and restores and maintains optimal bowel function.

7. It contains extra chromium—a full 1200 micrograms per serving—necessary for protection against blood-sugar disorders in a society where high-carbohydrate diets are contributing to rampant diabetes.

8. It contains astragalus, a superb Chinese herb that enhances immune-cell effectiveness and antibody production, as well as inhibiting suppression of immune function by tumors.

9. It contains therapeutic doses of saw palmetto and soy isolates, shown to enhance immunity, help prevent prostate and breast disease, and regulate both male and female hormones.

10. A therapeutic level of ginkgo biloba helps inhibit platelet aggregation and adhesion, *and* decrease fibrinogen and plasma thickness. Translated, that means it has blood-thinning activity. Ginkgo also helps protect cell membranes, and quench free radicals. Plus it famously improves blood circulation in the brain.

11. There are three QuickStart products. One is formulated without any animal products for strictly vegan diets. Another formula features a base of microfiltered, un-denatured whey protein isolate. This material is rich in antibodies, glycomacropeptide (GMP), and lactoferrin. GMP stimulates the release of cholecystokinin, a potent hormone that signals satiety to the appetite control centers in the brain; and lactoferrin binds free iron in the body, thereby reducing iron-induced free-radical production. A third formula contains prebiotic herbs to help re-establish a healthy microbiome (intestinal bacterial balance).

12. The formula also benefits the heart and contains potent nutritional elements known to reduce the risk of cardiovascular disease. The unique combination of antioxidants, B_6, B_{12}, chromium, DHA, folic acid, niacin, phytosterols, and soluble fiber improves insulin sensitivity and lowers LDL-cholesterol, triglycerides, and homocysteine levels.

13. All of the nutrients in QuickStart are organic and GMO- and gluten-free.

Directions for Taking QuickStart

Since QuickStart is formulated to duplicate the composition of a perfect food, I recommend taking it as a breakfast replacement.

Start with a half scoop or less. The formula is quite strong and your body may take a while to get used to it. Add one teaspoon of Super Fats or flax oil. This is very important. You'll hear more about Super Fats in a moment. Many of my patients add extras, such as protein powder and/or fruit, but you can make it up any way you want. Then add water or ice, according to your preference, and blend it in a blender.

When traveling, just shake it up in a container with some ice water. Don't bother with the oil on the road, because it requires refrigeration. Just take two fish oil capsules instead. After you've grown adjusted to a starting dose of QuickStart, gradually increase the daily dose to the recommended two scoops. After loading your body up for three months on two scoops per day, you can lower the dose to one scoop per day to maintain.

When you first start taking the formula, you may experience a warm, prickly feeling on your neck and face and under your arms. Don't be alarmed. This is just a cleansing reaction from the niacin. The feeling will gradually disappear as you continue the program. Think of QuickStart as your breakfast, and even your lunch as well. It is an extremely good way to pave the way to high energy levels all day long.

Super Fats™ for Super Health

I hope by now you are convinced that eating enough of the right fats is critically important for energy production, as well as every single other cellular function. But from a nutritional point of view, making sure you do this can be more than a little challenging.

NINE REASONS FOR TAKING SUPER FATS

1. Super Fats is a balanced source of all the essential and non-essential polyunsaturated fats that are so critical to health. It includes both the omega 3 and omega 6 fats. I don't know where else you get all these fats in one product.

2. The essential fats in Super Fats need to be present in a particular balance for optimum results. Research has shown that the optimum ratio of the omega 6 fats to the omega 3 fats is 6:1. Super Fats maintains this ratio.

3. Super Fats contains a supply of many of the most important but non-essential fats that you may not get enough of from your diet. These include alpha-linolenic acid, oleic acid, palmitoleic acid, palmitic acid, myristic acid, octacosanol, squalene, and both alpha and beta tocotrienol.

4. Super Fats is loaded with a full supply of natural antioxidants. That's very important, because polyunsaturated fats need to be taken together with the proper fat-soluble antioxidant nutrients in order to protect them from oxidation both in the bottle and in your body.

5. Super Fats has the entire spectrum of vitamin E components. These are known as alpha, beta, delta, and gamma tocopherol. This is exactly the way vitamin E is found in nature, and research has shown that it may be unsafe to take vitamin E in any other way. Furthermore, although most vitamins contain only alpha tocopherol, the evidence is that the other tocopherols are equally important.

6. Super Fats contains the important fat-soluble nutrient lycopene. Lycopene helps to prevent bladder, colon, breast, cervical, and prostate cancer. Lycopene has this effect due to its ability to interfere with the way cancers use growth factors to stimulate their proliferation. Lycopene is also instrumental at preventing macular degeneration.

7. You have already heard much about coenzyme Q_{10}. it is critical for energy production, and is the most important intracellular antioxidant. Super Fats contains a significant dose of CoQ_{10}. CoQ_{10} is a fat-soluble nutrient, and the fact that the CoQ_{10} in Super Fats is dissolved in other fats supports its absorption and uptake in the intestinal tract.

8. Super Fats contains one of the most important of all nutrients, lipoic acid. Lipoic acid has the unique ability to replenish vitamin C after it has been used up. This is a critical reaction, since humans cannot synthesize nearly enough vitamin C for the body to be completely protected from free-radical damage. Lipoic acid is also a crucial nutrient for the metabolism of fat, because it decreases insulin resistance. Lipoic acid protects the mitochondria from damage, and is critical for optimum energy production.

9. Super Fats contains vitamin D_3. This is the active form of vitamin D. From chapter 10, you know how important vitamin D is for cancer prevention, maximum immune function, and bone health.

Combining QuickStart with Super Fats and a healthy diet will provide almost everybody with all the supplementation they will ever need to produce maximum amounts of energy all their lives. There will always be certain people who because of their genetics will require higher doses; but for most, this is as complete as it gets.

My Three-Month Rule

Every cell in your body except the nerve and brain cells reproduces itself within three months. This means that every three months you get to have a brand-new body. If these new cells are bathed in all the nutrients found in QuickStart and Super Fats combined with a healthy diet, guess what? They are much healthier cells than their parents were. And the cells produced over the next three months will be even better. This rejuvenation phenomenon will continue until you feel as good as you've ever felt. At that point, continue to take QuickStart on a regular basis for maintenance.

MY RECOMMENDATIONS TO YOU

* Remember, supplements are there for you to improve on an already-good diet. They guarantee a state of super nutrition, but in no way will they replace a healthy diet.
* Basically, keep it simple. Start off each day with a QuickStart and Super Fats smoothie.
* If you don't want to keep it that simple, then take a copy of all the nutrients listed in the Appendix to a health store and get them separately. Take them in divided dose with some food.

* 12 *

SECRET FIVE—FOOD

Although the right supplements can be critical for optimal energy production, a healthy and complete diet is even more so. There have been many times when a serious decrease in energy production in one of my patients was completely turned around simply by correcting bad eating habits. This is especially true of the younger set, but it is a big factor in all ages.

I recently read an anti-aging book that emphasized the importance of hormone replacement, supplements, and exercise. The entire discussion of food was limited to one paragraph that basically repeated the worn-out mantra of keeping fat intake below 30 percent and cholesterol intake below 200 milligrams. Giving food such a low level of importance does a great disservice to the reader.

Healthy eating is essential to a healthy body, and all the hormones and exercise in the world will not make up for an unhealthy, unnatural diet. Chemical-free natural foods provide essential nutrients, fats, and proteins, without which the body would be unable to efficiently produce energy.

The fact is, today's Standard American Diet (SAD) puts the body under siege from a barrage of antibiotics, artificial colors, drugs, food additives, GMO toxins, pesticides, preservatives, and radiation by-products.

Simply limiting fat and cholesterol intake does not cut it. This information—I prefer the word *mis*information—doesn't come close to relating what eating healthily is all about.

I have great compassion for the poor consumer shopping in the supermarket. What confusion. What choices. The work of Madison Avenue reaches out with cute product names, radiant packaging, claims of fortified ingredients, and a lot of bad information to earn your purchase. In this fashion, the food industry is producing more and more man-made "foods" that are supposed to be every bit as good as the real thing.

The human liver and the intestinal tract have never seen these so-called foods before. *New and improved foods* inevitably means unbalanced, man-made concoctions packed with synthetic oils and processed, fragmented nutrients. Foods that are lacking in amino acids, fiber, healthy fats, nutrient balance, and trace elements. *These patented creations have absolutely nothing to do with real food.*

Whether it's a 40–30–30 energy bar or a Pop Tart, a much better description for these manufactured products of food technology would be industrial waste. Even real foods, milk, for example, have been so industrialized that they are no longer obtainable in their natural, raw state.

Unless you go out of your way to learn about real food, most of what you learn about nutrition comes from the same people who make the junk.

Confused? Sure you are.

Fortunately, I have a simple rule that can eliminate the confusion.

Shallenberger's Simple Guide to Food Selection

Don't Buy Anything with an Ingredients Label!!!!!!!!!

Another way of saying this is to avoid anything not made by nature. If nature made the food, it doesn't need an ingredients label. If nature didn't make it, then the FDA requires a food label—that's how you can tell.

Eat foods without added ingredients. That's a huge world of selection, in case you're worried. Your choices include grains, dairy, eggs, fish, vegetables, legumes, meats, nuts, poultry, quinoa, seeds, unprocessed oils, whole fruit, and on and on.

A diet high in non-labeled foods will ultimately be the best one for you.

Okay—Now Read the Label

There's a slight catch in the simplicity of this concept. It's this: not all foods have been created, or at least grown and marketed, equally. By this, I mean that many natural foods, including fruits, meats, and vegetables, are being increasingly irradiated with X-rays, and then contaminated with additives, antibiotics, dyes, and hormones. This is a big problem, especially for children. It's one thing to dose up an adult with hormones, but it's quite another to expose infants and young children to these substances.

Moreover, there is evidence to suggest that the rampant infertility among young men, and the endometriosis, menstrual disturbances, and obesity so common in young women originates largely from the estrogen contamination of beef, eggs, milk, and poultry. Fortunately, non-radiated and hormone-free foods are available if you look for them. Look for "Hormone-Free" on the label.

Up until now, the FDA has not required special labeling of foods irradiated with radioactive materials. This is a travesty, because irradiated foods have been shown to contain unnatural molecules that are foreign to our immune systems. Since the long-term effects of irradiated foods are not yet known, I recommend they be avoided as much as possible. Unfortunately, manufacturers who are radiating foods will probably not disclose what they are doing until this is required by the FDA. Unless you grow your own food, this makes it crucial to buy your produce from sources you trust.

The Fiber Connection to Health

Humans are omnivores. That means that we are designed to consume both animal and vegetable food sources. The word *vegans* is used to describe those people who choose to eat only plant-based foods. Although it is practiced by a great many people, this is an abnormal diet. It not only doesn't make any sense to be a vegan, for most people it is downright unhealthy. A number of studies have shown that people on vegan diets often have several deficiencies of vitamins, minerals, and amino acids. Vegans typically, although not always, test out terribly on Bio-Energy Testing.

But neither is it healthy for most people to be a 100 percent meat eater. All life is about balance, and diet is no exception. And although animal foods contain many critical and wonderful nutrients, they do not have any fiber. You have certainly heard about fiber, and now you're about to hear more.

Dietary fiber, also known as roughage, is the portion of plant food that human digestive enzymes cannot break down. It is most readily available in beans, fruits, nuts, seeds, vegetables, and *whole* grains. Fiber absorbs moisture, acts as a natural laxative, gives the muscles in the intestinal walls something to grip on, increases stool size, and makes the stool softer.

Fiber also helps to detoxify the liver. When the liver removes toxins from the blood, it excretes many of them into the intestines in the form of bile salts. Fiber, especially the soluble fiber found only in fruits and vegetables, acts like a sponge to absorb these toxic salts and escort them out of the body in your bowel movement. That's why regular bowel movements are so important to health. Without regularity, accumulated toxins build up in the intestines and the rest of the body.

But that's not all that fiber does. Much overlooked is the fact that the friendly bacteria in our intestines feed on fiber. These beneficial micro-organisms perform a wide array of services, including the elimination of harmful bacteria, and the production of vital enzymes, acids, and vitamins. Even more important, they contribute to the efficiency of the immune system. When they become depleted, your ability to fight off infections is affected.

Hundreds of studies have linked low-fiber diets to just about every condition and disease there is. These include acne, cancer, diabetes, epilepsy, gallbladder disease, heart disease, hypertension, atherosclerosis, infection, kidney stones, learning disabilities, lupus, obesity, and ulcers. There's not a lot more that can go wrong with you than that.

So make sure your diet emphasizes foods that are high in fiber. But not just any high-fiber foods. Focus primarily on the high-fiber foods that are low-glycemic (see chapter 5). Because many of the foods that are high in fiber, such as root vegetables (tubers like potatoes and carrots) and many fruits, are also so high in sugars and other carbohydrates that they are high-glycemic. And that means that they create way too much insulin for most people.

The best overall high-fiber foods are those that are also low in sugars and carbohydrates. I'm talking about vegetables. Specifically, vegetables that grow above ground such as broccoli, cauliflower, lettuce, spinach, string beans, zucchini, Brussels sprouts, cabbage, etc. Ideally, when you look at your plate, you should see that three quarters of it are covered with above-ground vegetables, and one quarter with animal proteins.

Although above-ground vegetables are the best source of fiber, there is no reason why most people can't also have some of the middle- and low-glycemic foods at least every now and then.

The least-desirable foods are the *refined* carbohydrate items, namely flour products and sugar. These fractured foods have very little or no fiber, and are the highest of all glycemic foods. Filling your stomach with these kinds of man-made foods is about the worst thing you can do for your health. It is an invitation to low energy and weight gain, as well as bacterial imbalance in the intestines and increased toxicity.

One last word about flour and sweets. When you do indulge yourself, definitely avoid doing so on an empty stomach. The negative effects of these foods are maximized when eaten by themselves. Eat them only after you have already ingested some fat and protein, as with a dessert. That minimizes their insulin stimulating effects.

Fat—More Than Just Energy

Whenever I start discussing diet with my patients, the first thing out of their mouths is that they are really trying to cut down on the fat.

What a great brainwashing the food industry has accomplished. Almost everybody thinks of fat as something to be avoided like the plague. The majority of the population has long been convinced, and even experts buy into it, that for the sake of health we should invest our food dollars in industrially altered food that has had the fat removed.

People are repeatedly told that fat is the enemy. And, like the cavalry, the food manufacturers are riding to the rescue carrying low-fat and non-fat substitutes to protect everyone's health and correct the mistakes of nature.

I used to buy into this nonsense as well. Years ago, I believed that dietary fat raised blood fats and created atherosclerosis, heart disease, and hypertension. I was convinced that dietary fat was the cause of obesity. I even remember one expert who wrote that dietary fat caused diabetes.

I began putting all my patients on low-fat programs. Guess what happened? Nothing. Almost nobody lost weight. Heart disease and hypertension didn't improve, and my patients continued to complain of depressed immunity, fatigue, insomnia, and so forth.

Then I learned that I was being too flexible: I was not sufficiently restricting fat. "No more than 15 to 20 percent of your dietary calories should be in the form of fat," came the word from the experts. So, still convinced, I clamped down and recommended that my patients eat even less fat.

Regardless of what the studies and the experts say, there really is no better litmus test than patient feedback. They live in the real world, not in laboratory cages. Physicians should always keep up on the literature. But when a study leads to recommendations that just don't work with actual patients, it should be ignored, and something else should be tried. That's my attitude.

Not only did my patients not improve on the low fat, but they were beginning to resent me for putting them on a diet that was extremely difficult to follow and did not taste good. The lack of results and the negative reactions caused me to do a lot of re-thinking.

I was indeed practicing medicine by placing my patients on an abnormal diet. The human body was not designed to be on a low-fat diet. Anthropological studies overwhelmingly concur that the original human diet was filled with meat and fat. Studies on Inuits (formerly known as Eskimos) who actually ate nothing but meat and fat revealed a complete absence of diabetes, heart disease, or hypertension. It was only when these Inuits began eating flour and sugar that they developed these diseases.

I began thinking about the diets of my patients when they first came to me, and asked myself how many obese patients ate a diet high in fat. I checked the dietary records. The answer—none.

How many of my patients with heart disease actually ate a diet high in fat? Again, very few.

How many of my patients with eating disorders gorged themselves on fat? Yet again, none.

People do not develop diseases or obesity from eating too much fat. It can't be done. You can't eat too much fat, even if you try. I once experimented on myself. I broiled a well-marbled steak, then covered it with butter. I quickly discovered I was stuffed before I had even finished half of it.

Compared to carbohydrates, fats and proteins sit a long time in the stomach in order to be digested. The result is that you feel full for a long time. As I researched this further, I learned that fat induces the release of a hormone called cholecystokinin that causes the brain to rapidly register satiety. It turns out that it is literally impossible to overeat on a diet high in meat and fat. Add that to the fact that a diet high in fat stabilizes blood sugar and many disorders of the stomach and bowels.

I've talked about fat as a basic energy food. But it is so much more. It is definitely something *not* to be avoided. All our cell membranes are made from fat. And over half the energy our cells produce goes into maintaining the integrity of these membranes. Research has shown that when cells become diseased or poisoned, the very first pathological findings occur in the membranes.

Think of the cell as an exclusive club. The cell membrane is like the front door. Nothing gets in or out without going through this door. It takes proper functioning of the membrane to allow entrance into the cell of all the vitamins, minerals, fat, glucose, and proteins needed as raw materials to fuel activity. And located on the membranes are receptor sites for hormones. This is where hormones, which are messenger proteins, transfer their regulatory commands to cells. Without healthy membranes, the hormones cannot do their jobs.

Your nervous system and your brain are almost completely composed of fats. Fats also serve as the building blocks for all the steroid hormones, such as cortisol, DHEA, and the sex hormones.

Fats make up prostaglandins, compounds that are intricately involved in the function of the immune system, the cardiovascular system, and the healing process after an injury.

From this, we can understand why we were designed to eat fat, and why fats should be appreciated and not avoided. Without an adequate supply of fat, we could not even begin to maintain our mental and physical health.

Not All Fats Are Created Equal

Having said this, my last statement needs to be qualified. I should say: without an adequate supply of the *right* fats. Nature has given us fat to eat, but so too has man. And once again, it is the man-made foods, this time fats, that cause enormous problems.

Take one guess as to which fats lead to decreased energy production, arthritis, diabetes, heart disease, hormonal deficiencies, immune suppression, macular degeneration, and premature aging. The answer is: the very fats the food industry has been pushing.

Decades ago, food manufacturers encountered a problem transporting and storing *processed* foods because the fats in their products quickly became rancid. In order to make their merchandise more widely available, the industry had to figure out how to get around the rancidity issue. Food scientists provided the answer in processes known as hydrogenation and partial hydrogenation. This technology altered naturally occurring fats in such a way that they did not become rancid. Moreover, these new fats were so foreign to nature that even bacteria and insects could not feed on them.

And the ideal commercial fat was created. A fat that could be stored for years without rancidity or attack from nature's predators. Food science had improved on the old-fashioned natural animal and vegetable fats, which, alas, became rancid if not refrigerated. Now there was margarine, which could sit on the countertop and thumb its nose at the oxygen in the air that causes rancidity. People could now have a cornucopia of new foods with enormous shelf life simply by using the hydrogenated and partially hydrogenated fat technology in breads, breakfast cereals, mayonnaise, peanut butter . . . ad infinitum.

The only problem with the breakthrough was that these synthetic fats are alien to the body. They can't perform all the healthy functions that fats are supposed to perform. Instead, they actually interfere with the function of natural fats. They don't adequately maintain cell membranes. They adversely affect the cell-membrane receptors that are basic to hormone function. They create imbalances in the body's inflammatory response—and, in fact, increase inflammation. They block the activity of plasmin, the enzyme whose function is to dissolve platelet clots. This increases the risk of developing blood clots, which can cause life-threatening heart attacks.

Recent publications have also demonstrated that these artificial fats are contributing to cardiovascular disease by actually damaging the inner walls of the arteries. Researchers have documented that the increased consumption of margarine exactly parallels the current epidemic of heart disease. Other studies have shown that these unnatural fats change the composition of the cell membranes in the heart, and that these changes are associated with heart disease.

And, worst of all, hydrogenated and partially hydrogenated fats have been shown in several studies to damage mitochondria and dangerously decrease energy production—causing you to age faster and become much more likely to develop chronic diseases of every kind. They do this by becoming part of the mitochondrial membrane where energy production occurs.

And once these destructive fats get into your mitochondrial membrane and disrupt your energy production, how long does it take your body to get rid of them? On average, it takes from six to nine months of eating none of them at all to clear them all out of your membranes and replace them with healthy fats. These man-made fats are poisons that take forever to get rid of, so do everything you can to be sure you don't eat them, ever.

The bottom line on fat? *Don't be concerned about how much fat you eat, just* ***which*** *fat you eat.*

High Fat and Low Fiber

What about medical reports showing an increase in cancer among people who eat high-fat diets?

First, let me say that many of these studies are seriously flawed. Total caloric intake and the incidence of obesity are almost never taken into account. The numbers of people monitored in these studies are relatively small and the supposed increase in cancer is modest at best. Moreover, there are many contradicting studies.

For example, breast cancer is often said to be strongly associated with excessive dietary fat. In a long-term study monitoring the health and habits of 90,000 nurses, some 601 cases of breast cancer developed. However, there was no evidence of any relationship to fat intake.

In another study, published in the *Journal of the National Cancer Institute*, it was pointed out that while obesity and excess calorie intake have been implicated in cancer in both human and animal studies, fat intake per se has not. In that study, rats that had been exposed to an agent that caused breast cancer were fed either a diet high in fat but restricted in calories, or one low in fat but with a much higher level of calories in the form of carbohydrates. Only 7 percent of the rats on the high-fat diet developed breast cancer, compared to 43 percent of those on the carbohydrate diet.

Unlike the supposed dietary-fat connection, when you review the medical literature you will find many impressive studies linking deficiencies of fiber, vitamins, and other nutrients to cancer. I believe that any possible fat connection can be explained by the fact that diets excessively high in fat tend to be low in fiber and nutrients. It is not the high fat, but rather the low fiber and deficient nutrient intake that presents a risk. Such deficiencies arise from diets lacking fresh vegetables.

Protein—What You Are Made Of

While fats and carbohydrates serve the body as sources of energy, protein forms the structural material of most of your body. Protein is also involved in much of the biochemical business going on around the clock.

Your cells need enough protein to make muscle tissue, repair damaged organs, and produce enzymes, hormones, immunoglobulins, and brain neurotransmitters.

Unfortunately, due to the popularity of vegetarian eating, many health-conscious people have been led to believe that dairy, eggs, and meat are unhealthy for them. Additionally, since nature designed that meat and fat would travel together, the low-fat frenzy has also resulted in a decrease in protein intake.

An insufficient amount of high-quality protein in the diet has many negative consequences, including arthritis, attention deficit syndrome, chronic infections, hormonal deficiencies, immune deficiencies, low blood sugar, osteoporosis, and many other degenerative diseases associated with aging.

The preferred protein sources are dairy, eggs, fish, poultry, and meats. These can be supplemented with protein from beans and soy. For the most part, make sure you eat a significant amount of protein with every meal. And keep in mind that the more you exercise or exert yourself, the more protein you will need.

The newest biggest problem in the food industry—GMO "foods"

GMO stands for genetically modified organisms. GMO foods are foods that have had the genetics of either insects or bacteria inserted into the genetics of the natural plant. This results in decreased nutritional value and also causes the formation of various proteins in the plant that act as toxins in animals and humans. However, as bad as that is, it may not be the worst thing about these foods.

Let's take a look at the most common GMO food out there: GMO soy. Given soy's centrality to our food and agriculture systems, the findings of an article published in the peer-reviewed journal *Food Chemistry* are required reading for all health-conscious Americans.

The authors noted that the main reason that the food chemistry industry embraces GMO foods is because they are designed to withstand highly toxic levels of the herbicide Roundup, which contains the poison glyphosate. Remember that name: glyphosate. Because of the glyphosate resistance of GMO soybeans, farmers growing GMO soybeans are able to dose those beans up with extra glyphosate without killing them. Naturally, this means that GMO soy contains significantly more herbicide residues than non-GMO soy. The authors also found that the GMO beans are nutritionally inferior.

In the study, the researchers examined three kinds of soybeans grown in Iowa: GMO beans, natural beans, and organically grown beans. They found glyphosate and aminomethylphosphonic acid in every GMO sample. Aminomethylphosphonic acid is the compound that glyphosate breaks down into as it decays. What about the normal beans? No evidence at all of any of these toxins. How high were the toxins? And should we be concerned?

The GMO soy contained glyphosate levels as high as 20.1 ppm. The Environmental Protection Agency and the European Union limit safe levels to below 20 ppm.

Soybeans are no exception. All GMO foods are loaded up with extra glyphosate. When you eat any GMO food, you are eating a food that is much more contaminated with glyphosate than a non-GMO food. And that means that you and your family are going to be consuming a much higher amount of glyphosate. It also means that the environment is progressively being contaminated by more and more glyphosate. Even our water and air have become contaminated. In one of the articles that you are going to read below, you will see just how serious this has become. So serious that all of us—yes, I said all of us, including babies—have blood levels of this chemical, even those of us who avoid Roundup and GMO foods. And the data look like that can't be good.

As the consumption of glyphosate has increased over the past twenty-five years, so have many diseases. One paper estimates that chronic disease has increased by 25 percent since glyphosate was first introduced into the market. Specifically, the disease rates of Parkinson's, Alzheimer's, diabetes, autism, anxiety and panic disorders, inflammatory bowel disease, and thyroid cancer have risen at the same rate as the use of glyphosate.

Is glyphosate a factor in the increase in all these and other diseases? We can't say for sure, but the statistical and scientific data look very suspicious. So now with that background, let's look at some new information on glyphosate. First, whether you like it or not, the odds are getting better all the time that you are going to be drinking and breathing glyphosate today.

One recent study published just two years ago looked at the amounts of various pesticides and herbicides in air and rain samples collected during the 2007 growing season in the Mississippi Delta agricultural region. The samples were taken within three miles of the farms using the chemicals. Here's what they found:

Glyphosate and its degradation product, aminomethylphosphonic acid, were detected in more than 75 percent of all of the air and rain samples. In the authors' own words, the overall amount of herbicides in the air and water in 2007 was greater than it had been in previous decades and was "dominated by glyphosate." These data go against the propaganda that we hear from the GMO people claiming that glyphosate completely disappears from the environment upon contact with air and water.

Of course, the contamination mentioned in the above study was only evaluated in an area close to agricultural sites. Perhaps it's not such a problem in urban areas? Think again.

In another review article published in 2013 titled "Glyphosate and its formulations—toxicity, occupational and environmental exposure," the authors analyzed and reported on a series of recently published papers (2010–2013) looking at the environmental impact of glyphosate and its formulations. Here's what they discovered.

"Initial reports about alleged biodegradability of glyphosate in the environment turned out to be wrong. It has been shown that glyphosate remains in the soil and can reach people by spreading along with groundwater."

Recent publications have shown that glyphosate is detected at low concentrations in the human blood. In 2013, people in eighteen countries across Europe were found to have traces of glyphosate in their urine by a test commissioned by Friends of the Earth Europe. And that's not all they reported on.

The authors also discussed the evidence that glyphosate induces cancerous changes in cells exposed to it. Like other environmental toxins, it also has been shown to cause hormonal imbalances and possibly interfere with reproduction and sexual function. Not surprisingly, it increases the formation of free radicals and changes what is called the redox balance of our cells to one that leads to oxidant stress, chronic disease, and premature aging. The researchers concluded their paper with the statement: "The discussed problems clearly show the need to evaluate the toxicity of glyphosate and its formulations and related potential threat to humans." And nobody is completely safe from glyphosate. Not even babies on breast milk.

Recently, a pilot study from Moms Across America and Sustainable Pulse analyzed the samples of breast milk from ten women across the country. The results are shocking. Three of the samples had detectable levels of glyphosate in their breast milk. The highest glyphosate level was detected in a mother from Florida. Her level was 166 μg/l, which is 1,600 times higher than the maximum detectable limit allowed in drinking water in Europe! The other two mothers with "positive" results were from Virginia (76 μg/l) and Oregon (99 μg/l).

The last paper I want you to be familiar with is titled "Evidence that glyphosate is a causative agent in chronic sub-clinical metabolic acidosis and mitochondrial dysfunction." Listen to the words of the authors of this latest review on the adverse health effects of glyphosate.

> "Many types of chemicals, including pesticides and pharmaceutical drugs, cause metabolic acidosis and mitochondrial disorder. We provide evidence from the scientific literature that glyphosate can be metabolized by humans, that it disrupts the intestinal microbiota [healthy intestinal bacteria], causes severe metabolic acidosis when ingested in high doses, and leads to mitochondrial dysfunction by uncoupling of phosphorylation."

This "uncoupling" phenomenon they are talking about is what causes the decreased E.Q. that I have been talking about. The authors continue:

> "The symptoms and diseases associated with metabolic acidosis and mitochondrial dysfunction compare well with those attributed to glyphosate. Taken together, this evidence suggests that glyphosate, in the doses equivalent to allowed residues in food ingested over a long period of time, causes a low-grade, chronic acidosis as well as mitochondrial dysfunction. We also provide evidence from the literature supporting the biochemical pathways whereby this occurs. We then extract the reports for symptoms and diseases associated with glyphosate from the U.S. Food and Drug Administration's Adverse Event Reporting System database. These are compared to the symptoms and diseases reported in the database for drugs that are known to cause mitochondrial dysfunction. The results are startlingly consistent."

Dear readers, here's the really scary part: I'm not making this up. You can read the entire paper, complete with 130 references, at the website listed in the Reference section of this book. The first thing is always to be informed. This information is published and fully available.

Eat Less More

One of the major rules of dietary adjustment with age is to lower the percentage of calories you get from carbohydrates. The dietary carbohydrate content for most twenty- to thirty-year-olds is often as high as 50 to 60 percent of the total calories. However, as you approach fifty, most will need to reduce the dietary carbohydrate content to between 30 and 40 percent. Additionally, since every human system is unique, some people will need to adhere more strictly to these guidelines than others. You will know how well your diet is working in several ways.

The first is how you feel. Are you as strong and energetic as always? A diet too high in carbohydrates will cause you to feel tired, especially in the afternoon. It can cause you to gain weight easily and have a tougher time keeping the weight off. Headaches are also more common. Another manifestation of eating too many carbs is in your cholesterol testing. If your cholesterol is too high, particularly if your triglycerides are greater than 110, chances are that you are eating too many carbs.

Of course, the best way to assess your level of carb intake is through Bio-Energy Testing. If you are overdoing the carbs, you will test out with a low E.Q. and a low C-Factor. This combined finding indicates that your carbohydrate intake is suppressing your fat metabolism. The lower the C-Factor, the greater the problem.

Another thing that will need to decrease as you get older is . . . everything. So, while you are busy getting your carbohydrate intake down, please keep in mind that with age, fewer total calories are required. This is true even if your lifestyle and exercise level remain in a youthful fast lane. For example, a sixty-year-old man with the exact same activity level as a forty-year-old requires fewer calories to fulfill his energy needs.

So, a major golden rule of eating as you age is to eat less. Especially less carbohydrate, but also less fat and protein. Fewer calories in general. Bio-Energy Testing can determine exactly what your daily calorie needs are, so that you don't have to just guess about it. But in general, know that eating fewer calories is a hallmark of any program designed to keep you living longer and healthier.

The Power of Fasting

As long as you are healthy, you can help keep yourself that way with regular short fasts. Animal studies have conclusively proven that fasting can significantly extend lifespan.

Basically, any time you don't eat for two or three hours, your body begins to go into a fasting mode. Fasting, and even just skipping meals, has been shown to elevate growth hormone levels by as much as 400 percent, a very significant result. (See chapter 15, Secret 8.)

Regular short fasting is also a superior way to detoxify the body. Many toxins, particularly heavy metals, organic acids, and substances known as advanced glycosylated end products (AGEs), become lodged in the interstitial space. The interstitial space is the space in between the cells. These toxins are removed during fasting.

The interstitial space is not just a domain of empty space. It is an active and systemic-wide production field where many important regulating systems operate. One of those systems is the one that forms collagen.

Collagen is the major protein molecule that makes up the basic substance of all tissue. Collagen is what holds our blood vessels, bones, joints, and skin together.

The presence of toxins in the interstitial space not only interferes with the formation of collagen; it also results in a very undesirable process known as cross-linking.

Cross-linking is a general organic-chemistry term that refers to what happens when one chain of molecules is chemically linked to another one. Plastics are made through this process. And it is the effect of cross-linking that gives plastics their hard and inflexible qualities. Plastics that are harder and more inflexible are more heavily cross-linked. Those that are soft and pliable are minimally cross-linked. When two biological molecular chains, such as two collagen molecules, are joined through this process, they also become hard and inflexible. The result of too much collagen cross-linking is a tendency for the tissues to easily break down.

An example of collagen cross-linking can be seen in what happens to leather. Over time, even the best leather will show the classic signs of collagen cross-linking: it becomes dry and wrinkled, and it ultimately cracks. A certain amount of collagen cross-linking is natural and necessary to provide structure and form to our bodies. It is excess and/or unintended cross-linking that is the culprit.

Just like with the leather, as the collagen in our skin and other tissues becomes cross-linked, they become less flexible and less able to fulfill normal functions. The most obvious example of collagen cross-linking can be seen as we get older—wrinkles. One of the major causes of wrinkles is the collagen cross-linking that occurs as a consequence of excessive sun exposure. That's why when you are enjoying all the health benefits of sunbathing, be sure to protect your face. The skin there is thin and is very prone to solar-induced collagen cross-linking.

But collagen cross-linking is more than just skin-deep; its nasty effects are widely distributed. As the collagen in the arteries becomes cross-linked, they will become hardened and much more likely to cause high blood pressure and strokes. Bones become more brittle. The same process happens to all the organs, including the liver, kidneys, intestinal tract, eyes, muscles, tendons—everything.

Fasting helps eliminate many of the toxic molecules that contribute to cross-linking. Exercise and saunas also have the same effect, but fasting is very special in its own way. Except in unusual circumstances I'm not an advocate of extended fasting, because there is too much protein lost from the body, and after two or three days fasting starts to lose many of its effects. Moreover, I believe the same detoxifying benefits reaped from long fasts can also be achieved by a series of regular short fasts. The principle is called intermittent fasting. Below is what I recommend.

My Intermittent Fasting Program

Pick one day a week, and on that day eat a large, high-protein, high-fat, low-carbohydrate breakfast. Have lunch around noon. But after lunch, eat nothing until breakfast the next day. Make sure that you drink at least 1 quart of water during the day. You may squeeze the juice of a lemon in the water if you want to. After lunch, you may have coffee or tea, but nothing added that has any calories.

On the same day the next week, eliminate not only the dinner but also the lunch. So, on that day, you will be fasting 24 hours until breakfast the next day.

For many people, this simple one-day fast will increase detoxification and improve weight control, blood-sugar levels, blood pressure, and energy production. For others, it would be good to have the same intermittent fast on another day. The maximum number of days for intermittent fasting on any kind of a regular basis should be limited to one or two days. More than that can be counterproductive.

The benefits of fasting also extend to the emotional area. Even though we may not always be aware of it, almost all of us eat for many emotional reasons that have nothing to do with hunger or nutrition. We often eat simply because the regularity of timed meals confirms a sense of safety and security. As long as the meals are there, our unconscious minds can relax, knowing that all is well in the world. We also eat for social reasons; to squelch uncomfortable emotions; and to reward ourselves for one thing or another.

For all these reasons, it is very common to confront uncomfortable feelings, such as anger, anxiety, boredom, guilt, insecurity, low self-esteem, and sadness, when going on a fast. Sometimes these emotions can be intense. They indicate the emotional connections with eating, and for many this revelation will become an eye-opener. I know it was for me.

Many people either eat too much, or eat foods they know are poor choices, simply to make them feel better emotionally. Fasting presents a wonderful opportunity to examine just how much these suppressed emotions may be running our lives without our really realizing it.

And for those who like personal insights, a fast offers the impetus to deal with emotions in a healthy way, rather than continuing to suppress them under binges of chips, chocolate, crackers, or other goodies. Fasting can also instill a sense of gratitude for living in a country where hunger is rare. Gratefulness is surely one of the healthiest anti-aging emotions.

Another really amazing thing about fasting is the amount of extra time you will have during the fasting day. It is just amazing to me how much time we spend around meals. We spend a lot of time buying the food, preparing the food, eating the food, and cleaning up afterward. On my fasting days, I find that I have about two extra hours that day. It's like getting a twenty-six-hour day one or two times a week.

My Diet

My patients always ask me how I eat. So, in case you are curious too, here's the kind of diet I generally follow.

I drink a 12-ounce glass of water with a teaspoon of organic apple-cider vinegar as soon as I get out of bed. Right after my shower, I drink a cup of organic green tea.

For breakfast, I down some QuickStart and a teaspoon of Super Fats. If I have the time and the inclination, I get fancy and make up a smoothie with cream, yogurt (high-fat!), and frozen berries. To this I will usually add some steel-cut oatmeal with whipping cream, berries, and nuts. On alternate mornings, I will have eggs (saturated in butter and olive oil) and some beans. I finish it off with a beautiful cup of organic espresso.

For lunch, I have one of several options: (1) leftovers from dinner the night before; (2) a salad with blue cheese dressing, cheese, and meat; (3) a bowl of soup; (4) a meat sandwich; or (5) a bean, cheese, and meat burrito.

For dinner, I eat a salad, fresh vegetables, and some form of meat, poultry, or fish. I don't usually snack or eat sweets, but maybe once or twice a week I'll have a sweet or some fruit right after dinner.

My goal is to eat at least two servings of vegetables a day, and at least one fresh salad. Since every vegetable has its own unique nutrient content, I make sure I eat a variety.

I try to keep the bread, cereals, rice, and pasta to a minimum—probably no more than 1 or 2 times a week will I have anything from that list.

I am not concerned about eating too much fat or protein, and I strictly avoid nonfat or reduced-fat foods.

I eat very slowly, thoroughly chewing my food (very important for good digestion), and am usually the last one at the table to finish.

I avoid overeating. I never want to leave the table stuffed in the least.

Just to be real, I break all these rules every now and then. It's not the occasional indiscretions that kill us; it's the regular ones.

MY RECOMMENDATIONS TO YOU

* As much as possible, avoid man-made foods, particularly nonfat or reduced-fat foods.
* Avoid the regular intake of high-glycemic foods (see page 90). Eat them as you would chocolate cake. I consider them strictly treat items.
* Limit your intake of organic coffee to 4 to 8 ounces a day. This amount of coffee is actually very beneficial for those who can tolerate it, but too much coffee is hard on the intestinal tract. Moreover, too much java creates an acid condition in the tissues and acts as a diuretic. This combination contributes to osteoporosis because, when the level of acidity rises in the body, the system responds by pulling calcium out of bone tissue to buffer the acid. If you enjoy the stimulant effect of coffee, you might want to give green tea a try. Not only is it a strong stimulant, but it has anti-cancer properties.
* For these same reasons, limit alcohol to 1 or 2 drinks a day. In small amounts, alcohol has a beneficial stimulatory effect on the liver, as can coffee.
* Mass-production milk has been ruined by the homogenization and pasteurization processes. Even in small amounts, it often triggers allergies. In larger amounts, it often causes bowel and liver problems. If you live in a state where raw milk is available, you are lucky. Raw milk has very few of the problems that pasteurized milk has. You can use the internet to go to http://www.realmilk.com/where2.html. There you will find a state-by-state listing of raw milk suppliers. Milk is a good source of calcium, but you can get more calcium per gram of weight from spinach and many other vegetables than from milk. Children do not need milk at all. Children who don't drink milk have bones just as strong as their milk-drinking friends, and they avoid the common problems associated with pasteurized milk. Dr. Frank Orski, director of the Department of Pediatrics at Johns Hopkins Hospital, has pointed out that milk contributes to anemia, constipation, diarrhea, ear infections, hyperactivity, and skin rashes in children.
* Avoid fast food, junk food, sodas, sugar, and sweets.

* When you do eat sweets, eat them in the form of a dessert: that is, after a meal. Avoid cakes, cookies, or any sweets on an empty stomach. By eating them after a meal, you dilute their sugar content with the other foods already in your stomach.

* Artificial sweeteners are okay in small amounts.

* Use butter, lecithin, olive oil, or Pam when you cook. Avoid deep-fried foods. Learn to lightly sauté foods in a little olive oil or butter.

* Never use margarine, shortening, or hydrogenated or partially hydrogenated oils. Never! They are poisons.

* Forget fruit juice. It is not a health food. Drink juice only sparingly, as a treat. Why? It has no fiber, and it is high in sugar. Did you know that a glass of most fruit juices contains as much sugar as a cola?

* Keep your dinner on the light side. And avoid going to sleep for at least three hours after dinner. This means eating dinner early, say around 6:00. Three hours is enough time for your body to digest the meal. If you are tired before that time, lie down and rest, but try not to fall asleep. You cannot fully digest your foods while you sleep, and sleeping soon after dinner on a regular basis will lead to increased toxicity and weight gain.

* Be consciously grateful for the blessing of the good food and water you have.

* Chew your food well. Eat slowly. And enjoy what you eat.

* ***My favorite recommendation:*** Feel free to break all the above rules periodically. It's how you eat over the long term that counts, not the transgressions you commit now and then. A healthy body can handle a toxic situation periodically, and besides, it gives you something different to look forward to.

✳ 13 ✳

SECRET SIX—EXERCISE: THE MOST IMPORTANT SECRET OF ALL

First, let me make this completely clear: For the over-fifty set, there is nothing you can do to increase your energy production, prolong your life, decrease your risk of disease, and slow down your rate of aging that is anywhere close to being as powerful as regular, correct exercise. Nothing. It alone sits on the throne of health.

What you eat, what supplements you take, what hormones you replace—as important as these are, none of them can do what exercise can do. Over the years, after doing hundreds of Bio-Energy Tests on people between the ages of fifty and ninety, this fact has become abundantly evident. Those people who improve their energy production inevitably are the exercisers. Those who don't exercise as a rule never improve. Of course, the ones that do the best are those who exercise and also follow all the other secrets in this book.

But if for some reason you have decided to try only one of the secrets, make it exercise. By the way, it has the added advantage of being free.

It's Not for the Young

Few things, perhaps, are more misunderstood than exercise. In this country, people have the concept completely backward. Let me explain: on the one hand, parents are almost obsessed with making sure their kids get plenty of it. They demand regular physical education classes—if you've had children in the school system, you know that getting them excused from Physical Education (P.E.) classes usually requires something akin to a letter from the Pope.

Parents go to great expense to make sure that schools offer a large and diverse sports program, and they enthusiastically encourage participation. The irony of this is that, while exercise is obviously good for children and adults under thirty-five, the primary needs in these age brackets are good nutrition and adequate rest—exercise per se is not all that important. Somewhere around the age of thirty-five, however, the physiology starts to change in significant ways. And with the changes and the years comes an increasingly greater need for exercise.

But go into a health club, and who do you see? Not many seventy-year-olds. Mostly you see the younger set getting ready for their next date, while the majority of the older generation is home actively pursuing some version of couch behavior. Why?

According to what I hear, most older folks have developed the idea that they're too old for that stuff. They're at that point in life in which they need to slow down. Despite what they read in the popular press, which more and more is espousing regular exercise, many still don't get it. I think many people in this time of their lives just can't believe that jogging, calisthenics, and lifting weights can really do anything substantial for them. *The truth is that they're not only not too old to do that stuff, they're too old NOT to do that stuff.*

Exercise has been accepted by most as just a good way to look and feel great. But so many older folks say "I don't need to look great, and I don't feel all that bad. So why shoul,d I waste my precious time exercising?" But those who want to slow down the aging process and be fully functional for as long as they live need to understand that exercise is *absolutely essential*. There is no way around it. No matter how many anti-aging hormones and supplements a person takes, without the correct exercise program they are wasting their time.

Exercise Cuts Your Disease Rate

Two-thousand four-hundred years ago, Aristotle said, "A man falls into ill health as a result of not caring for exercise." He was right on the money. Many gerontologists (medical experts specializing in treating older people) regard properly focused exercise as perhaps the closest thing there is to an anti-aging pill. They believe that a regular program of high-intensity interval training can go far in slowing or reversing virtually all the physiological changes and illnesses associated with aging.

As a longevity elixir, exercise has been the focus of an ongoing world-famous study conducted by Stanford researcher Ralph Paffenbarger Jr., MD. With updates published over the years in leading medical journals, the study tracks exercise habits and longevity among more than 17,000 Harvard alumni. In a 1986 report for the *New England Journal of Medicine,* Paffenbarger said his findings show that "for each hour of physical activity, you can expect to live that hour over—and live one or two more hours to boot."

But exercise does so much more than just extend your life. It also dramatically improves the day-to-day quality of life. Here's a sampling of the evidence:

* According to Dr. Ken Cooper, MD, of the Cooper Institute of Aerobic Research, there are 40 percent fewer heart attacks among women who exercise and 60 percent fewer among exercising males. In another study, he determined that individuals in the lowest 20 percent bracket of cardiovascular fitness had a death rate three times higher than the fittest group. The study also indicated that men who started exercising, even after the age of sixty, increased their life expectancy.

* Among post-menopausal women, osteoporosis can be reduced by weight training twice a week. This increases bone density; plus it improves strength and balance, which can reduce the risk of falls in older people. This lowers the mortality rate, because in the over-seventy group, fractured hips from falls are associated with a fairly high death rate.

* A 1994 study in the *Journal of the American Medical Association* (*JAMA*) points to a decreased incidence of gastrointestinal hemorrhage among older people who exercise regularly.

* An article in the *Archives of Internal Medicine* demonstrated that men who were physically unfit were almost three times as likely to die from all causes, including cancer, even after the researchers accounted for age, alcohol use, and smoking.

* Studies have shown that exercise reduces the incidence of colon cancer by 50 percent, and of breast and ovarian cancer by a very significant margin.

* Impotence occurs in 25 percent of all men over the age of sixty-five. Researchers say, however, that men who regularly exercise have a much lower incidence of this problem. If you like sex, you're going to love exercise.

* Exercise is the healthiest way to treat depression. A 2000 study reported in *Psychosomatic Medicine* concluded that exercise provides as much effectiveness against depression as the latest medications—and with no side effects. Additionally, people who exercised actually had better long-term results than those on medication. After six months, those on medication had a three times greater relapse rate than those who exercised.

* Exercise also helps keep Alzheimer's at bay, as well as the usual mental decline associated with aging. It is also a very effective treatment for insomnia.

Exercise—It's Addictive

Getting sedentary people to exercise is often a challenge. Sometimes it's harder than getting them to make any other lifestyle change. But just try to get them to stop once they've been into it for a few months. Once you are in great shape, you just don't want to go back. It is truly addicting.

Are You Exercising Too Hard?

Some people, especially those who find it hard to control their weight, are actually exercising too hard for their level of fitness and genetics. Often, they rely on calculated heart-rate formulas that are notoriously inaccurate. If you calculate your exercise level in this manner, the odds are high that you are wasting much of your effort.

Currently, the formula that is most widely used by exercise experts to compute proper exercise zones is 208 – (.7 x age). Many exercise experts use this formula to calculate a person's maximum heart rate.

I'll apply that formula to forty-five-year-old Mary, one of my many overweight patients. It estimates that her maximum heart rate is 176 beats per minute. According to another, commonly accepted, standard formula, her maximum fat-burning rate (FBR) would occur at 65 percent of her estimated maximum heart rate, or 176 x .65 = 114 beats per minute, and her anaerobic threshold rate (ATR) would be equal to .85 of the estimated maximum heart rate, or 176 x .85 = 150 beats per minute. The trainer she was going to had therefore instructed her to exercise at a heart rate of between 114 and 150 beats per minute.

In fact, though, when we measured Mary's actual zones using Bio-Energy Testing, we discovered, not surprisingly, a very different picture from that predicted by the equations. First of all, her FBR turned out to be 95 beats per minute, not 114. And her ATR was measured at 110 beats per minute, much lower than the predicted value of 150. When she was working out in the zone given to her by her trainer, she was not only completely wasting her time; she was in fact exercising at a rate that was unhealthy and damaging for her. Let me explain.

Burning Carbohydrates Instead of Fat

Her trainer had predicted that her FBR, the rate at which she burns maximum fat, was 114 beats per minute. But Bio-Energy Testing determined that when she worked out at this predicted FBR, she was actually exercising above her ATR. The ATR is where no fat is being burned, only carbohydrate stores. And so for her entire exercise period, Mary was not burning any fat at all. Instead of training her body to burn fat, all she was doing was depleting her carbohydrate stores.

Technically speaking, according to the books, after exercise her carbohydrate stores should eventually be replenished by her fat stores. And in this way she should burn at least some fat. But this breaking-down-fat-stores-to-replenish-carbohydrate-stores idea turns out to be a bit of a myth for Mary for one simple reason: the metabolic hallmark of most people with weight disorders is that they are unable to mobilize fat stores to replenish anything. The only way an overweight person is able to replenish carbohydrate stores is by eating carbohydrates. And, of course, that only decreases fat metabolism even more.

Since Mary's carbohydrate stores had become depleted from the way she was exercising, she had to immediately eat some carbohydrates in order to recover and feel well. In actuality, therefore, it's not her fat stores that are replenishing her depleted carbohydrate stores; it's her diet. All this was reflected in what she said when she first saw me: "I don't understand. No matter how hard I exercise, it does no good at all. All I do is get sore, and I can't lose weight." I can't tell you how often I have heard this refrain.

Pain = No Gain

The reason Mary is so sore after exercise is because her trainer had also instructed her to spend half her exercise time at her supposed ATR of 150. But from her Bio-Energy Testing results, we were able to determine that her real ATR was 110, not 150. Any time she spent exercising above 110, which she had been doing for twenty-five to thirty minutes every day, she was going into lactic acidosis.

Lactic acidosis not only gives her needless pain (this kind of pain equals no gain), but also causes her muscles to be sore and increases the free-radical damage to her entire body. So, exercising above a heart rate of 110 not only doesn't help her lose weight or enhance her health at all, it actually makes her more susceptible to disease and injury. Mary was suffering from over-training. Because her trainer had been using completely inaccurate formulas to predict her exercise zone, her *entire* exercise time had been wasted.

Getting Your Zone Right

As soon as Mary completed her Bio-Energy Testing, I explained to her why she had been so unsuccessful. "You mean I have been exercising too hard for my own good?" I told her that was the case. I then explained how research is continually showing that for her, spending most of her exercise time at or below the ATR is the most effective way to lose weight and stay healthy. Much better than the old push-it-to-the-limits approach.

Mary needed to lose fat. But her body composition analysis indicated that besides having too much fat on board, she also had much too little muscle mass. I told her that her biggest problem was not that she had too much fat, it was that she did not have enough muscle. Whatever exercise program she went on, it would have to emphasize muscle gain. With this in mind, I started her on an aerobic program that emphasized fat burning called high intensity interval training, or HIIT for short. I then had her alternate her HIIT program with circuit training. Both of these methods are described below.

Mary only spent thirty minutes a day exercising. This is really all anybody needs to stay healthy. I knew that she was going to get great results, because using the other information from her Bio-Energy Testing, I also put her on an individualized dietary and supplement program. Although the intensity of her exercise programs seemed like nothing after all she had been through, she did finally start to lose some weight to the tune of one pound a week. More importantly, she was feeling more energetic, sleeping better, and losing her craving for carbohydrates.

In six months, she had lost all her excess fat, and we examined her Bio-Energy Testing results again. This time, her FBR turned out to have

improved to 112 beats per minute, and her ATR had risen to 130 beats per minute. While these numbers were not yet where they needed to be for optimal anti-aging, they did demonstrate that Mary's overall program was working. Of course, her new FBR and ATR determined a different exercise zone, which she immediately began to incorporate into her exercise program.

Living in Lactic Acidosis

Many trainers accustomed to using fitness formulas instead of Bio-Energy Testing may find Mary's case hard to believe. They think it would become quickly obvious to anyone that they were in lactic acidosis, since lactic acidosis in healthy people characteristically causes rapid breathing and muscle aching. But my research has shown me that a large percentage of people, particularly those with weight-control issues, have trained their bodies to be so used to lactic acidosis that they don't usually develop these symptoms.

Because their E.Q. is so low, they may spend a considerable part of their day in lactic acidosis simply from everyday exertions such as walking. Some of my patients go into lactic acidosis simply from getting out of a chair. The livers in these people have often developed an extraordinary ability to convert lactic acid back to blood sugar with incredible efficiency, allowing them to be in lactic acidosis without having the characteristically severe symptoms. This conversion in the liver happens in what is called the Cori cycle.

Mary was one of these people. Under the advice of a trainer who used the standard formulas, she had regularly been exercising in lactic acidosis for more than two years. Exercise was not fun for her, and she had to force herself to do it. She was chronically tired and achy; but because her doctors could find no reason for these symptoms, she had just learned to live with it. Mary was a determined woman. Most women after this experience just give up exercise entirely.

Being in the Zone Is Fun

Not long after Mary's Bio-Energy Testing discovered her correct zones, she called me up complaining about her new exercise program. "This is much too easy," she said. "It can't possibly work. I'm sure I'm wasting my time." I assured her this was because for the past two years she had been overdoing it, and naturally this one felt too easy. I told her to enjoy the fact that she would no longer have to dread her exercise periods, and she would actually begin to look forward to them. Exercising in the correct zone is fun and enjoyable. When she came to the clinic two months later, she was smiling and finally seeing the light. This was the first non-dieting weight loss she had ever seen.

Mary's case exemplifies the importance of exercising in your real zone, not an imaginary one deduced from wholly inaccurate one-size-fits-all formulas. I have seen so many cases like Mary's over the years that I often wonder if these formulas actually work for anyone at all. Knowing your *real* FBR and ATR are invaluable keys to getting the most from your workouts.

In twelve months, Mary's numbers became optimal and she settled into an easy maintenance program consisting of exercise for twenty to twenty-five minutes three or four times a week. She will be doing this for the rest of her life. And at the rate she is going, that should be a really long time.

Your Optimum Exercise Zone

One of the many advantages of Bio-Energy Testing is that instead of having to rely on an erroneous calculated formula, it is able to determine your unique exercise zone. This is important. So, let me just repeat myself. When you are exercising above your ATR for longer than a few minutes, your body will increase its level of free-radical damage, and it will actually age faster. When you are exercising at a level of exercise that is below your FBR, your exercise will be inefficient, and you will be wasting your exercise time. *So, whenever you exercise, be sure to wear your heart rate monitor, and keep within your zone.*

There are two basic ways to exercise that really work: *High Intensity interval training,* and *circuit training.* HIIT emphasizes increasing both your ability to burn fat and your total aerobic energy-producing capability. Circuit training accomplishes both of these goals as well, but also adds in the element of resistance training to increase muscle gain. Both are valuable, and I generally recommend that each be done on alternating days. Let's talk about interval training first.

HIIT Interval Training

To do HIIT, you will need some exercise equipment. The only equipment I don't like for this purpose is the treadmill, because there is too great a chance for injury. Anything else is good, including stationary bicycles, rowing machines, stepper machines, elliptical trainers, etc. If you are working, it's great to have your own equipment in the house. That saves a lot of time driving to and from the gym.

HIIT involves alternating longer intervals of time at your FBR with shorter times at your ATR and very brief spurts above your ATR. The time spent at your FBR is called your recovery time. It is where your mitochondria can recover from the more intense exercise that you are doing the rest of the time. It is also where you will train your body to burn fat more efficiently.

A typical interval-training session begins by exercising hard enough to raise your heart rate up to your FBR. This is a warm-up period. After a few minutes warming up, start exercising at a pace that keeps your heart rate at your ATR, and leave it there for two minutes.

Next, go all out for twenty to thirty seconds. This is called an "anaerobic burst," because during it your heart rate will climb way above your ATR, and you will be producing energy anaerobically—without oxygen. I have already told you in three or four places in this book that exercising above your ATR is bad, but now I am going to fine-tune that statement.

It's true. Extended time exercising above your ATR is harmful. Athletes need to do it to win races, but nevertheless it is not good for their health. However, brief spurts of exercise in this zone is actually quite stimulating for the mitochondria. If you are a competitive athlete, you can extend the anaerobic burst to as long as two to three minutes. But for non-competitive people, twenty to thirty seconds is perfect. And go hard—really hard. So hard that by the time you hit that 20–30 mark, you are pretty well spent and have to stop.

After this short anaerobic burst, your heart should be pounding, you should be breathing very hard, and you should be really happy that you don't have to do it any longer. At this point, either get off the equipment and sit on a chair or decrease the pace way down to barely moving until your heart rate comes down to your FBR. This may take from three to five minutes.

Once you reach your FBR, that is your signal that your cells have completely recovered from what you just did to them and are ready to go again. Just remember this: your recovery period is *every bit as important* as the ATR interval and the anaerobic bursts. It may feel easy, and you may think that it is a waste of time, but it isn't.

As soon as you reach your FBR, repeat another interval of two minutes at your ATR followed by an anaerobic burst. According to the latest findings, all you need to do is two of these cycles. It will take about five or six minutes per cycle, or a total workout time of fifteen to twenty minutes. Just do this on a regular basis three times a week. That's all the aerobic workout you need. I guarantee that you will love this form of exercise. It changes enough so that it is not boring, and it is so much easier than continually overtaxing your body's reserves. And more than any other form of exercise, it will improve your E.Q.

Many people erroneously think the only good form of exercise is hard and fast. That may be a great way to win a race, but it is not the best way to stay healthy. It is very important to always exercise in intervals, spending time at both your FBR and your ATR. Although it is easier than spending your entire exercise time at your ATR, interval training is much more effective than any other form of exercise. It is also healthier, not to mention more fun.

Circuit Training

Circuit training involves the use of multi-set, high-repetition, non-stop weight resistance training. It's easy to do once you learn, and it has the advantage of strength training while at the same time offering an aerobic workout.

The first thing to do is to get a personal trainer to instruct and follow you for the first few months. Have the trainer set up a circuit of resistance exercises for you that work all the major muscle groups in your body. Make sure to show your trainer the instructions given below. The weight-lifting movement should be slow, so as to avoid injury. In circuit training, the weight resistance of the weight is set such that you can just barely lift the weight fifteen times.

The procedure goes like this: After you put on your heart rate monitor, perform the first fifteen repetitions. Check your heart rate. If it is below your ATR, immediately go on to the next set and check your heart rate again. Keep on doing this until your heart rate is at or above your ATR. Once this happens, sit down and rest. You can read a magazine while you are waiting. I like to answer my email then.

As soon as your heart rate has come down to your FBR, start in with the next set of exercises. Keep on exercising with this pattern, going on to the next set when your heart rate has not reached your ATR, and resting when it has. Do this for thirty minutes, and your exercise is over. Do this two or three times a week.

My 1–2 Rule

How many times have you arrived at your regularly scheduled exercise time, only to find that you just don't feel up to it? I don't know about you, but this happens to me almost all the time. My inner voice is rebelling: "I'm too tired," or "I just don't feel like it right now."

A long time ago, I decided I had to develop a way of dealing with this in order to pursue any semblance of a regular exercise schedule. So, I came up with what I call my 1–2 rule. It works for me. See if it works as well for you.

When it's time for your regularly scheduled exercise period, no matter how you feel, start your exercise. No excuses allowed—just start it. Put on your exercise outfit, get on the machine, and start the two minutes at your ATR.

If, after the first interval cycle, you actually feel worse than you did when you started, you get to call it quits for the day. If not, then finish the second cycle.

I can honestly tell you that when you use this yardstick, you'll end up quitting only a very small percent of the time. It just reaffirms in my mind the incredible value of exercise on both the physical and mental levels.

MY RECOMMENDATIONS TO YOU

* Find out what your FBR and ATR are, using Bio-Energy Testing. You can find practitioners offering this at www.bioenergytesting.com.
* Unless you plan on serious competition, there is no benefit in exercising harder than described above.
* If your exercise equipment doesn't have a good heart rate monitor, you can purchase one online or from a sporting goods store. You can buy a good device for about $50. Use it every time you exercise.
* Find a personal trainer to work with for the first three to six months. This is very important for your success. Go on and spend the money. It's not that much, and you are definitely worth it. As a bonus, give him/her a copy of this book so that your trainer will be on the same wavelength as you.
* Do you want to get started right away? Fantastic! Until you find out your exercise zone via Bio-Energy Testing, a good estimate of your ATR is that it's going to be the heart rate at which you start becoming breathless. Once you are on the exercise equipment, for example, start gradually increasing your speed. Very soon, you will start needing to increase your breathing rate. At this point, look at your heart rate monitor. The reading is close to your ATR. Multiply this estimated ATR by .80 to guesstimate your FBR.
* If you need to lose weight, exercise for at least thirty minutes every day in addition to cutting back on the calories. Alternate between interval training and circuit training.
* Also be sure to check your Bio-Energy Testing values at least once a year. The chances are, as you get in better shape, both your FBR and your ATR are going to change.
* My advice is to get your own exercise equipment and schedule your exercise time right after you wake up. I find that if I don't take care of it then, the odds are that either something later on in the day will come up and get in the way or I'm going to be too tired to do it. So, on my exercise days, I wake up forty-five minutes earlier than I really need to, and get it over with. It's a great way to start the day.

✳ 14 ✳

SECRET SEVEN—BREATHING RIGHT

Breathing is elemental—like eating. You do it, or else. Obviously, since breathing is how we get oxygen, poor or incomplete breathing will dramatically affect energy production in a way that nothing else can.

Contemporary science has provided the details of the exchange of oxygen for carbon dioxide that occurs in the breathing process, but ancient thinkers put attention on this issue long before anyone had such a detailed understanding. The ancients quite naturally reasoned that, since *not* breathing was synonymous with death, breathing itself must be pretty important. They furthermore concluded that there must be both proper and improper ways to breathe.

It turns out that this is very true. There is a right way and a wrong way to breathe. And all too frequently, it is done the *wrong* way. After years of seeing people diagnosed with problems such as chronic anxiety and panic disorder, I am firmly convinced that many of them result from improper breathing. It is, in fact, a major—and widely ignored—cause of anxiety, low energy, panic attacks, premature aging, and overall stress.

The Right and the Wrong Way to Breathe

There are basically two different ways to breathe.

Chest-Wall Breathing

Chest-wall breathing uses the chest, neck, and shoulder muscles to lift up the chest in order to inflate the lungs. As you inhale, the chest expands. The abdomen is sucked in.

This is the classic *chest out, abdomen in* form of breathing taught in the military and reinforced all throughout youth. To determine if you are a chest breather, just sit and rest quietly in a chair, breathing easily, and observe how your chest and abdomen move when you inhale. If your

Manny's Problem and the Solution

Shortly after I began routinely using Bio-Energy Testing in my clinic to examine the energy status of my patients, it became very clear that many of them were shortchanging themselves, from an energy standpoint, because of the way they breathed.

A primary example was Manny, a forty-three-year-old man who made his living installing drywall. In order to be successful in a very competitive field, he worked hard for long hours. He first consulted me about low energy and episodes of panic attacks. His previous doctor had told him that his tests were normal, and that the drop in his energy level was caused by his anxiety.

When the panic attacks occurred, Manny felt as though he could not catch a complete breath. His heart would beat rapidly, and he would become fearful of passing out. These episodes occurred suddenly and without warning. Although he had stopped drinking his daily pot of coffee, the problem persisted.

He was soon prescribed an anti-depressant medication. When that didn't work, he was told to work at a less stressful occupation. Since that wasn't going to fly, he came to our clinic looking for another answer.

His Bio-Energy Testing revealed a fairly significant decrease in energy production. The test also showed that it was an insufficient delivery of oxygen at the capillary level that was causing this. During testing, we noticed that his respiration rate at rest was between fifteen and eighteen breaths per minute. That is way too high. A normal resting breathing rate is less than twelve.

Most importantly, Manny breathed by expanding his chest, even when lying down. This is fairly unusual because most people automatically breathe with the abdomen while they are lying down. Breathing with the abdomen is known as diaphragmatic or abdominal breathing. I'll stick with the term abdominal breathing. When we asked him about it, Manny said he didn't feel short of breath. He said his breathing seemed normal for him.

Immediately following the test, my technician spent a half hour with Manny, teaching him some proper breathing techniques. When his Bio-Energy Testing was re-examined afterward, his respiration rate had come down to under twelve breaths per minute. Along with this, his energy production had increased 20 percent—almost to an optimum level.

This turnaround had occurred in less than an hour, simply because Manny had started breathing properly. The most significant development, however, came later in the form of decreased feelings of anxiety. After three weeks of continuing his breathing exercises for fifteen minutes twice a day, Manny's anxiety symptoms completely disappeared. And he had his energy back. It's amazing what can happen when causes are treated instead of just symptoms.

Such dramatic results, and in such a short period of time, show just how powerful an influence breathing habits can be. Manny's problem was not all that unusual, either. Like a great many people, especially those with chronic anxiety, he was a chronic chest-wall breather. This method of breathing aggravates, and most times causes, chronic anxiety.

abdomen does not go out every time you inhale, and/or if your chest expands, you are chest-wall breathing. This is not the preferred style.

Abdominal Breathing

If your abdomen goes out when you inhale and your chest remains still, this is abdominal breathing. You are pulling out the diaphragm muscles in your abdomen to draw in air. You are doing this instead of raising up your chest to draw in air. This is the preferred style.

The Shortcomings of Chest-Wall Breathing

Chest-wall breathing fails to draw in as much oxygen to the lungs' air sacs as abdominal breathing. Here's why: the lungs have what is known in pulmonary physiology as dead space. This refers to the space taken up by the tubes (airways) through which the air passes en route to the lungs' air sacs. The air sacs are where oxygen is delivered to the bloodstream. These airways leading to the tubes are called dead space because they don't participate in the actual exchange of oxygen.

Dead space is more prevalent in the upper part of the lungs than the lower, and chest-wall breathing selectively fills the upper part of the lungs. This means that when you chest-wall breathe, a greater proportion of your breath is being wasted in the dead space. On the other hand, abdominal breathing selectively fills the lower part, where there is less dead space. This leads to greater oxygen absorption.

In order to make up for the decreased amount of oxygen acquired per breath, chest-wall breathers automatically compensate by increasing their respiratory rate. Before Manny's breathing was reorganized, his rate at rest was typical of this—fifteen to eighteen breaths per minute. By comparison, an abdominal breather usually needs only six to eight breaths per minute to acquire the same volume of oxygen.

Chest-wall breathers are obviously working harder to acquire the same amount of oxygen as abdominal breathers. But that's only part of the downside. The other part stems from the fact that every time you breathe, you exhale carbon dioxide. Thus, if you're breathing fifteen times a minute, you are exhaling two times more carbon dioxide than when you breathe seven times a minute. This condition can easily be detected by Bio-Energy Testing, because it results in an excessive excretion of carbon dioxide.

The excessive loss of carbon dioxide shifts the pH (acid balance) of the blood into a state called *alkalosis*. Alkalosis has immediate and dramatic effects on the brain. It often leads to an edgy, anxious sensation. Try it yourself. Take three or four rapid deep breaths, and you will feel the difference. When people do this all the time, the condition is known as *chronic sub-acute hyperventilation*. Chronic sub-acute hyperventilation often leads to panic attacks and chronic low-level anxiety. Because of its effects on the blood pH, it also results in a decreased oxygen delivery to every cell in your body. Let me explain how.

When you breathe in oxygen, it gets taken up by the hemoglobin molecule contained in your red blood cells. Hemoglobin has an incredibly strong attraction for oxygen. It holds tightly to the oxygen as it passes through the arterial network and down to the level of the cells, where the oxygen is finally delivered to the cells.

The hemoglobin molecule is triggered to release its oxygen cargo in response to the acid pH it encounters at the cellular level. However, when the normal acid pH becomes disrupted due to the alkalosis caused by chest-wall breathing, the hemoglobin molecule is effectively prevented from releasing its oxygen payload. The result is a decrease in available oxygen to the cells, and a decrease in energy production.

If you have ever gone through a very stressful period (and who hasn't?), you may have noticed that afterward you feel drained and fatigued. One reason for this is that stress almost always puts people into a chest-wall breathing mode, which, as noted, contributes to low energy through the alkalosis effect.

Since your body is designed to operate more efficiently through abdominal breathing, you might wonder why do we even have chest-wall breathing. The answer lies in the unconscious, primitive part of the brain that regulates breathing. Under emergency situations, in times of danger, the body requires additional oxygen. In the distant past, you would have needed a major injection of oxygen to flee from a lion that had you in mind as its next meal. To meet such threatening challenges, the body kicks into a double-breathing mode—chest-wall combined with abdominal breathing. This sucks in a quick oxygen increase. In intense situations like these, where exertion is at an ultra-peak level, alkalosis does not occur, and oxygen uptake and delivery are maximized. This is the only time the body will benefit from chest-wall breathing.

Although survival and escape from life-threatening predicaments may not be part of daily existence for most, the everyday variety of mental stress so common to modern life is often enough to switch on the chest-breathing response. The unconscious part of the brain reads the stress reaction as a sign of an impending emergency and triggers a subtle but slightly increased breathing rate.

You may just be sitting in your car knowing you are running late for an appointment when, whammo, quite suddenly your body goes into that emergency mode. You may then experience a panicky feeling, which is all the more stressful because there is no apparent reason why you should have such a reaction. It's at times like these that it becomes all that much more important to make sure that you are breathing from your abdomen.

The Nitty-Gritty on Sighing

Before closing the case on chest-wall breathing, I'd like to make a few comments about sighing. Although you may associate sighing with the sight of a heartthrob or another romantic imagery, the body has other primary reasons in mind.

A sigh is a distinct physiological event characterized by a deep full breath, using both abdominal and chest-wall breathing. Sighs occur naturally about every ten to fifteen minutes, allowing the lungs to completely fill up. It works like this:

When you are *not* exerting yourself, you use very little of your lung capacity. At these times, the body creates the sigh response—a quick, deep breath—to help expand and engage areas of the lungs not being used. If it were not for an occasional sigh, the lungs would eventually start collapsing. The medical word for this is *atelectasis*. Sighing prevents atelectasis.

You've probably had many occasions to notice the wonderfully relaxing effect of a sigh. It often seems to automatically occur when you are stressed. The problem with chronic chest-wall breathing is that, due to its associated hyperventilation and alkalosis, it acts to prevent the sighing mechanism. When this happens, it can be very disturbing.

Sometimes a person who desires the calming benefit of a sigh, but can't do it secondary to chronic chest-wall breathing, will call me quite concerned and say, "I can't get a deep-enough breath, and I think something must be wrong with my lungs." Of course, the mere thought that something is wrong with their lungs is enough to agitate most people and perhaps trigger an anxiety attack. At times like these, I just tell them to relax, and explain some basic facts on sighing to reassure them that their lungs are really okay.

The first fact is that you can only sigh a maximum of once every ten minutes. Second, you can't force a sigh. You just have to be patient and wait for it to happen. Third, not being able to initiate a sigh at will does not indicate that there is any problem with your lungs.

Don't be nervous if you can't sigh on demand. Just be patient and wait. It will come soon enough, but only to the degree that you are breathing with your abdomen.

Breaking the Vicious Cycle

By now, it's obvious that chronic chest-wall breathing generates a vicious cycle with a number of negative results:

* Increased respiration
* Alkalosis
* An emergency mode in the body
* Feelings of tension
* Interference with the sighing mechanism

These all promote even more chest-wall breathing. And as this progresses, you can readily see how an anxiety attack can develop.

When anxiety becomes chronic, most people will run to the doctor and get a prescription for a sedative. The medication slows down the respiratory rate and seems to correct the problem. However, the sedative only takes care of the symptoms, and does not correct the root problem. Even more damaging, it often creates new problems in terms of side effects and dependency.

A healthier way is to teach yourself to breathe with your diaphragm. The information below tells you how to do this.

How to Breathe the Right Way

Diaphragmatic breathing is one of the very first techniques that singers and musicians are taught in order to provide them with enough air for those long notes. I learned the method years ago in a yoga class, and it gave me a significant advantage later when I was involved in competitive cycling.

The technique is quite simple, but you may need guidance because it is somewhat subtle. Once you've got the idea, it just takes a little practice over a few months to fully perfect it and make it automatic.

When I started learning the technique, I made up little signs saying "Breathe!" I put them everywhere—on my bike, my dashboard, my mirror, my watch. The signs were reminders to check how I was breathing. And when I checked, I was usually breathing with my chest. At that point, I would just take a few good abdominal breaths and try to concentrate on breathing this new way as much as possible. The other thing I did, which helped enormously, was to spend a few minutes every morning and evening performing breath meditation, which I will describe in the next section.

Here are a few simple points to help you learn the diaphragmatic technique. Many people can grasp the basic movement within a few minutes.

* Lie down on your back. It's hard to chest-wall breathe while lying down. Even the most die-hard chest breathers tend to breathe with the diaphragm in this position. Make sure that you are breathing through your nose and not your mouth.

* Now place your hand on your abdomen. Notice how it rises slightly when you inhale and goes down when you exhale. This movement is the hallmark of breathing with your diaphragm. If you breathe with your chest, your hand will not elevate during the inhale, it will drop

down instead. If you are naturally breathing with your diaphragm while lying down, you are well on your way. If it isn't coming naturally, don't worry. Just give it a bit more time. You'll get it soon enough.

* After a few moments of noticing how your abdomen is moving during diaphragmatic breathing, you will start to get the idea. At that point, while you are still lying down, I would like you to exaggerate the breathing pattern by contracting your abdominal muscles inward (sucking in your gut) as you exhale the air from your lungs.
* Then expand the same muscles outward as you inhale.
* Keep practicing this technique until you can breathe fully without moving your chest. When you are doing this really well, you can literally put a belt around your chest to prevent any movement, and you will still be able to breathe comfortably.
* If the movement doesn't come easily, ask your spouse, or a friend or yoga instructor, to help you.
* Once you have learned to do this lying down, try the same thing while sitting in a chair, and then while standing. Finally, to perfect your newly discovered talent, try doing it while you are singing in the shower or lightly exercising. You can then proudly announce to friends and family that you have finally learned to breathe correctly.

There are additional benefits to abdominal breathing that should inspire you. One is that it often helps the neck pain and tension commonly caused by chronically raising up the chest during chest-wall breathing. Abdominal breathing does not create any neck and shoulder strain, since it moves with gravity instead of against it. It also strengthens and tightens the abdominal muscles. And finally, it often benefits those with asthma or other lung conditions.

Breath Meditation

Perhaps nothing is as powerful as the mind to either make you sick or keep you healthy. But how does one learn to harness and direct that power? One tried-and-true method is breath meditation.

This meditative exercise is particularly effective for hypertension, insomnia, and other stress-related disorders. It will also generate more energy and stamina. In addition, it's a very effective way to train your mind to work better for you. That means increased clarity, memory, and speed. Another bonus is that breath meditation is completely devoid of side effects. And there are no gyms to join or pills to take. The little time it takes to do it can lead to many wonderful rewards.

First, it's a good idea to get the concept straight. Meditation, at least the way I'm using the word here, refers to mental exercise. Meditation and prayer are not the same thing. Praying is a different concept. So even if you regularly pray, please be sure to practice some form of meditation as well.

Breath meditation trains the conscious mind to focus better and the unconscious mind to relax better. It works the same way that training your muscles makes them function better.

Most of the time, your meditation session will be relaxing. But there can also be days in which emotions or stresses may preoccupy your mind, and you may find yourself expending more effort to meditate. You don't need to worry about that. It's normal. Just take it as it comes and apply the simple guidelines I'll be giving you. What's important to understand here is that no matter how relaxing a meditation session may or may not be, it doesn't matter: the time spent will still serve to improve your overall relaxation potential and strengthen your powers of concentration.

Your mind is like a puppy. It wants to wander around and experience everything it can. This is a wonderful thing, but it can also limit the mind's ability to focus. And mental power is directly related to focus. Breath meditation trains your mind to better focus. In so doing, it strengthens your mental power, which increases the ease at which you do everything.

The process takes fifteen to twenty minutes. And if you can do it regularly, once or twice a day, it may be the most productive fifteen or twenty minutes of doing nothing that you can possibly imagine. Just follow these easy steps, and you'll be on your way.

Step 1—The Setting

You ideally need some quiet space, a room where you can meditate without interruptions. Leave your cell phone in another room with the ringer off.

- You need a comfortable chair, one with arm rests if possible.
- Sit comfortably in it. Don't cross your legs.

* Take three deep, relaxing breaths through your nose, and when you exhale the third time, let your eyes close.

Step 2—Breathing in Squares

* Use the abdominal breathing technique you just learned. I want you to breathe in squares. By that, I mean pausing to hold your breath at the end of both your inhale and your exhale. The pauses should be the same length of time you use to breathe. For example, if you inhale (expanding your abdomen in the process) over a two-second period, hold your breath for a two-second pause before you begin to exhale. Then exhale (sucking in your abdomen) over a two-second interval. At the end of your exhale, pause for two seconds before you begin your next breath. If you inhale over a three-second count, then just make sure the other intervals are three seconds long.
* Keep repeating this process for each and every breath. It's as simple as that.

You can count the seconds to yourself as you go along, but after a while you will probably find that you are able to naturally keep the intervals the same without counting. Just remember to breathe only with your abdomen. Keep your chest free of movement. While you go through this routine, there are several things you should be aware of.

Sighs and yawns. As mentioned above, most people experience the need to sigh about every ten minutes. During meditation, when you feel the urge to sigh, just go with it. Remember that sighing invokes both chest wall and diaphragmatic breathing. After the sigh, simply return to the abdominal breathing in squares. Sometimes you may feel the urge to sigh, but it just doesn't develop. This just means your body doesn't need one yet. Sighs are relaxing, but don't force them. Be patient. One will come along soon enough.

Don't be bothered by yawning. I can remember many times when I have yawned more than twenty times in a meditation session. Just go with it; and as soon as the yawn passes, simply return to abdominal breathing in squares.

Altering your breathing rate. One thing sure to happen during breath meditation is that you will need to alter your breathing rate to accommodate

Nasal Breathing vs. Mouth Breathing

Did you know that there is a world of difference between the effects of breathing through your nose versus your mouth? In a way, it makes sense. Why would we have been designed with a nose if we weren't supposed to be breathing through it? That's where we smell. The hairs in the nose along with the special epithelial mucosa clean the particles out of the air and alert the immune system as to what is in the air. Mouth breathing does none of that.

Nasal breathing during sleep is especially important because it acts to 1) stimulate adequate ventilation, 2) activate reflexes that help maintain the action of the muscles that stabilize the upper airway, and 3) avoid the airway instability that results from mouth breathing. In addition, nasal breathing stimulates the parasympathetic (rest and digest) part of the autonomic nervous system. Mouth breathing instead stimulates the sympathetic (fight or flight) part of the nervous system—therefore, it can result in hyperactivity, fragmented sleep, rapid heart rate, and the like.

The problem with mouth breathing is that it does none of the good things that nasal breathing does. Instead, mouth breathing limits the flow of air during breathing. It's because when the mouth is open, the soft palate and the tongue fall. This acts to decrease the airway opening. In addition, an open mouth causes the mandible (jaw bone) to open up, which also exerts pressure on the airway opening, further compromising it. It all adds up to lower oxygen levels. This is especially true during sleep. Mouth breathing during sleep is associated with sleep apnea, snoring, and light sleep with frequent arousals and all of the complications that come with those problems. During the day, mouth breathing can result in decreased energy levels and behavioral and cognitive problems.

So, examine yourself. If you find that you are breathing through your mouth more than occasionally, you need to shut that mouth down! Start training yourself to breathe through your nose even when exercising.

If you suspect that you are a mouth breather, and you can't train yourself to breathe through your nose, you may have an airway problem. In that case, I recommend you read an excellent book by James Nestor titled *Breath*. You will be amazed at how chronic mouth breathing can lead to mitochondrial dysfunction, high blood pressure, diabetes, and other health problems.

how you feel. If you feel breathless while you are pausing at the end of exhalation, you will need to increase the rate. When you notice this, simply up your breathing rate by decreasing the pause length until you are comfortable and no longer feel in need of air.

As the session progresses and your body becomes more relaxed, you will usually need to decrease your breathing rate. If you start to feel a little dizzy, like you are hyperventilating or breathing too fast, just decrease your breathing rate accordingly by increasing the pause length. You may have to adjust your breathing rate a few times during a session in order to keep feeling comfortable.

Step 3—Training the Puppy

A crucial part of breath meditation is your mental focus. While you are just sitting there comfortably using your abdominal muscles to breathe in squares, it is important to keep your mind entirely focused on your breathing. You can focus on your breathing rate, how the air feels in your lungs, or how your abdomen feels as it moves in and out. It doesn't make any difference exactly what you focus on, as long as it has something to do with your breathing.

But the mind, as I mentioned above, is like a very inquisitive and active puppy. It may not always reconcile itself with the drill called meditation. Imagine having a puppy on a leash and training it to sit comfortably by your side. As soon as you place the puppy on the floor next to you, it will immediately begin to wander in one direction or another. Without becoming upset—after all, you are only training it—just gently retrieve the puppy and put it next to you again.

Your mind is going to stray the same way. No matter how hard you try to keep your attention on your breathing, your mind will wander off into this or that thought. And, as with the puppy, the minute you become aware that your mind is wandering, gently retrieve it and refocus on your breathing.

This repetitive cycle of concentrating, straying, and refocusing again is the nature of breath meditation. The more you practice this retrieving and refocusing, the stronger your power of concentration and sense of relaxation will become. After only six weeks of regular practice, you will begin to notice that your mind is wandering less, and you are retrieving your awareness more easily. Although your mind can be an extremely stubborn puppy, it will eventually learn.

Breath meditation contributes to a longer, healthier, more enjoyable, and more productive life. People who continue meditating in this fashion see an improvement in almost every health function measured. Don't underestimate the power of this simple way to enhance your mental speed and concentration; improve your mood, sleep, and emotional state; and increase your energy levels.

MY RECOMMENDATIONS TO YOU

* During the day, and especially when you exercise, check your breathing regularly to see if you are breathing correctly. Be patient, and keep working at it. It took me about two years before I was consistently breathing correctly without thinking about it.
* Make it part of your daily routine to practice breath meditation fifteen minutes once or twice a day as your schedule allows. The best time for most people is before and after work. At first, it may seem a little intimidating, but after a few months you will actually prefer it over any previous thing you might have done to unwind and relax.

✳ 15 ✳

SECRET EIGHT—BIO-IDENTICAL HORMONAL REPLACEMENT

It would be impossible to discuss the topic of optimal energy production without discussing bio-identical hormonal replacement. This is because mitochondrial function is intimately tied to hormonal stimulation. In the absence of adequate hormonal encouragement, our mitochondria will just sit around and do the minimum.

Undoubtedly the single most important contribution to the new explosion of anti-aging medicine has been the availability of natural *bio-identical* hormones, and the growing research regarding their effects. *The efficacy of all the secrets I discuss in this book is greatly limited in the absence of proper hormonal replacement.*

Ever wonder how it is that young people can get away with everything? They can eat terrible diets, experience huge amounts of stress, fail to get enough rest, smoke, and otherwise carry on, and still do better than older folks on a health program. Well, wonder no more—it's all about hormones. Youth is a time of boundless levels of hormones. And as people navigate through the years, their hormone tanks become drained.

Refilling the tank has become an exciting new frontier in medicine, which I am thrilled to be part of. And refilling the tank—replacing drained hormones—often produces such startling reversals in energy production and overall health that people can't believe all the good things that are happening to them.

Here are some of the improvements to be had as a result of this approach.

* Better mood and sleep
* Built-in resistance to illness and infections

* Enhanced healing
* Enhanced sexual performance
* Fat loss without dieting
* Increased muscle mass without exercising
* Fortified brain, heart, kidneys, liver, spleen, and other organs that atrophy with aging
* Improved cardiac function
* Increased exercise capacity
* Increased mental function
* Lower blood pressure
* Lower LDL cholesterol, the bad cholesterol that contributes to harmful plaque when it becomes oxidized
* Reduced wrinkles, and tighter and thicker skin
* Strengthened bones
* Youthful energy production

Thirty-one years ago, Daniel Rudman, MD, of the Medical College of Wisconsin, published a landmark study in the *New England Journal of Medicine*. Dr. Rudman gave human growth hormone to nine men between the ages of sixty-one and eighty-one for only six months. In that short period of time, he was able to show that their physiological age could be reversed approximately 10 percent. They put on muscle and bone, their skin became thicker, and their bone densities improved. All this without any change in anything else. No change in diet, exercise, alcohol consumption, or even smoking. These changes were entirely from the growth hormone.

A decreased muscle-to-fat ratio, thinning skin, and decreased bone density are all hallmarks of aging. So what Rudman concluded is that he *reversed the functional age of his patients ten to twenty years simply by restoring their growth hormone levels to youthful levels*. As hard as it is for many to believe that result, Rudman's conclusion was based on results he obtained from sound scientific principles that were verified by a placebo-controlled medical study.

Growth hormone is, of course, only one of the hormones that become deficient as people age. How much better his results would have been had he simultaneously replaced the other deficient hormones, and placed his patients on an optimum diet, supplement, and lifestyle program.

Hormonal Replacement is the Key

Hormones are molecular messengers that operate between the brain and the cells. They control just about every aspect of human functioning. This includes energy production, body composition, digestion, healing, immune function, memory and mood, sexual function, skin thickness, strength, and tissue regeneration—everything.

> ***The major difference between you at age 70 and you at age 25 is hormones.***

After the reproductive age, say around thirty-five (but in some cases even earlier), the body's production of hormones starts a steady decline. It's a dirty trick that nature plays on us. It's as if to say, "Well, you have reproduced to ensure the perpetuation of the species, so you're not really needed anymore. You can go now."

The question is not *if* you are going to become hormone deficient, it's *when,* and *how significant* the deficiencies will be. The rate at which these deficiencies develop determines your risk for chronic disease and how fast you will age. The major determining factors are genetics and lifestyle. More than any other single factor, the hormonal deficiencies that routinely occur as you get older are one of the major causes of a low E.Q.

Both Men and Women

Hormonal deficiencies affect both men and women. Specifically, there are twelve different hormones in women, and eight in men, that become deficient over time. The symptoms they create include anxiety, bladder disorders, decreased bone mass, decreased muscle mass, decreased sexual drive and function, decreased stamina, declining immune-system function, depression, fatigue, hair loss, increased fat mass, insomnia, reduced equilibrium, reduced mental function, weakness, wrinkles, and, above all, decreased energy production.

Hormone deficiencies can occur even in younger people—especially thyroid hormone deficiencies. Occasionally, I even see them in children. But they don't usually show up until people are in their forties or fifties.

Besides making us age faster, hormone deficiencies also play a major role in the development of most age-related diseases, including Alzheimer's, dementia, arthritis, cancer, depression, diabetes, heart disease, osteoporosis, and strokes.

Now, that's the bad news. The good news is that there are safe, easy, and inexpensive ways to replace the sagging levels with bio-identical hormones.

By the term "bio-identical," I mean hormones that are exact molecular replicas of the hormones they are replacing. With this bio-identical ability, hormone replacement joined the twenty-first century.

While there are definite and significant problems with the synthetic hormonal drugs that are still widely used, several long- and short-term studies with both men and women demonstrate the safety of bio-identical hormone replacement. Not surprisingly, people maintaining youthful hormone levels by using bio-identical hormone replacement live longer and have a much greater quality of life than those not supplemented. The problems that have been seen and widely publicized with the synthetic hormone drugs have just not been seen with bio-identical hormone replacement. Thanks to this new generation of bio-identical hormones, hormone deficiencies can now be safely diagnosed and treated as they develop.

It's Never Too Late

Jane had many health problems when she first came to me as a new patient. Although she was only seventy-four years old, she had severe chronic lung disease from years of smoking and could barely walk across the room without help. Her heart was starting to fail, and her bones had become quite osteoporotic. Besides her chronic shortness of breath, her main complaint was profound weakness. She took several medications to help her breathe better and was dependent on a supply of oxygen at all times.

Jane had been treated the same as most older people by her medical doctor. According to Jane, he had told her to learn to live with her problems, because "at your age, you should be content just to be alive." Sad to say, too many physicians and their patients subscribe to the concept that being weak and feeble are just inevitable features of growing older.

When I first saw Jane, I had to tell her that despite her serious lung disease, it was still possible to improve her energy production, and hence her overall health, by giving her body back the hormones it had been missing for thirty or more years.

I started Jane on a comprehensive bio-identical hormonal replacement program that included DHEA, estrogens, growth hormone, melatonin, progesterone, testosterone, and thyroid. I also placed her on a high-protein diet with a broad-range program of nutritional supplements. Three short months later, she showed considerable improvement in energy, pain, strength, and sleep. She still needed to take her oxygen bottle wherever she went, but she was finally able to easily ascend the same flight of stairs at home that had previously been extremely difficult for her.

Three years down the road, Jane had made significant across-the-board improvement. Her lung condition had not degenerated. Her bone density was better, as was her heart function. Had it not been for hormone replacement, it is quite possible she would have been either dead or institutionalized. Such improvements, even in someone with the poor health that Jane had, are not unusual. One of the characteristics of natural hormone replacement is that the natural deterioration associated with aging seems to go into reverse gear.

Bless her heart, Jane died peacefully at home seven years later. Her body could no longer subsist on the meager amount of oxygen that her lungs could deliver. While hormonal replacement could never have helped Jane's serious lung disease, it did give her an extra seven years. Seven quality years. During that time, she was fully functional right up until twenty days before she left us.

How Are Hormone Deficiencies Determined?

Hormone deficiencies are determined in three different ways. First, a detailed history and physical examination can often diagnose a specific deficiency. After this diagnosis, laboratory testing can confirm the condition. And finally, a therapeutic trial can be initiated to see if specific symptoms resolve with proper replacement.

One thing is for sure: diagnosis of a hormone deficiency should *never* be done solely based on any lab test. There are two reasons for this.

One, hormones work through what is called receptor molecules on the surface of the cells. In order for a hormone to have its effect on a cell, it has to interact with a receptor molecule on that cell that is specific to that particular hormone. Let's look at the example of testosterone to see what this means.

In the case of someone who has enough active testosterone receptors, it is not necessary to have as much of the hormone. The fact that there are plenty of receptors and that they are active means that the person can easily get by with less testosterone. However, in a person who only has a few receptors for testosterone and/or receptors that are not very active, the same amount of testosterone will not be enough. That person will need much more testosterone to make up for the fact that she/he has less receptors. And here's the thing: we can't measure receptors. Therefore, people who have poor receptor activity and who are functionally hormone-deficient can still have levels that are in the so-called normal range. And guess what? Hormone receptors lose activity the older we get. If simply looking at hormone levels is all that is considered in such a person, they will be underdiagnosed.

Two, there is an enormous amount of variation between how much hormone one person needs and how much another needs. Let's look at testosterone again.

The laboratories report a "normal" blood level of testosterone for men between 250 and 1000 ng/dl. The average is about 650 ng/dl. So, say I am treating a sixty-year-old man who has many of the symptoms of testosterone deficiency but whose testosterone levels are 300 ng/dl. It's easy to imagine that even though his 300 ng/dl is in the normal range, the optimal level might be much higher. So, in that case, what can a doctor do?

Well, I can either say too bad, you have symptoms pointing to a deficiency of testosterone; but unfortunately for you, your lab tests fall in the statistically normal range. Or I can say, even though your levels are in the statistical range, since you are not a statistic, and since there is sufficient reason to believe that you need testosterone replacement, let's give you a trial of testosterone to see what happens. This second choice is called a clinical trial.

Doctors do clinical trials all the time. For example, if a patient has high blood pressure, the doctor gives him a blood-pressure pill as a clinical trial. If the pill works, then the clinical trial indicates that he guessed right. If it doesn't, then he can try another pill. In the same way, doctors can give their patients with symptoms of a hormone deficiency a clinical trial of the hormone to see if the symptoms go away. If they do, then the diagnosis was right. If they don't go away, the diagnosis was wrong. It's as simple as that.

But you might object and say, "But if I don't really need the hormone, won't it hurt me to take it?" The answer is yes, but only if you take it for a long period of time. A short-term use of it to determine if your symptoms go away is not a problem even if you don't need it.

In short, the best way to diagnose any hormone deficiency is as follows:

* Take a good history of the symptoms that commonly occur from a deficiency of that particular hormone.
* Perform a physical examination to see if there are any signs of a deficiency.
* Get a baseline laboratory level of the hormone.
* If the symptoms and/or signs or lab tests indicate a possible deficiency of the hormone, even though the lab tests may be in range, give the patient a one- to two-month trial of the hormone.
* If the patient's symptoms go away from the trial, then the diagnosis is confirmed, even though the levels were in the normal statistical range.
* Continue to monitor the patient to make sure the dose is right. The correct dose of any hormone is the lowest dose that works.

What's So Different about Bio-identical Hormone Replacement?

Synthetic hormonal therapy, the conventional way hormones have been replaced, has some serious drawbacks.

Drawback 1

Synthetic hormones are not really hormones at all; they are drugs with hormone-like effects. These commonly prescribed substances are not found in the human body. They are molecularly different from the hormones they are replacing.

Since they are foreign to the body, synthetic hormones not only cannot function properly, they are also treated as toxins by the liver. According to several studies on the use of these synthetic hormones, side effects prompt up to 30 percent of all the people placed on these modern wonders to stop using them within twelve months.

All this begs the question, "If I am deficient in a particular hormone, why isn't the deficiency treated with that exact hormone?" Unfortunately, the reason has nothing to do with good medicine, or even common sense. The answer lies in the economic fact that molecules, such as hormones, that occur naturally in the body are not patentable. This means that they are therefore not profitable for the drug companies to sell.

The good news, however, is that bio-identical hormone therapy—using hormones that are molecularly identical to the hormones they are replacing—is now readily available and is being used by many doctors all over the world.

Drawback 2

The conventional approach completely ignores the fact that hormones work together as a team. Although each individual hormone has its own specific actions, it also requires other hormones to be present in order to function properly. *Since any given hormone can enhance the action of one hormone while suppressing another, too much or too little of one hormone can create an imbalance in other hormones.*

The system of hormonal checks and balances is the way the body regulates itself. If a person is deficient in two hormones, she or he should replace both hormones. If deficient in seven hormones, for optimum results, all seven should be replaced. Conventional replacement strategy ignores these important interrelationships.

Drawback 3

The conventional approach tends to embrace a one-size-fits-all mentality. Individual hormone deficiencies vary greatly. Therefore, the correct dose for one person with a particular hormone deficiency may be very different from the correct dose for another person. *In the conventional approach, it is quite common for people to take either too much or too little of a hormone drug.* That's because the Big Pharma drugs do not come in adjustable sizes. It's like a shoe store that only has three or four sizes.

My Three Golden Rules

To avoid these problems, I follow three golden rules in regard to hormone replacement, and they have worked well for me over the years.

Golden Rule 1

I use only bio-identical hormones. The exact same hormones that occur naturally in the human body. It has never made any sense to me to replace the human hormone estradiol with the pharmaceutical Premarin, the most commonly prescribed estrogen replacement for women.

Similarly, since natural progesterone is available, and is identical to the body's own progesterone, why substitute the drug Provera, which is a synthetic form of progesterone? Why not use the real thing? Foreign substances, such as Provera, set off immune responses in the body that frequently cause complications. These complications simply don't occur when bio-identical hormones are used.

Golden Rule 2

I replace all hormone deficiencies present. Not just the ones that give the effect I'm looking for. This helps maintain a youthful balance of hormones, and allows me to use much lower individual hormone doses and still get the same effects.

Golden Rule 3

I individualize all doses, and prescribe just enough, not too much, of each hormone. One size definitely does not fit all. Even twins may have widely divergent levels of hormones.

Customizing Dosages

Because of the need for individual dosing, standardized capsules or creams are never used in bio-identical replacement. All bio-identical hormone-replacement capsules, drops, creams, or pellets are made up individually for each person.

The process of making a customized hormonal replacement for a particular person is called compounding. These customized medications can be obtained only from one of the many compounding pharmacies located throughout the country. Compounding pharmacies specialize in making hormone prescriptions, and other preparations, directly from raw materials and according to the exact recommendations of your doctor. Because of this, they are able to customize the exact ratio of hormones that your particular body needs. At regular, non-compounding pharmacies, the only bio-identical hormones you can get are the standard one-size-fits-all dosages supplied by drug manufacturers.

Is It Safe *Not* to Replace Hormonal Deficiencies?

The most frequent question I hear from my patients regarding bio-identical hormone replacement is the obvious one: Is it safe? I have been prescribing bio-identical hormones for over forty years now, and I believe it is among the safest of all medical treatments. Every single study that has looked at the safety of bio-identical hormones has shown that the men and women who take them are not prone to the same side effects and complications that doctors see with synthetic hormones. Moreover, I tell my patients that the most significant danger regarding bio-identical hormonal replacement is *not* replacing them.

And so let's look at the other side of that question: Is it safe *not* to replace hormones when there is a deficiency? Although the scientific and clinical data on this issue can be criticized from all sides, the evidence strongly suggests that denying a person bio-identical hormonal replacement is dangerous. Just as dangerous as denying appropriate treatment to a person with high blood pressure.

For example, in every long-term human study that has looked at estrogen replacement therapy, those on estrogen replacement lived longer, had a lower incidence of disease, and had a higher quality of life than comparison groups who did not take the hormone.

According to one published study of 8,881 post-menopausal women, "Current users with more than 15 years of estrogen use had a 40-percent reduction in their overall mortality." That's a lot! The users also had reduced mortality from cancer.

The same kind of data is available for men as well. Several studies evaluating older men on testosterone replacement therapy have found no side effects or dangers of any consequence. Some doctors are still concerned about what might happen to the prostate of men on testosterone replacement therapy, but so far, no problems have been encountered.

These gratifying results occurred in spite of the fact that most of the research was done with synthetic hormones, not bio-identical hormones.

I can only wonder how much better the results would have been had the treatment been bio-identical.

There have been two recent studies that specifically looked at large groups of post-menopausal women who were either not replacing their hormones, replacing them with bio-identical hormones, or replacing them with synthetic hormones. Both of these studies have shown that the risk for breast cancer in women on bio-identical hormones is the same as the risk for women not on any hormone replacement therapy. The only increase in breast-cancer risk was seen in the groups on the synthetic hormones.

The Players

There are basically two different categories of hormones: the catabolic hormones and the anabolic hormones. Both are major players in total energy production.

Catabolic hormones directly stimulate the mitochondria to produce more energy. The process is called catabolism. The thyroid hormones, and the adrenal hormones cortisol and adrenalin, are the most potent catabolic hormones.

The anabolic hormones increase energy production in a different way. They don't directly stimulate the mitochondria to go to work. Instead, by stimulating protein synthesis, organ repair, and other cellular processes, they use up the energy that the mitochondria produce. By using up energy, they then create the need for more energy. This is critical to mitochondrial function. Mitochondria are not able to produce energy unless there is an energy demand. The anabolic hormones supply this demand.

The most important anabolic hormones are estrogen, progesterone, testosterone, growth hormone, DHEA, and melatonin. Let's take a look at how properly replacing both catabolic and anabolic hormones increases longevity and decreases disease by keeping energy production at more youthful levels.

About Estrogen

There are two forms of estrogen that are used in estrogen replacement therapy (ERT), not just one: estradiol and estriol. The most powerful form is estradiol—almost every cell membrane has receptor sites specific for estradiol.

Estradiol affects everything from the way a woman thinks to the way she looks. It exerts a profound influence on the arteries, bladder, bones, brain, fat cells, liver, soft tissues of the joints and muscles, thyroid gland, and cellular metabolism in general.

Estradiol decreases the clotting tendency of the blood, keeps the blood thin, and causes a marked improvement in the HDL/LDL cholesterol ratio; it is the reason that heart attacks and strokes occur much less frequently in women. It is also an extremely powerful antioxidant, and in this way retards the aging process in general.

Since estradiol stimulates the synthesis of choline acetyltransferase, an important brain enzyme that is lacking in Alzheimer's disease, a deficiency of estradiol is regarded as a primary cause of this disease in women. Even without the extreme condition of outright Alzheimer's disease, a deficiency in estradiol can result in mood swings, forgetfulness, and difficulty in concentration.

The wrinkles that begin to develop after menopause are primarily secondary to a deficiency in estradiol. That's because this hormone enhances the production of collagen and keeps the skin thick and hydrated.

Estradiol also prevents the facial-hair growth that is common after menopause. A deficiency of estradiol not only paves the way for osteoporosis but is also behind many of the other diseases associated with aging women. According to gynecologist Uzzi Reiss, MD, who authored the excellent book *Natural Hormone Balance for Women*, women with estradiol deficiency often experience a decreased sense of *womanness,* and report a diminished self-image, sensuality, and sexuality.

Half the Death Rate

One of the most famous studies on the benefits of estradiol replacement came out of the Oakland Kaiser Permanente Medical Care Program in 1996. The study monitored 232 women who for years had been taking estradiol. These women were compared with a control group of other women who did not take any hormones. The results showed that women taking the estradiol had only about half the overall death rate of those who didn't. Deaths from cancer were essentially the same in both groups.

Despite this study and others like it, ERT has received a rash of criticism it doesn't deserve. The criticism stems mostly from the fact that ERT, as it is conventionally administered, uses a synthetic version of estradiol. *In my practice, I routinely recommend ERT to my female patients, but never conventional ERT.* It's been proven to be too dangerous.

As I have already pointed out, conventional ERT isn't replacement therapy at all. It's drug therapy. The definition of replacement therapy implies that a molecule found deficient in the human body is replaced by the identical molecule. But conventional ERT does not follow this maxim. Conventional estradiol "replacement" uses patented drugs like Premarin, for example. Premarin is a drug. It does not contain bio-identical estrogens. It contains horse estrogens made from the urine of pregnant mares. As my friend Jonathan Wright, MD, a pioneer in the science of bio-identical hormonal replacement, has been saying for years, "Premarin is replacement therapy for horses, but it is drug therapy for humans." It's no wonder Premarin and other synthetic estrogens cause problems in humans. They don't belong in the human body.

A reasonable person might ask, "If human estrogens are available, why are physicians prescribing synthetic estrogens?" As I explained earlier, the answer has nothing to do with good medicine. The reason is not medical, it's economic. It stems from the fact that the law does not allow the drug companies to patent a *naturally occurring substance.* And without a patent on a medication, there is no way for a drug company to make a decent profit from it. The pharmaceutical industry is a multi-billion-dollar, for-profit corporate industry. There's nothing wrong with that. It's just that like any other industry, its primary interest is the bottom line.

And since the FDA demands very extensive tests and clinical investigations before any pharmaceutical treatment can be approved, it does not make good business sense to market a non-patentable substance. The sad result of this situation is that so many women are being prescribed a patentable combination containing horse estrogens or other synthetics instead of the real thing.

It's a Balancing Act

Another problem with conventional prescriptions of estrogens relates to lack of balance. Although estradiol is the most powerful estrogen in the body, the less-powerful estriol interacts with it and keeps it in check. This is the body's intelligence at work. It's a balancing act. And balance is critical to hormones because they have such major effects in the body. That is why there is more than one estrogen in the body.

To replace an estradiol deficiency with estradiol but neglect to replace an estriol deficiency doesn't make good sense. Moreover, it can be dangerous.

The pharmaceutical companies have patented a delivery system called the estradiol patch to enhance the introduction of the compound into the body. There has been much advertising hoopla about this new form of ERT because they are actually using the bio-identical form of estradiol. The problem with the estradiol patch, however, is that it's not balanced with estriol.

When I give ERT to my patients, I prescribe both estradiol and estriol in a balanced formula. They are natural and bio-identical to what a woman normally has in her body. And I always individualize the dose for each woman, based on testing and retesting her hormonal status.

Creams versus Pills

Another important consideration concerning natural ERT is how the estrogens are being administered. Estrogen taken in pill or capsule form upsets the balance of other hormones, such as the growth hormone IGF-1, testosterone, and the thyroid hormones.

Since oral estrogen goes immediately to the liver after it is absorbed, very high concentrations build up in the liver. This high level of estrogen has several effects on the way the liver regulates hormones. For example, the growth hormone IGF-1 is made in the liver. These high concentrations of estrogen cause the liver to make less IGF-1, thus creating a growth-hormone deficiency.

The next problem with oral estrogen has to do with a hormone-carrying protein called sex-hormone-binding globulin (SHBG). SHBG is a carrier protein that is formed in the liver. It binds to both estradiol and testosterone. The good news is that SHBG preserves healthy levels of estradiol and testosterone, because as long as they are bound to SHBG they will not be lost in the urine. The bad news is that when hormones are bound to SHBG, they cannot exert their hormonal effects. It's as if they weren't there, as far as the body is concerned.

So, when too much SHBG is present, the hormones are excessively bound up and can't work. And that's the problem with oral estrogen. Because so much of it is concentrated in the liver, the liver responds by making too much SHBG. The excess SHBG also binds up so much testosterone that the body experiences a lack of testosterone activity. Testosterone is an important hormone not only for sexual functioning but also for muscle maintenance. One study points this out:

The researchers looked at forty-six post-menopausal women who were taking oral estrogen and compared them to women not taking any hormones. The SHBG levels of the women on the oral estrogen were so high that their testosterone levels were excessively bound up. This caused them to have a significant reduction in their muscle mass.

Oral estrogen has a similar effect on the thyroid hormones. It causes the liver to make too much thyroid-hormone-binding globulin. This globulin binds up the thyroid; therefore, just like with testosterone, it can't exert its effects. The result is low thyroid function.

For all the above reasons, I much prefer to use topical creams, sublingual drops, patches, or pellets over estrogen capsules and pills. This way of supplying estrogen bypasses the liver and does not cause any increase at all in SHBG.

About Progesterone

Progesterone is a critical hormone in the reproductive cycle. After a woman ovulates, she produces progesterone in the ovaries to prepare the uterus for conception and the development of a fertilized egg.

But progesterone plays many other important and protective roles in a woman's body:

* It contributes to a healthier LDL/HDL cholesterol ratio.
* It enhances the activity of the thyroid hormone on energy production.
* It has a calming effect on mood.
* It helps balance the estrogen compounds.
* It helps prevent abnormal blood clotting.
* It helps stabilize blood sugar.
* It improves the sex drive.
* It is a natural diuretic, and as such decreases edema and subsequent cellulite formation.
* It supports healthy sleep.
* It is a powerful antioxidant.
* It provides hormonal security against the development of breast and uterine cancer.

* It stimulates formation of new bone tissue. Estradiol decreases bone loss. Progesterone promotes new bone growth.

The list could go on, but this is enough to show you what an extremely important hormone this is. Unfortunately, however, the progesterone level generally starts to decline when a woman reaches her mid-thirties. And by the time a woman reaches the age of forty-five, the decline accelerates so fast that it quickly becomes deficient. Because of all the remarkable benefits listed above, women in this category should consider replacing deficient progesterone levels as soon as they occur.

Estrogen Dominance

Estrogen and progesterone oppose each other. Whatever one does, the other un-does. This is very common in the body. One hormone does one thing, and another does the opposite. It is in this way that the body can regulate itself. A deficiency of progesterone is equivalent to an excess of estrogen. When either the progesterone levels decline or the estrogen levels increase, the condition is referred to as estrogen dominance.

Estrogen dominance causes a lot of havoc in a woman's body. Breast and uterine cancer, cellulite, endometriosis, fibrocystic breast disease, PMS, water retention, and weight gain are all side effects of estrogen dominance. And it can be just as big a problem with young women as it is with the older set.

The most common manifestation of estrogen dominance is PMS, with its symptoms of anxiety, breast swelling, depression, insomnia, irritability, loss of libido, pelvic pain, and water retention. This is low progesterone at work, and it can be corrected with progesterone replacement therapy. But what causes estrogen dominance in the first place?

Estrogen dominance initially stems from a combination of decreased liver function and an excessive environmental exposure to *xenoestrogens*. Xenoestrogens is a term referring to synthetic chemicals that can act like human estrogens. These compounds are used everywhere—in fungicides, herbicides, pesticides, solvents, paper, and plastics. You can't escape them.

Over the years, xenoestrogens have thoroughly infiltrated the food chain. Every time you eat, you're getting a barrage of these estrogen-like compounds. The highest exposures come from beef and chicken because they are routinely dosed up with estrogens to increase their weight and fat content. You can buy hormone-free meats, but you have to look for them in the supermarket.

Make no mistake about it, xenoestrogens are a real problem. They are believed to contribute to the rise in sterility so commonly seen in our young. And many researchers feel they are also behind the growing incidence of premature secondary sex characteristics developing in children.

Ovulation refers to the moment that the ovaries release an egg to be fertilized into a person. Ovulation occurs about ten days after the menstrual period begins. It triggers the production of progesterone. As xenoestrogens build up in the body, however, they can suppress normal ovulation, causing progesterone production to dramatically decrease. The result: estrogen dominance.

Suppressed Ovulation—More Common Than Is Realized

Traditionally, doctors have always thought that as long as a woman was menstruating, she must be ovulating. It was thought that suppressed ovulation occurred only rarely in regularly menstruating women. But recent research shows it is much more common than previously realized: it can easily occur in a menstruating woman.

Birth-control pills also suppress ovulation; and inasmuch as they contain strong synthetic estrogen compounds, they act to increase estrogen dominance. This is the reason for most of their side effects.

And, as women approach their mid-forties, suppressed ovulation becomes even more commonplace. And the estrogen dominance that ensues causes cellulite and weight gain around the hips, and increases the risk of breast and uterine cancer.

The solution to this would be for everyone to avoid the *-cides* (pesticides, fungicides, and herbicides), and eat only hormone-free beef and chicken. An additional measure should also include not storing foods in soft plastic wraps. Soft plastics are loaded with xenoestrogens, and they can easily be absorbed from the plastic into the food wrapped in the plastic. But this is not a perfect world, and the chances of avoiding all exposure to xenoestrogens is slim. So, what else can you do?

Another very accessible and powerful strategy to combat the buildup of xenoestrogens is to take the nutrients in QuickStart. This particular combination promotes detoxification and gives significant nutritional support to the liver. It is the liver that is ultimately responsible for removing the xenoestrogens you have been exposed to from your system. And it needs all the help you can give it. Along with these nutrients, regular exercise and a high-fiber diet will help the cleanup process.

But My Doctor Says

Doctors often tell their patients that a woman who has had a hysterectomy doesn't need progesterone replacement. I guess if a woman were simply a large uterus with legs, they would have a point. But the truth is, such a statement disregards the fact that almost every organ in a woman's body has progesterone receptor sites. Bones have receptors. So does the brain. So do the breasts, and the liver, the bladder, and the skin—every cell. And progesterone is just as important to these cells as it is to the uterus.

A woman needs progesterone whether or not she has a uterus. Furthermore, this fact is greatly exaggerated in the presence of estrogen dominance, because you will remember that estrogen opposes progesterone. When all those cells have decreased levels of progesterone activating their receptors, it causes a whole host of problems. Problems that so many otherwise normal healthy women often experience. Problems such as anxiety, cellulite, endometriosis, fatigue, fibrocystic breasts, gallstones, insomnia, irritability, menstrual pain, migraines, panic disorder, PMS, uterine fibroids, water retention, and weight gain. Give these women progesterone, and a wonderful thing happens. Most of the time, it all goes away like magic.

Provera Is *Not* Progesterone

One more comment about progesterone. More specifically about Provera, a drug masquerading as progesterone. Provera, even though it is not progesterone, is routinely prescribed by doctors as a progesterone replacement. Provera is a drug, not a hormone. As has been previously stressed in this book, if it were a hormone, it would not be patentable, and it would not be nearly as profitable for drug companies to manufacture. But since it is a drug, it *is* patentable, and, as such, it has been heavily promoted for years as a viable substitute for the real thing.

Make no mistake about it, though—it may be a pharmaceutical best seller, but it is a nightmare for the human body. If there is some legitimate use for this drug, I don't know what it is. Like any physician, I appreciate that some of the drugs developed by the pharmaceutical industry have saved lives. But Provera is not one of them. It should be taken off the market, because it is one of the worst drugs currently available.

If you take a look at the *Physicians' Desk Reference* (*PDR*) and check out the common side effects of this drug, you would wonder why anyone would prescribe it. The list reads like a who's who of symptoms: acne, birth defects, blood clots, fatigue, breast cancer, breast tenderness, depression, strokes, dementia, heart disease, diabetes, facial hair growth, fluid retention, head-hair loss, pulmonary embolism, rashes, and weight gain. And these are common side effects. They occur to some degree or another in just about every woman who takes the drug.

Bio-identical progesterone has none of these problems. So why would anyone want to take this drug—or any other drug in this class of progesterone substitutes called progestins—when real, natural progesterone is readily available?

The answer is, they take the drug because that's what their doctors prescribe. Hard as it is to believe, I have talked with many doctors who don't know that Provera is not progesterone. Many doctors are just unaware of the natural option. Still others mistakenly believe that bio-identical progesterone doesn't work because their drug detailers are not pushing it. And many of their patients, particularly those not up on the latest in medicine, don't know about it.

I find that a topical progesterone cream works best for the majority of my female patients. This is because progesterone is notoriously poor at being absorbed when taken orally. There are some excellent bio-identical progesterone creams available over the counter. If you decide to use one of these creams, be sure to find a physician who is familiar with their use. Also be sure to check your progesterone levels after you are on it a few weeks, just to be sure you are taking the correct dose.

Thyroid Hormones—The Master Hormones

And this conversation is not just limited to the significant benefits gained by restoring deficient levels of estrogen or progesterone for menopausal women. I am talking about the replacement of many different hormones in both women and men as they get older.

Normally, when we think of hormones, we think of the sex hormones. And we tend to think of hormonal replacement as something that the older crew needs. And this is generally true. But many young people also have undiagnosed deficiencies of hormones, particularly the thyroid hormones. And as you will soon see, the thyroid hormones are the most critical to energy production.

The thyroid gland has the primary responsibility for stimulating your trillions of cells to produce energy. All aspects of energy production are dependent on the actions of the thyroid hormones. Cells are like little factories. Their mitochondria take in oxygen, carbohydrates, fat, protein, and nutrients, and from all these raw materials they produce the energy that enables us to function.

Without adequate energy production, the cells would cease to work and you would cease to live. To keep this fundamental process running on full steam, it takes an adequate amount of the thyroid hormones T_3 and T_4. It's no wonder then that the symptoms associated with a malfunctioning thyroid read like a litany of what can go wrong in the human body.

The most common problem encountered in the aging thyroid is when it doesn't produce enough hormones, a condition called hypothyroidism. More than half of American men and women older than forty experience *three or more* symptoms related to hypothyroidism. And past the age of fifty, I find it is fairly uncommon to have an optimally functioning thyroid.

The thyroid gland, wrapped around the front of your windpipe just below the Adam's apple, produces these master hormones. They are called master hormones for a very simple reason: *All the other hormones are dependent on them for their own optimal functioning*. Even if you have optimal levels of other hormones, they will not work properly if you are deficient in your levels of T_3 and T_4.

Broda Barnes, MD—Master Clinician

Years ago, when I first began to study alternative medical treatments, I read an important book. It was on the unrecognized prevalence of hypothyroidism and the importance of thyroid replacement. The book was written in 1976 by Broda Barnes, MD. Dr. Barnes was a veteran physician who went way back to the days when medicine was practiced as a clinical art, instead of just a recitation of laboratory tests. He felt the best way to determine the presence of a thyroid deficiency was to monitor the body temperature using a basal thermometer.

Why temperature? It's because 60 percent of all the energy your cells harvest from oxygen goes to producing heat. It's what keeps us warm. So Dr. Barnes, being the brilliant clinician he was, thought that checking body temperatures would give a better look at what the thyroid was doing than the notoriously inaccurate blood tests. He was right.

Dr. Barnes's procedure was simple enough. He had his patients take their underarm temperature when they awoke in the morning. A normal underarm temperature is between 96.6 and 98 degrees. A measurement less than 96.6 degrees, particularly if it was less than 95 degrees, is a fairly good indication that the cells are not producing enough energy. But here's the problem:

After I was doing this temperature test for a few months to all my over-forty patients, I realized that probably no more than 5 percent of my patients had a normal reading. If Barnes was correct, the great majority of my patients needed thyroid replacement. This was despite the fact that almost all of them tested normal for thyroid when using standard laboratory tests.

I was confused. And to make matters even more confusing, Barnes said the correct thyroid dose was one that restored temperatures to an optimum level. In order to accomplish this, though, I would have to give many of my patients thyroid doses that were much higher than what was considered by some to be the maximum output of an adult thyroid.

But I decided to try the Barnes approach anyway. It was, after all, based on his thirty-five years of clinical experience with thousands of patients. Soon, *my* patients started telling me the same things Barnes's patients had reported to him—that they had never felt so good in all their lives. And that many of their long-standing and unresolved symptoms had simply vanished.

Barnes, the old master clinician, had apparently discovered something very profound that was completely perplexing to me. How was it possible that almost everyone I tested using the temperature test was found to have low thyroid function? And how could so many patients do so well on thyroid doses that most experts would regard as excessive? It wasn't until almost twenty years later, when I began using Bio-Energy Testing, that I was finally able to answer these questions.

Why Does Almost Everyone Need Thyroid?

No one really knows exactly why the decline in the thyroid axis function is so common. Perhaps it is simply the effect of aging. The levels of all the other hormones decrease with age: why not the thyroid hormones? There are few things more certain than a decline in the metabolic rate associated with aging. And since thyroid hormones control the metabolic rate, it seems very probable that decreased thyroid function is just what happens as we get older.

But thyroid hormone decline can also occur from fluoride supplementation, selenium and zinc deficiency, iodine deficiency, viruses, gluten intolerance, autoimmune disease, pregnancy, silver dental fillings (they contain mercury, which is highly toxic to the thyroid gland), and chiropractic, dental, and medical X-rays. These are commonplace factors that compound the problem.

The female hormone estrogen interferes with thyroid hormone function. Women always have a lower metabolic rate than men because of this effect of estrogen. That's why they tend to be more sensitive to the cold than men. Estrogen dominance decreases thyroid function even more. Paradoxically, a thyroid decline also results in lack of ovulation in women, which is a primary cause of estrogen dominance.

Why Do People Sometimes Need Excessive Thyroid Doses?

The answers lie beyond the thyroid itself—with the hypothalamus (an area in the brain), and our old friend the liver.

The hypothalamus is the hormone thermostat for the body, and it is very sensitive to the body's need for thyroid hormones. When it senses that the body's resting metabolic rate (the M-Factor on Bio-Energy Testing) is too slow, it sends a signal to the pituitary gland to release thyroid-stimulating hormone (TSH). TSH then goes to the thyroid and stimulates it to make T_4, an inactive form of the thyroid hormone. By "inactive," I mean that T_4 is not able to stimulate energy production.

T_4 then circulates through the bloodstream to the liver, where it is converted into T_3. T_3 is the active thyroid hormone. It is responsible for stimulating the cells to increase their energy production so that they can function properly.

The liver converts T_4 to T_3 on a demand basis. When there is a greater need for a stepped-up metabolism—for example, to support increased activity, such as exercise or fighting an infection—the liver responds by converting more T_4 to T_3. As more T_3 is made, it exerts what is known as a negative feedback to the hypothalamus, which turns down the production of TSH. This in turn causes the thyroid to decrease its production of T_4. This prevents too much T_3 from being produced. This elaborate and complex control mechanism is called the thyroid axis. Here is a graphic representation of it.

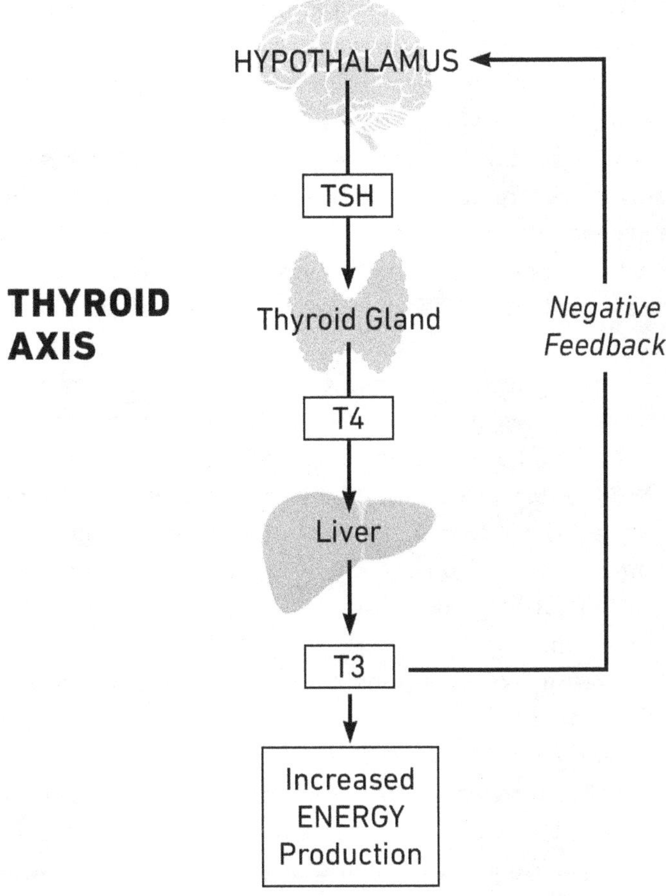

I believe the reason some of my patients thrive on high doses of thyroid is that there is a breakdown in one or more aspects of this axis.

In many cases, the problem may be a sluggish liver. In that case, a revitalization of the liver will allow lower thyroid doses to be just as effective. In other cases, the problem may lie in the hypothalamus.

Loretta's Problem Solved and Re-solved

Loretta is one of many people I have treated over the years who dramatically demonstrate the heavy, unreliable dependence many physicians have on thyroid blood testing.

Loretta was fifty-two years old and "healthy" according to her previous physician. This, despite the fact that she had been complaining of dry skin, fatigue, intolerance for cold, lack of energy, and weight gain for eight years. She also had an increasing cholesterol level.

Loretta had done her homework. She knew that her symptoms and her elevated cholesterol are often related to low thyroid. Over the years, she repeatedly asked her doctor to give her a trial dose of thyroid hormone. Her doctor, however, was wedded to the thyroid blood tests and refused to do so because her results had always been in the normal range.

Finally, she came to my clinic because she had read an article that I wrote regarding the inaccuracy of thyroid blood testing. Using Bio-Energy Testing, I checked her M-Factor. Remember that M-Factor is a percentage representation of the resting metabolic rate, the best way to analyze thyroid function. I was not at all surprised to find that she was running at about 60 percent of optimum. Since she had many of the symptoms of hypothyroidism, I started her on a trial of thyroid hormone replacement.

Loretta lived out of town. She called me in about four weeks to say, elatedly, "I feel like I've been given a second chance at life." Her symptoms were gone, and her cholesterol readings were improved.

A couple of years went by before I heard from her again. She had sprained her ankle a few months before and had seen her regular doctor for treatment. When he learned that she had been taking thyroid replacement, he became quite upset, insisting that all her tests failed to show a need for the hormone.

Loretta explained the results of her testing, but like many physicians he was unfamiliar with Bio-Energy Testing. He took some blood tests again, and they were still in the normal range, but that didn't keep him from insisting that she discontinue the thyroid. He never explained why her blood test results were within normal limits both on and off thyroid replacement. Of course, the reason is that they are just not as accurate as actually looking at the resting metabolic rate.

Because of his insistence, she stopped taking the thyroid. Predictably, within two weeks she began to notice a return of her symptoms. When she saw her doctor two months later, she was back to feeling as bad as ever. In spite of this rather obvious clinical example of thyroid hormone deficiency, her physician continued to maintain that she didn't need any replacement therapy because the "blood tests are all still normal." He appeared happier with a miserable patient who had normal tests than with a well patient who also had normal lab tests.

It may seem strange, but some physicians are more devoted to laboratory results than they are to how their patients are feeling. Needless to say, Loretta had had enough. She was smart enough to listen to her body, and so she called my clinic. I restarted her on the hormone replacement she so obviously needed, and she immediately began to regain her health.

Bio-Energy Testing to the Rescue

Many people are relegated to permanent misery simply because they have what is described in the medical literature as sub-clinical hypothyroidism.

This means people such as my patient Loretta, who have low thyroid function in the face of lab results that fall within the statistical normal range. A 1983 study published in *Postgraduate Medicine* and titled "How to Detect Hypothyroidism when Screening Tests Are Normal" covered this issue.

In the study, sixty-five women like Loretta were examined because of their many symptoms suggestive of hypothyroidism. In all cases, the blood tests were within normal range. Using a sophisticated stimulation challenge test, the researchers demonstrated that forty-seven of the women, 72 percent, did in fact have hypothyroidism despite the normal tests. It's no surprise that when they were treated with thyroid hormone, they improved.

Other studies have revealed that in any given age group, somewhere between 5 and 15 percent has subclinical hypothyroidism. One of the great advantages of Bio-Energy Testing is that since it measures resting metabolic rate, it is the most sensitive way to determine the presence of low-thyroid function—even when subclinical hypothyroidism is present.

Testosterone

Testosterone is considered the male sex hormone. But it doesn't belong exclusively to men. Women's bodies also make a small, but important, amount that greatly contributes to their health. In women, a testosterone deficiency leads to apathy, depression, a diminished or lost sex drive, fat gain, joint aches and pains, loss of exercise endurance, and osteoporosis. There is almost always a deficiency in women who have had a hysterectomy.

But back to the men. Unlike women, who have been studied for sex-hormone deficiency for decades, testosterone deficiencies in men have largely been ignored in this country. Women experience a rapid decline of sex hormones, but the loss of testosterone in men is often quite slow, taking effect very gradually over ten to fifteen years. And because it occurs so slowly, men often do not realize what has happened to them. Fortunately, that is starting to change.

Another reason why men just haven't gotten equal treatment is related to the male ego and the nothing-is-wrong mentality. I routinely see this attitude among my male patients. Sometimes, because I'm like that myself, it is almost comical. Here's a typical example of an interview in my office with a fifty-five- or sixty-year-old man.

ME: "So how's your sex life?"

HIM: "Not a problem."

ME: "Okay, how about your memory?"

Him: "Not a problem."

ME: "Great. How about your moods?"

HIM: "Seem fine."

ME: "And how's your strength and stamina?"

HIM: "No complaints there either, Doc."

ME: "Okay. Now, I want you to compare how all these things are to how they were ten or fifteen years ago."

He thinks for a few moments.

"Of course, I'm not the man I used to be," he admits. "Those were the days. Nothing could get me down. I could have sex all the time, stay out all night long, and get up in the morning and. . . ."

Often, it's only when men honestly compare their current level of function to their peak years that they realize there has been a definite decline.

Grumpy Old Men

Few things in medicine are as rewarding to me as replacing a man's depleted testosterone. Few things seem to be as rewarding to the man's wife as well.

I vividly remember the morning I walked into the clinic and saw a gorgeous arrangement of roses on the counter. Being a big lover of flowers, I immediately asked, "Well, who did what to get those?" The answer from the staff was, "That's what we'd like to know. They're for you."

The card was from one of my female patients and read as follows:

> "Roses are red,
> Violets are blue,
> My husband's a stud,
> All thanks to you!"

It wasn't just his renewed interest in sex, a result of testosterone replacement, that had this lady so pleased. It was also his remarkable improvement in mood.

Testosterone has a marked uplifting effect on the mood of both men and women. The positive enthusiasm, passion, and risk-taking so characteristic of men is mediated by testosterone. As men age and their testosterone levels decrease, they tend to become grumpy, irritable, apathetic, and listless.

Tiberius Reiter, MD, first reported the benefits of testosterone replacement for men back in the early 1960s. After twelve years, and 240 patients who complained of premature aging, he described the following results: "Men who were stooped, slow moving, slow thinking, and considering retirement like old men, came back for a check-up at two months looking quite different. They walk well, hold themselves erect, and talk and act like very young fifty-year-olds instead of very old sixty-year-olds. There is even a change in the voice, manner, and handshake."

Testosterone and Your Heart

Testosterone and the heart is a connection that is often missed. The fact is, testosterone exerts great protective and therapeutic effects on the heart.

This shouldn't seem too strange, because the heart is a muscle, after all, and testosterone exerts a powerful effect on muscle function. The benefit is particularly significant for men who have diabetes, but it also applies to all men with heart disease.

Testosterone deficiency causes an undesirable decrease in the HDL/LDL cholesterol ratio, which is associated with atherosclerosis. In addition, it contributes to coronary artery blockage, elevated blood pressure, elevated triglycerides, an increased tendency for blood clotting, congestive heart failure, and insulin resistance.

Testosterone replacement reverses these negative developments. Men report improvements on many fronts, including blood clotting, cardiac function, chest pain, glucose control, cholesterol profiles, treadmill testing, and weight management. Men (and women) with heart disease should definitely explore testosterone replacement therapy.

Testosterone and Your Prostate

Fearing it will aggravate the prostate, many doctors shy away from testosterone replacement. This fear persists despite the reality that both prostate cancer and prostate enlargement only develop in older men who have lower testosterone levels.

I carefully monitor the prostate status of my patients on testosterone replacement, just as I routinely do with all the men I treat who are over fifty. With proper testosterone replacement therapy, the only effect I usually see on the prostate is *improvement*. PSA tests improve. Bladder function improves. I have never seen the opposite occur. Perhaps this is because I also carefully monitor the estrogen level.

Yes, men have some estrogen, just as women have some testosterone. Here's how that works:

Older men's bodies tend to increase the production of an enzyme called aromatase. Other factors that tend to increase the production of aromatase are too much alcohol, obesity, and insulin resistance. This enzyme acts to convert testosterone into the estrogen estradiol. So, when a man is replacing his sagging testosterone levels, what can happen about two or three months later is that his elevated aromatase levels will start converting the testosterone into estradiol. This does two things:

First of all, it decreases his testosterone levels, and the replacement doesn't seem to work anymore. Secondly, it increases his estradiol levels, and the extra estradiol starts to have all kinds of negative effects. The elevated estradiol levels can then cause swelling in the prostate (called benign prostatic hypertrophy) so common to men as we get older. It can also cause breast development and sexual dysfunction. Fortunately, if this is happening to a man on testosterone replacement, there are very effective ways to decrease the activity of aromatase.

But what about prostate cancer? In his 1998 book *Maximizing Manhood,* British physician Malcolm Carruthers describes his experience treating more than a thousand men with testosterone replacement. He writes that after a half-century of testosterone treatment for men with low testosterone levels, there is no evidence of any associated rise in prostate cancer or benign prostatic hypertrophy.

Men, understand this: testosterone does not cause prostate cancer. However, men that have prostate cancer need to know that testosterone replacement will induce the cancer to grow at an accelerated rate. With this in mind, I do not administer testosterone to any of my patients with prostate cancer.

But many men have prostate cancer that is so small that they don't know they have it. So just in case, for the first year that I give testosterone replacement to any man, I check the PSA test every three months. If he has an undiagnosed prostate cancer, its presence will become apparent, because we will see the PSA steadily climb. I have had a few cases like this. In each case, we were glad that we gave testosterone, because if we hadn't, we would not have discovered the cancer as early as we did.

The Amazing Human Growth Hormone

The longer I use human growth hormone (hGH) replacement, the more amazed I am. More than any other hormone, hGH has the most stunning and wide-ranging anti-aging properties. It significantly influences all aspects of aging, including the production of other hormones.

According to Daniel Rudman, MD, the pioneering physician I mentioned earlier, "The overall deterioration of the body that comes with growing old is not inevitable. . . . We now realize that some aspects of it can be prevented or reversed."

In a 2000 article published in *Hormone Research,* the author concludes that life without growth hormone is poor in quality and quantity. hGH is produced in the pituitary part of the brain. Rudman makes the point that typical growth-hormone levels of men in their sixties are "indistinguishable" from people with documented diseases of the pituitary gland.

hGH is named after the growth spurts synonymous with the teenage years. An enormous increase of hGH sparks this high-growth period. During this time of life, hGH blood levels can soar to as much as 2,000 mcg/L per day.

Documented Benefits of hGH Therapy

- An 8.8 percent increase in muscle mass in six months without exercise
- A 14.4 percent loss of fat mass in six months without dieting
- Enhanced sexual performance
- Faster healing
- Higher energy levels
- Improved brain function
- Improved cardiac output
- Improved cholesterol levels
- Improved immune function
- Improved sleep
- Improved vision
- Lowered blood pressure
- Mood elevation
- Reduction of cellulite
- Reduction of wrinkles
- Re-growth of hair
- Re-growth of shrunken organs
- Stronger bones
- Tighter, thicker, more hydrated skin
- PLUS: Enhancement of effects generated by replacement of other hormones

What goes up must come down; so after the sharp rise during the growth spurt, there is a falloff. The average amount of hGH produced at age twenty is about 600 mcg/L; at thirty, about 400 mcg/L; and by forty, the level is down to 250 mcg/L. From here, it tends to decrease very slowly over the next forty years to a lowly average of 25 mcg/L per day.

The elevated levels seen in the teenage years drive the systemic growth. The lower levels in adulthood serve to maintain that growth.

As you grow older, when your hGH levels start sagging below 200 mcg/L, your body will also begin to sag—and shrink as well. Ever so slowly. That's right. Your brain, heart, liver, lungs, and all the rest actually reduce in size.

This downsizing is referred to as atrophy. You see it most noticeably as sagging muscles and skin. And you feel it most noticeably in the form of diminished functioning.

- As the bones atrophy, you become shorter, and your face actually begins to shrink, causing many of the facial changes we can expect with age.

* As the brain shrinks, you are not able to think as quickly and as clearly as you once could.
* As the heart atrophies, you won't have the stamina and endurance you had.
* As the hormone-producing glands atrophy, you will have lower and lower levels of hormones.
* As the immune system atrophies, your resistance will suffer and you will be more likely to develop infectious illnesses and cancer.
* As your skin atrophies, you will develop wrinkles.
* As your muscles atrophy, you will start to lose your strength and your physique.

hGH can slow down such central losses and, in many cases, even reverse the process, as the Documented Benefits of hGH Therapy indicate.

When to Start hGH

The original studies on hGH were performed on men aged seventy to seventy-two. As a result, many physicians and their patients regard this general period as the appropriate time to start hGH replacement. But more recent data now indicate that the optimum time to start is much earlier. And it makes sense. Why start hGH therapy after all the damage has been done?

Early physical signs of growth-hormone deficiency include skeletal muscle loss, as evidenced by sagging skin in the face, arms, and buttocks. These signs are normally seen as people enter their fifties, and are often pronounced by the time they reach sixty. The blood test known as IGF-1 is an excellent indicator of your level of growth hormone. Optimum levels of IGF-1 should be greater than 150 ng/mL.

The effects of hGH are mediated primarily through the action of the liver—once again, the all-important liver. For this reason, I recommend that anyone using hGH be sure to also include all the vitamins, minerals, and herbal supplements found in QuickStart. This, along with the other steps in this book, will guarantee optimal liver function.

Other Ways to Increase hGH Levels

In the old days, when hGH was $200/month, I was good about taking it. And then the cost suddenly increased to $700/month, and I was having a hard time justifying the expense. Was it really worth it?

It was then that I saw a report in one of the anti-aging magazines about seven men and women in their seventies. The researchers took these men and women, none of whom was an exerciser, to the gym. In the gym, each person had a physical trainer put them through a fairly grueling forty-five-minute weight-lifting session. The researchers checked the hGH levels before and right after the session. Remarkably, the levels had doubled in each case. That's when I had the "Aha!" moment:

Why should I spend $700/month for hGH injections, when I can make the real thing for free and save the money for that new motorcycle I have been looking at? So, back in 2010, I upped my weight training regime, stopped with the hGH injections, and am now riding a beautiful Harley. But that is not all I have been doing. It turns out that there are all kinds of other ways to stimulate the body to increase hGH production.

One way is with peptides. Peptides are messenger molecules that the body uses to regulate tissue regeneration, among other things. Peptides have anti-aging, anti-inflammatory, and muscle-building properties. There are special peptides that doctors can prescribe that stimulate hGH production. You can learn a lot about the various peptides that are good hGH stimulators online.

Another way to stimulate hGH is to use large doses of what are called freeform amino acids. Amino acids are the breakdown products of the protein in our diets. The body uses specific amino acids to signal it to produce more or less hGH. The amino acids that tend to work best are glutamine, arginine, and lysine. Take about 4 grams of one or all three on an empty stomach about an hour before bed. And one last thing:

We make hGH almost entirely when we sleep. So, disturbed sleep can be a real problem. Do everything you can to make sure you are sleeping like a baby. And that brings me to one of my most favorite of all hormones: melatonin.

Melatonin—More Than Just for Sleeping

Melatonin. As a result of front-cover magazine treatment and the 1995 bestseller *The Melatonin Miracle*, most people have heard about this celebrated hormone. Most of these people think of melatonin as a sleeping and jet-lag aid, which it certainly is. But its influence extends far beyond putting you to sleep. Let me cover a bit of the sleep connection first, and then I'll move on to the other exciting effects of melatonin.

Studies have shown a consistent and progressive decline in melatonin production starting in your early twenties. By age fifty, your melatonin level is half what it was in your early adult years. By seventy, it is less than half of what you had at fifty, and so on and so on, in a continuing decline.

Insomnia associated with aging? That's a direct effect of this decline. Twenty-year-olds sleep an average of ten hours a night. Sixty-year-olds only get in six hours or so of sleep, much of it restless.

In 1995, one of the first scientific studies reporting this effect was published in the British medical journal *The Lancet*. This was a double-blind controlled study, considered the most reliable kind of study design. The researchers demonstrated a direct relationship between the amount of melatonin being produced and the quality of sleep. They concluded that melatonin deficiency seems to be a key factor in the sleep disorders so common in older people.

Melatonin turns out to be a key element in the induction of a sleep cycle known as slow-wave sleep. This is the restorative stage of sleep when the body repairs the damage that has occurred during the day. Ever wonder why you don't heal as well from the stresses and strains of exercise or injury as you did when you were younger? You can blame much of that on a decreased level of melatonin. Austrian researchers have found that people who take a melatonin supplement spend a much longer time in slow-wave sleep than those who do not.

It is interesting to note that hGH is released by the pituitary during the slow-wave stage of sleep. A study published in the *Journal of the American Medical Association* (*JAMA*) revealed that sleep deprivation resulted in significantly lowered levels of growth-hormone production. This study once again serves to point out the close relationships between hormones.

The melatonin-sleeping connection, however, is really only the tip of the iceberg. There are many other talents of this extremely important hormone.

You've Got Rhythm

Melatonin is a major player, perhaps *the* major player, in your natural biological cycle known as the circadian rhythm. This inner intelligence acts like a clock, controlling your sleep/wake cycle, blood pressure, body temperature, brain and hormone neurotransmitter production, energy level, immunity, mood, and weight gain or loss.

Melatonin is secreted in the pineal gland, a part of the brain behind your forehead. This gland is extremely sensitive to sunlight. It releases melatonin in direct relationship to our sunlight exposure. I've covered the importance of obtaining adequate sunlight (see chapter 10, Secret 3); now here is another reason you need to get enough sun into your life. And, of course, get enough sleep, which melatonin supplementation can enhance.

The natural circadian rhythm is central to biological functioning. This fact was demonstrated by Walter Pierpaoli, MD, the world-famous Italian researcher, in a series of dramatic and elaborate laboratory

How Robert Regained the Use of His Knees

When Robert first came to me, he was sixty-two years old. Years of hard living had resulted in both good and bad effects. He had been a hard drinker until he was fifty-five, at which time he realized it was a problem and stopped. He told me, "I've never been happier in my whole life than I have been since I stopped drinking. The older I got, the more I realized how important my kids are to me. The drinking was ruining my relationships."

On the good side of the equation was the fact that he had been a rancher all his life. He had always eaten real food, and spent hours each day doing hard work. He appeared thin and reasonably healthy, but he looked about ten years older than his stated age—all the years of drinking had definitely accelerated the aging process for him.

He was complaining of moodiness, no sex drive, and insomnia. He also said he just did not have the energy to work around the ranch the way he used to. He was only sleeping five to six hours "on a good night," but his major concern was his knees. "An orthopedist told me my knees had been so deteriorated over the years, from arthritis and hard work, that the only solution available was joint replacement." Indeed, as he struggled to get out of the waiting-room chair and then walk slowly into my office, it was apparent that his knees were a serious impediment.

Robert's symptoms were so characteristic of testosterone deficiency that I didn't even wait to get the tests back before starting him on replacement therapy. Because of his Bio-Energy Testing results, I also got him experiments in the early 1990s. Working with Vladimir Lesnikov, PhD, a Russian researcher, Pierpaoli surgically exchanged the pineal glands of young mice with those of old mice. Since the rodents were genetically identical, there was no rejection of the transplants.

As expected, the younger mice with the old pineal glands soon began to show unmistakable signs of accelerated aging. Meanwhile, the older mice with the transplanted young glands appeared rejuvenated. At the end of the experiment, the old mice ended up living twice as long as the young ones. In terms of human years, the old mice with the young glands lived more than a hundred years. These experiments have led many experts in longevity medicine to regard melatonin as something of a fountain of youth.

on QuickStart, DHEA, lipoic acid, an exercise program, and a low dose of thyroid. And I made sure he was following all the other important steps outlined in this book.

When he returned six weeks later to go over the test results, he was already starting to notice more energy, but his other symptoms were still very much in evidence. His tests revealed that he was extremely deficient in growth hormone. After I explained the many beneficial effects of hGH to him, he agreed to give it a try.

Two months later, he reported back that "My energy level is starting to get much closer to the way it has always been, and best of all I am starting to really sleep well." He also said his knees were starting to feel better, and I noted how much more quickly he was able to get out of the chair.

Six months down the road, after nine months of therapy, he was "feeling as good as I ever had in my life, maybe even better." Particularly important was the fact that his knees were almost back to complete functioning. He was walking normally and was able to hike up hills he hadn't even considered in years.

Robert's case is an excellent example of two important effects of hGH replacement. First, many of the beneficial effects of testosterone and DHEA replacement simply will not occur in the absence of adequate growth-hormone replacement. Testosterone is a hormone that requires the presence of growth hormone in order to be fully effective. Second, growth hormone can literally regenerate the lost cartilage in knees damaged by years of osteoarthritis and wear and tear.

Melatonin and Cancer

Some very convincing studies have shown that melatonin can help in the treatment and prevention of breast and prostate cancer, and several other cancers. For example, in one study researchers first grew estrogen-positive breast cancers in culture. They then supplied some of these cultures with the blood of women with high melatonin levels. The other cultures were exposed to the blood of women who had low levels. What they found was striking.

The cancer cells divided much more rapidly when they were exposed to the lower levels of melatonin. When the researchers spiked the low-melatonin blood samples with synthetic melatonin, it removed their capacity to promote cancer, and inhibited the growth of the cancer cells by 30 to 40 percent. According to one of the researchers, these results show "close to conclusively" that low melatonin levels promote breast-tumor growth.

It also shows that taking melatonin supplements may be effective in treating cancer. In one study published in the *British Journal of Cancer,* the use of melatonin supplements in women with breast cancer was effective in 28.5 percent of the women. What is most impressive about this small study is that all of these women were not responding to the conventional treatment they were getting.

Another study examined the levels of melatonin in the first morning urine of 147 women with invasive breast cancer and 291 women without cancer. They then divided both groups of women into four groups, depending on how high their melatonin levels were. Those in the highest-melatonin group had about half the risk of having breast cancer that those in the lowest group had.

Since melatonin is formed during sleep, some other researchers took a slightly different approach. They looked at a group of 7,396 women over a period of six years. One hundred forty-six of these women developed breast cancer. What they found was that those who had the shortest amount of horizontal time, and therefore presumably had the lowest levels of melatonin, had almost three times the chance of developing cancer compared to the other women.

Other studies on melatonin and prostate cancer have been just as remarkable. Given these studies and others, it seems very prudent to supplement with melatonin once you hit your fifties.

Priming the Immune System

Melatonin also exerts a marked effect on the immune system. This is because melatonin enhances the immune activity of the thymus gland, located in the upper chest just below the neck. The thymus is a repository of first-line immune cells called lymphocytes. And it is here, in this gland, that immature lymphocytes go through a conditioning process—a kind of immune-system boot camp—that turns them into disease-fighting units that protect your body.

As people age, alas, the thymus gland also atrophies and increasingly loses its ability to churn out the mature immune cells called T-lymphocytes. This results in the lowered immune response so common in older people. And it is specifically why older people are so much more likely to die from viral infections that seem harmless to the young.

Receptor sites for melatonin have been found both on thymus cells and lymphocytes. In 1993, European researcher George Maestroni published the first study demonstrating that melatonin stimulated the production of T-lymphocytes in people with lowered immune function. He concluded that "the pineal gland might thus be viewed as the crux of a sophisticated immuno-neuroendocrine network."

But Wait—There's More

Melatonin also provides another major benefit to the body—as an antioxidant. As previously discussed, free radicals create much, if not most, of the deterioration that occurs in everyone's body as they age. Crucial antioxidant vitamins, such as vitamins C and E, along with CoQ_{10}, are the primary agents that snuff out harmful free-radical activity.

As an antioxidant, melatonin possesses its very own unique ability. An article by melatonin researcher R. Hardeland, which studied the antioxidant properties of melatonin, concluded that melatonin is an even more potent antioxidant than both vitamins C and E.

Additionally, researchers have discovered that melatonin penetrates all the way into the nucleus of cells. There, its antioxidant activity protects DNA from the type of free-radical destruction that can lead to cancer and neurological diseases. Because melatonin is the primary antioxidant in the nervous system, studies have shown that it can prevent the memory loss, Alzheimer's, Parkinson's, macular degeneration, and other brain disorders so common to older people.

According to Ray Sahelian, MD, author of an excellent book, *Melatonin, Nature's Sleeping Pill*, "Melatonin, taken as a supplement, could slow down the aging process and decrease the incidences of brain damage and cancer."

I recommend starting melatonin supplementation around the age of fifty. The only thing to consider is how much to take.

When I first heard about melatonin and cancer prevention, I called the world's leading melatonin researcher, a man by the name of Russel Reiter, PhD. Dr. Reiter has authored more papers and research into melatonin than anyone else on the planet. The last time I talked with him, he was eighty-four years old and still going strong. Here's more information on Dr. Reiter.

Dr. Reiter earned his PhD in endocrinology and radiation biology. He has also been awarded three honorary doctor of medicine (MD) degrees and one honorary doctor of science (DSc) degree. He has published 1,200-plus articles in scientific journals and books, and he has trained 140 postdoctoral fellows and 25 PhD students.

Dr. Reiter has received numerous awards for this research, including the A. Ross McIntyre Gold Medal, Alexander von Humboldt Award (Germany), Lezoni Lincee Award (Italy), and more. He is editor-in-chief of the *Journal of Pineal Research* (Impact Factor 5.855), and he is, or has been, on the editorial boards of twenty-six other journals. In short, Dr. Reiter is about as accomplished a scientist as you can get. Here's why this is important:

When I first talked with Dr. Reiter back in 2012, I learned some amazing things. First, melatonin is the safest of all hormones. Unlike all other hormones, melatonin is unique—there is no negative feedback inhibition with melatonin. This means that no matter how much you take, it will not interfere with your body's own production.

Secondly, melatonin is incredibly safe. Studies have shown that you can give animals extremely high doses for long periods of time with no negative effect. Amazingly, there is no LD50 for melatonin. That means it has never been shown, in over sixty years of study, to be toxic in any dose.

I take 180 mg of melatonin every night, about thirty minutes before bed. That is a whopping dose. Why do I take such a large dose? First, I do it because that is the human equivalent of the dose that has been needed in all of the animal studies that prevents virtually every kind of cancer tested, neurological diseases such as Parkinson's and Alzheimer's, macular degeneration, osteoporosis, and death from viral infections. Second, I do it because it is entirely safe. I, along with many other doctors, have been using this dose with all my patients for years.

I recommend 1 mg of melatonin taken before bed for every pound of body weight.

There are always people who are sensitive to anything. This is also true of melatonin. I find that about 10 percent of people will either have wild and uncomfortable dreams, or will wake up feeling drugged, when taking melatonin orally. For those people, the dose will just have to be cut back until we can find another route of administration that does not cause these symptoms.

DHEA

Of all the hormones supplemented for anti-aging reasons, DHEA (dehydroepiandrosterone) is perhaps the best known. A lot has been written and said about it. Considerable research has been conducted showing that a low level of this adrenal hormone is associated with almost every disease studied. This list includes AIDS, Alzheimer's, cancer, cardiovascular disease, diabetes, lupus, osteoporosis, and viral and bacterial infections.

Clinically, I don't see the obvious and immediate benefit from DHEA replacement that I routinely observe with estrogen, hGH, progesterone, and testosterone therapy. It is a very clinically subtle hormone. Nevertheless, I regard DHEA as an extremely important element in a total-disease-prevention strategy.

DHEA is the most abundant steroid hormone in the body. It is secreted in response to everything that stresses the body, from infections to allergies. By age seventy-five, however, you only produce about 10 percent of the amount you made as a twenty-five-year-old.

DHEA has been labeled as the "mother hormone," because it can be, and often is, converted by the body into other hormones as they become low. The rate of this conversion differs widely among individuals and is significant enough that anyone taking DHEA needs to have their other hormones monitored.

Many human studies involving DHEA supplementation mention the feeling of well-being that most people experience. I have found this generalized rejuvenating effect to be very consistent in my patients as well. I also see my older patients on DHEA recovering much more quickly from flu and colds. Only rarely do these infections last beyond a mild three or four days. This is partly attributable to DHEA's ability to boost the immune response in older people.

Animal studies have shown that DHEA protects the thymus gland from the normal shrinking that is associated with aging. This is the same thymus gland I mentioned in relation to melatonin. So here is another thymus-friendly hormone. Other promising animal studies have shown regression of tumors when animals were supplemented with DHEA.

MY RECOMMENDATIONS TO YOU

* If you are over forty, look for a prevention-oriented physician familiar with natural hormonal testing and replacement therapy. He or she can gently and safely escort you into an effective program that will revitalize your life. Do it now, even if you feel great.
* The best treatment is prevention. Don't wait until you are symptomatic. You can find a referral for an experienced practitioner near you by contacting the American Academy of Anti-Aging Medicine at www.a4m.com or by calling them at 1–888–997–0112.
* Use Bio-Energy Testing to determine if your energy production status needs help. Remember that energy production is the bottom line. If your M-Factor (basal metabolism) is low, be sure your hormone replacement program includes thyroid. Rely on thyroid blood testing only to help monitor your replacement dosing. As I said earlier in this book, that blood testing will miss low-thyroid states in a great many cases. That's why Bio-Energy Testing is the only way to go. You can obtain a referral to a Bio-Energy Testing certified healthcare practitioner in your area by going to www.bioenergytesting.com-.
* Many natural hormones are available over the counter or through the internet, but I always discourage people from getting their hormones this way. Many of the products are ineffective, and some do not contain the potency they say they do. A physician who is properly trained in natural bio-identical hormones is really necessary. And through the doctor, and the compounding pharmacy she or he uses, you can purchase the very best quality of natural hormones.

✳ 16 ✳

PUTTING IT ALL TOGETHER

It's all about energy. How efficiently you produce it, and how efficiently your body uses what you produce. My goal for you is that you live to be really old with youthful energy production. In that way you will maintain most of your youthful vigor and weight, avoid disease, and age at the slowest possible rate. You will enjoy a much more functional, happy life. There are few things worse than growing old and sick and dependent.

There's a huge amount of information in this book—and many guidelines. It's the same basic information I give my patients, only with them I don't have the time to go into all the detail I've included here. Don't be intimidated by everything you have read. Plan on incorporating this information into your life gradually over the next year. You will want to read the book several times and earmark those sections that seem the most important to you.

This is basic information. It will not grow old and obsolete with time. Certainly, we will learn many new and wonderful things in the years to come, but these basic tenets of health and longevity will always remain true.

I tell my patients I want them to eventually incorporate all the steps—all the secrets—into their everyday life. Bursting with energy isn't quite as simple as taking a single pill and voila—it's done. I wish it were, but it doesn't work that way. If I had that pill, I'd be the richest man in the world.

The anti-aging and detoxification program I've outlined is not just a temporary deal. It is something you are going to want to do until it's time for you to move on to the next world. Until then, the elements need to become routine.

After saying this to my patients, I very quickly add that I don't want them to feel overwhelmed. So I encourage them to apply my guidelines sequentially—one at a time.

For the very best results, all the elements need to be addressed—all the steps I have discussed. That's because they work together. In other words, how you eat affects how you exercise, how you exercise affects how you sleep, how you sleep affects hormone production, hormone production affects how you eat and exercise, and so forth.

In this book, I have laid out my recommendations—the secrets—in sequence, starting with the simplest steps. It's easy, for instance, to start drinking more water. And getting more rest. And going out into the sunlight. Those are my first three secrets.

Change is hard. Routine is easy. Once the changes I recommend become a part of your everyday life, they too will become routine and automatic. You will be replacing one routine with another one that is just as easy, but better for you. You may feel some resistance at first, particularly if you are used to eating a certain way, or going to bed too late, or not used to HIIT exercise. So here's my advice:

Just focus on a three-month turnaround time. At the end of three months, the resistance will be gone, and it will be replaced with the satisfaction that comes with feeling great and knowing that your future is looking better.

Whatever it takes, just give yourself time to adopt the changes. Don't rush and try to accomplish all the steps too fast. It's not in your interest, or in the interest of the program, to become overwhelmed and stressed while trying to fashion a healthier lifestyle.

My supplement secret revolves mainly around my use of all the ingredients and doses in QuickStart and Super Fats. The breathing recommendations can be applied easily, and when practiced over time can also become an automatic part of your life.

Weight loss is always a tough nut to crack. But the information I have provided will give you a new perspective on why you may be having a harder time than necessary trying to lose weight. Hopefully, knowing what is getting in the way of success will provide new inspiration. If you are very overweight, this is something you cannot put off. It is too critical to your energy, longevity, and quality of life.

Hormone replacement and Bio-Energy Testing can't be done on your own. You'll need to find a licensed practitioner to help you with that.

Another reason for needing some help is medications. Up until now, I have avoided this very unpleasant topic—and that is that many of the medications that doctors put patients on for the rest of their lives are toxic to mitochondria. They poison the mitochondria and cause a significant decrease in E.Q. and overall energy production. One review article titled "Drugs Interfering with Mitochondrial Behaviors" goes into this great detail. Here's a brief list of some of the more common drugs that are known to cripple mitochondrial function in susceptible people:

* Corticosteroids
* Seizure medications, including valproic acid, phenytoin, and barbiturates
* Anesthetics—it's why some people are never quite the same after a long surgery
* Nondepolarizing muscle relaxants
* Cholesterol-lowering drugs, including statins and fibrates
* Diabetes drugs, including biguanides and glitazones
* Beta-blockers
* Amiodarone

If you are taking any of these drugs and your E.Q. is low, it could definitely be the drug. The only way to find out is to either stop or substitute the drug for a few weeks and repeat the Bio-Energy Testing.

Dear reader, pretend it's New Year's Day and you are resolving to be healthier every year, instead of slowly going down the tube. To do that, start adopting all these guidelines as early as possible. Please don't "Put it off until I'm more ready." You may not be able to turn the train around once it has gone so far.

Make it a point to find a practitioner who can provide Bio-Energy Testing for you. It is the most amazing health-promoting technology that I have ever encountered. It alone can pinpoint your energy production deficits and speed the process of overcoming them.

If your doctor is not aware of Bio-Energy Testing, show him or her this book, and have them contact me through the phone numbers or website provided in the book. You can also refer them to a very technical dissertation on the science and clinical application of Bio-Energy Testing by going to my clinic website, clicking on the video tab, and watching the four-part series titled "Health, aging, and disease—It's all about energy."

By the way, if you have not already figured it out, I follow my own preaching. There is no way in the world that I want to risk having the problems that are so common in the elderly. I know first-hand that everything described in this book can be easily incorporated even in a busy lifestyle. And I know that it is actually quite easy, once you're used to it. I also know from my many patients that it works. When they follow the guidelines, their Bio-Energy Testing reveals energy levels that are typical of people much younger. They are literally bursting with energy.

Many of my recommendations are designed to make you feel better immediately, but a lot of what I say has prevention in mind. These preventive measures are also very, very important because, why would you want to feel better now, only to be sick later?

Medicine is changing as we speak. Soon, the days of "seeing your doctor means you are sick" will be gone. Now, physicians and their patients alike are finally getting the idea that seeing a doctor should be something you do *before* you are ill, in order to make sure you don't become ill. I've been seeing patients for almost fifty years now. And I can't tell you how often I see patients who are miserable with one problem or another that could have been completely avoided simply by following the advice in this book.

If your physician is already familiar with this concept, great. This is important, because you will not be able to implement some of the guidelines without the assistance of a prevention-oriented physician working with you.

Encouraging stories are always great. Here's one you will appreciate.

Steve's Success Story

What would you say about an eighty-four-year-old man, I'll call him Steve, who has the mitochondrial function of a thirty-four-year-old? What's the deal with Steve? Even though he is going to put eighty-five candles on his next birthday cake, from a functional standpoint he has not yet started to age—amazing! What in the world is he doing that could produce that kind of result?

Steve first came to see me nine years ago. He was disease-free. He was taking a blood-pressure pill, and other than the usual wear-and-tear symptoms that are typical of a man of seventy-six, he felt and functioned great. His intake form said, "I want to improve my general health."

His mitochondrial function was that of the average forty-eight-year-old. In fact, the only thing I could find wrong with him was that his thyroid was slightly off. His thyroid blood tests were perfect. But, as I have reported to you many times above, thyroid blood testing is notoriously unable to identify people with age-related thyroid dysfunction. So, I started him on a low dose of thyroid, and gave him an exercise prescription based on his Bio-Energy Test. But that was not all.

Initial testing showed him to be deficient in growth hormone and testosterone. And to make matters worse, his estrogen levels were sky-high. Estrogen is great for women, but high levels are not good for men. They interfere with testosterone and lead to muscle loss, decreased libido, moodiness, decreased brain function, and "man boobs." Steve confessed that he was having symptoms like this. I explained to him that although these findings were not at all surprising in a seventy-six-year-old man, the good news is that they can be corrected.

When I checked his heavy metals, he tested out quite high in mercury and moderately high in lead. Besides the usual environmental exposure to mercury, Steve had several "silver" dental fillings. These fillings slowly release mercury into the body, even decades after they were placed. I also asked him if he was getting flu shots, because they are also loaded with mercury. Fortunately, he had not fallen into that trap. The high lead was typical. Virtually everyone his age has levels as high, or higher. I had him see a biological dentist to have the mercury fillings exchanged for non-toxic fillings. And I started him on oral chelation therapy with DMSA. DMSA is an excellent chelator for both lead and mercury.

When he came back the following year for his annual mitochondrial testing, we were both happy to see that he was then testing out like a forty-three-year-old. He had gotten a year older chronologically, but he had gotten five years younger from a functional standpoint. It seemed like he was on a roll. But was he?

The following year, his Bio-Energy Testing had significantly declined to the point that he was now testing like a fifty-seven-year-old. What had happened? He continued to feel great. He had been faithful in working his program, and nothing had changed in his life. Nothing, that is, except one thing: he had gotten a year older. Not long ago, I reported on a similar case of a man who had great annual Bio-Energy Testing results until he hit his sixty-seventh birthday. That man was me. Both cases serve to illustrate two things.

One, the aging process is not necessarily obvious. It can sneak up on you while you're feeling great. Often, you don't even know there's something wrong until you find it out on Bio-Energy Testing.

Secondly, time takes its toll. Sooner or later it gets you. Sometimes even only one year can make a significant difference. The only way to stay ahead of it is to use Bio-Energy Testing to monitor your mitochondrial function on a regular basis. That way, you can be alerted to any changes long before they cause problems.

The other thing to remember is that depending on what's going on in your life, your mitochondrial function can change on a dime. Maybe I was just catching him at a bad time. Or maybe things were starting to unravel. The only way we were going to be able to figure it out was with follow-up testing the next year. Using the new data, I set up a different interval-training program for Steve. And that brings us to the end of this success story.

The last three years, Steve has consistently tested out like a man in his thirties. I still find it amazing that at his age of eighty-four, he is every bit as functional as he has ever been in his life. And he doesn't show any signs of stopping! His story is encouraging to all of us who want to live up to my motto: live long and live strong.

Get an Attitude

Getting old is the perfect time to get a positive attitude. Enough cannot be said about the importance of attitude. I haven't talked about this so far, because I wanted to save it for last. But it is probably the most important single component of life. Your attitude can make or break anything else you do. Attitude governs how happily or unhappily you live life—and perhaps how long you live it as well. And I think you will agree that how long you live is really inconsequential, compared to how well you live.

Did you hear the joke about the guy who goes in to see his doctor? After examining him, and checking out all the tests, the doctor says: "You're going to have to stop drinking, skiing, smoking cigars, and chasing women."

"Will it make me live longer, Doc?" the man asks.

"No, but I promise you it will seem longer."

Joking aside, I can promise you that sickness and pain will make life seem longer as well. And that, for sure, is not the kind of longevity you are seeking.

Growing old is just about the best thing that can happen to a person. It is a real gift. Make the most of it. Don't pay any attention to all the negative cultural messages implying you're over the hill. Sure, when you were younger, maybe you could do things twice as fast, but you probably enjoyed them only half as much.

Don't yield to aging. The senior years represent a time in your life when you are wise enough to really enjoy all that life has to offer. The key is, *while you grow old chronologically, you don't have to keep pace biologically.* You can have youthful energy levels and feel great even at very old ages. That's what this book is about.

Nor do you have to grow old psychologically. Think young. Ask yourself, "Is there anything I would do now if I were only younger?" If there is a positive answer to this question, my advice to you is to do it. This is your life: live it to the fullest until it ends. Now is a great time to rid yourself of any negative attitudes and assumptions that get in the way.

I have no great words of wisdom here, except to remind you that all things are possible when you open up your heart and let love in. Love is the ultimate vitamin. If you are not in love with someone or something, it's important to work on this. Ask yourself what it is that you love. Cultivate and value connections with people, animals, plants, mountains, lakes, bicycles, your car, whatever.

Appreciate all your good qualities, and work on developing more. Accept full responsibility for every aspect of your life. For what has gone wrong. And for what has gone right. This is what free will is all about. And the realization of this is the source of all your power, including the power to get well and stay well.

The four most important aspects of life are relationships, money, work, and health. All require some work. They are never dialed in. They constantly change, and they must be continuously reexamined. Get some professional counseling if you need it. There is no one who can't benefit from counseling every now and then.

Happiness is not a goal. It's a path. And so is contentment in who you are, and how you live your life. Don't compare yourself to others: it's a waste of valuable time. There will always be someone who is better, and someone who is worse; so what's the point?

Whenever you can, sing, dance, pray, rejoice, and laugh—especially at yourself. Don't you sometimes feel like one of the Three Stooges, only without the sophistication? Be forgiving with yourself. If you don't forgive yourself, you won't be able to forgive others.

Lastly, don't be afraid to try on new attitudes. It's okay to make mistakes at any age. Mistakes are how we learn. They actually aren't mistakes; they are lessons. You get them over and over until you learn. If you don't learn, you don't grow. Imagine how smart you're going to be after an entire lifetime of lessons.

Good luck!

✳ APPENDIX A ✳

DR. SHALLENBERGER'S SUPER IMMUNE QUICKSTART

Dr. Shallenberger is licensed both as a Medical Doctor and a Homeopathic Medical Doctor. He has been practicing nutritional and preventive medicine since 1978. During that time, he has analyzed the biochemical and nutritional needs of literally thousands of his patients. He discovered there were certain nutrients and herbs that all his patients needed, and he decided to put full doses of all these ingredients in one easy-to-take product.

While it is in no way a substitute for a healthy diet, the spectrum and doses in this mixture reflect the current state of the art in nutritional supplementation and detoxification. *When used in conjunction with Super Fats and a three-week detoxification program of exercise and abstention from alcohol, coffee, flour, milk, and sweets, Dr. S's QuickStart formula prevents and often solves many problems and disorders without any other intervention needed.*

Pills vs. Food

Because of the complex nature of digestive tracts, capsules and tablets are not the best way of delivering nutrients. There are four basic reasons for this.

First, some vitamin content may be decreased in the manufacturing process.

Second, tablets and capsules do not always adequately break down in many people, which means that much of their content may not be absorbed.

Third, it would require over forty horse-size capsules to get the same amount of nutrients found in the recommended amount of QuickStart.

Very few people are going to take that many capsules for very long, if they would even take them in the first place.

Fourth, Dr. Shallenberger has carefully formulated this product so that each vitamin, mineral, and herb is present in the exact form he has determined to be the most clinically effective.

All the nutrients in QuickStart are prepared as a fine powder. Not only are nutrient values maintained throughout the manufacturing process, but also the absorption rate is high, even in individuals with compromised digestive systems.

Immune Systems Under Siege

What causes one person to catch a flu and another to avoid it? Why does one person develop an immune-related disease while another living in the same environment doesn't? Why do some people have allergies? Why do serious outbreaks of infectious diseases leave some individuals untouched? The answers, of course, live within the immune system.

From viruses never before discovered to antibiotic-resistant bacteria, immune systems are being challenged in ways never before seen. These times require the most supercharged immune systems imaginable. Through diet, adequate rest, and the special nutrients in Dr. S's formula, you will harness your body's ability to do the job that nature intended—combat and prevent disease.

The Ultimate Prescription

Many people taking QuickStart have reported a noticeable improvement in a variety of conditions, despite the fact that QuickStart was often the only clinical intervention they were using. This is because the formula works on such basic levels, providing antioxidant protection and nutritional insurance, while at the same time enhancing immunity, alkalinizing tissues, improving brain function, improving circulation, detoxifying the liver and intestinal tract, stabilizing appetite and metabolism, and, most importantly, increasing energy production.

Consultants will appreciate the fact that QuickStart is not just another multi-vitamin using meaningless doses of many nutrients just to make the label look good. Every ingredient is clinically proven and is added in its full recommended amount.

QuickStart is the only product available that has the recommended amount of *all* the vitamins, minerals, and antioxidants, and

QuickStart Ingredients

Two Scoops (42.3 grams) provides:

- 30,000 IU beta carotene
- 10,000 IU vitamin A
- 2,000 mg vitamin C
- 400 IU vitamin E (d-alpha)
- 1000 mg hesperidin bioflav complex
- 120 mg ginkgo biloba extract
- 600 mg magnesium (citrate)
- 10 mg manganese (amino-acid chelate)
- 300 mg potassium (citrate)
- 200 mcg selenium (selenate)
- 1200 mcg chromium (picolinate)
- 16 mg zinc (picolinate)
- 2 mg copper (amino-acid chelate)
- 100 mg vitamin B1
- 50 mg vitamin B2
- 100 mg niacin
- 300 mg pantothenic acid
- 100 mg vitamin B6
- 1000 mcg vitamin B12
- 1000 mcg folic acid
- 500 mcg biotin
- 300 mg astragalus extract
- 6 gm spirolina Pacifica
- 750 mg L-glutamine
- 100 mg n-acetyl cysteine (NAC)
- 320 mg saw palmetto
- 5 gm psyllium husks
- 5 gm stabilized rice bran
- 5 gm soy protein isolate*
- 5 gm whey protein (undenatured)*

**NOTE: Some people are allergic to soy or whey. For them, there is QuickStart-HA (hypo-allergenic). QuickStart-HA provides the same nutrients found in regular QuickStart, except that the soy and whey have been replaced with pre-biotics.*

the full-strength detoxifying power of rice bran, psyllium, nacetyl cysteine, l-glutamine, and spirolina Pacifica. QuickStart also contains the hormone-balancing effects of soy protein isolates, the remarkable immune-enhancing power of astragalus and hydrolyzed whey protein, and the prostate- and breast-cancer prevention afforded by saw palmetto extract. Additionally, QuickStart offers the blood-thinning and circulation-enhancement power of ginkgo biloba extract.

Of course, QuickStart is completely organic and free of any GMO ingredients.

QuickStart Pre-Biotic

QuickStart Pre-Biotic also contains the following herbs that help to establish and maintain a healthy microbiome: chicory root, Jerusalem artichoke root, green banana flour, and galacto-oligosaccharides

Directions to Doctors

QuickStart forms the foundation for the entire Bio-Energy Testing program. All my patients are started on QuickStart unless their energy parameters are completely optimal.

Have your patients first begin taking QuickStart as a breakfast replacement in the morning, and again as an adrenal supporter in the afternoon, sometime between noon and 3 p.m. It usually takes patients a few weeks to get into the habit of remembering this afternoon dose, but once they see how much their energy levels improve, it will become second nature.

Always have them start with a half scoop or less. The formula is quite strong, and it may take a few weeks for the liver and the bowels to adjust to QuickStart. After patients have adjusted to the starting amount, have them gradually increase to the recommended amount of one scoop.

Although QuickStart can be taken simply by shaking it up with water, many people enjoy making a smoothie by adding extras, such as vanilla, yogurt, carrots or other vegetables, or fruit, along with water and ice, and blending it in a blender. When they do this, they can also throw in any other powders, capsules, or tablets they have been prescribed and blend it all together. Patients should also add one tablespoon of flax oil to the morning dose.

Super Fats Ingredients

One teaspoon provides:

* 3 cc fish oil concentrate
* 1 cc wheat germ oil
* 1 cc flax oil
* 135 mg mixed tocopherols, containing 20% gamma tocopherol
* 15 mg lycopene
* 50 mg CoQ_{10}
* 50 mg alpha lipoic acid
* 750 mg vitamin D

How to Order QuickStart and Super Fats

QuickStart can be ordered by calling this toll-free number: 1–866–376–0610. It can also be ordered online at http://www.bioenergytesting.com.

✷ APPENDIX B ✷

IS YOUR PATIENT EXERCISING TOO HARD TO BE HEALTHY?

Frank Shallenberger, MD, HMD, ABAAM

Townsend Letter for Doctors,
August/September 2004, 97–99.

Abstract

Context: Aerobic exercise is a documented and well-accepted measure to decrease incidence of degenerative disease, increase quality of life, and extend lifespan. However, exercising above anaerobic threshold is known to increase free-radical production, and exhausts both redox buffering and acid-base buffering capabilities. Both these latter phenomena are known to increase the rate of aging and tissue and organ degeneration. It is not clear whether exercising at levels of exertion consistent with the most popular current method of predicting anaerobic threshold is healthy.

Objective: To examine if the predictive formula, anaerobic threshold heart rate = .8 x (220 – age), is a safe formula to use in prescribing an exercise regimen for health and longevity.

Design, Setting, and Participants: Nineteen patients who were free of degenerative disease, and who were consulting a board-certified physician in anti-aging medicine for purposes of longevity and disease prevention, were randomly selected. Patients served as their own controls.

Main Outcome Measure: Heart rate at anaerobic threshold as determined, using respiratory gas-exchange analysis and a computer-driven algorithm known as Bio-Energy Testing.

Results: Among nineteen patients tested, sixteen (84%) had a measured anaerobic threshold heart rate which was significantly below, and two (10%) had a measured anaerobic threshold heart rate which was significantly above, that predicted by the formula, anaerobic threshold heart rate = .8 x (220 – age). Thirteen (68%) had a measured anaerobic threshold heart rate which was at least 10% less than that predicted by the formula. Furthermore, the point of anaerobic threshold could not be accurately determined by the classical clinical symptoms of anaerobic threshold, such as significant breathlessness and muscle pain.

Conclusion: Using either the predictive formula: anaerobic threshold heart rate = .8 x (220 – age), or the clinical signs of breathlessness and muscle pain, to prescribe an exercise regimen for health and longevity is unreliable, and in the majority of cases will result in patients exercising at dangerously high levels.

Introduction

Aerobic exercise is a documented and well-accepted measure to decrease incidence of degenerative disease, increase quality of life, and extend lifespan. (1) As the intensity of exercise increases, the rate of oxygen consumption increases in order to provide the necessary energy production for the increased exertional demand. In any given subject, as the intensity of exertion is steadily and incrementally increased, he/she will eventually come to a level of exertion which exceeds his body's capacity to consume oxygen. This point is referred to as the subject's *anaerobic threshold* because, if the level of exertion is increased beyond this point, he will no longer be able to meet his energy needs from oxygen metabolism, and he will begin to produce energy anaerobically.

It is important for every person who exercises to know at what level of exertion he will exceed his oxygen-consuming capacity and enter into anaerobic metabolism, because anaerobic metabolism is known to dramatically increase the production of powerful pro-oxidant molecules known as free radicals. Many, if not most, of the damaging effects that occur during the aging process and in degenerative disease are mediated by free radicals. (2) Most of these free radicals are eliminated by antioxidant enzyme buffering systems, such as glutathione peroxidase, catalase, and superoxide dismutase; but in the process of eliminating free-radical stress, these enzymes are consumed. Sustained exertional effort above anaerobic threshold produces such an abundance of free radicals that these redox buffering enzymes eventually become depleted. (3) This depletion results in an increased rate of aging and risk of disease secondary to increased oxidant stress.

Furthermore, exercising above the anaerobic threshold also produces an abundance of lactic acid. The lactic acid is either recycled in the Cori cycle, in which it is converted in the liver back into glucose, converted into carbon dioxide through the action of the enzyme carbonic anhydrase, or buffered by various acid-base buffering systems. The first two of these systems have limitations, however.

The Cori system requires ATP, which results in increased energy consumption at a time when energy needs are already being exceeded. The carbonic anhydrase system is limited by respiration, which is evidenced by the fact that as a subject exceeds his anaerobic threshold, his serum levels of both carbon dioxide and lactate increase. Because of these limitations, sustained exercise above anaerobic threshold results in increased demands on the acid-base buffering systems, which eventually deplete these systems. Similar to what happens when antioxidant buffering is depleted, a depletion of acid-base buffering results in a sustained increase in mesenchymal acid levels. Increased mesenchymal acidosis is known to dramatically mediate both acute and chronic disease, as well as most of the pathology associated with the aging process. (4)

Thus, exercising above anaerobic threshold results in an increase in oxidant stress as well as an increase in mesenchymal acidosis, and both of these phenomena increase the rate of aging and tissue and organ degeneration. Ironically enough, many people who exercise regularly may be actually increasing their rate of aging if they are exercising above their anaerobic threshold. This fact is well known, and to avoid doing so, subjects are advised to use the following formula to determine what their heart rate will be as they come close to their anaerobic threshold:

$$\text{Anaerobic threshold heart rate} = .8 \times (220 - \text{age})$$

Subjects are commonly advised to use this formula to avoid exercising above this determined heart rate in order to avoid exceeding their anaerobic threshold. Furthermore, many exercise experts feel that a subject will immediately sense when he is exceeding his anaerobic threshold because the increased production of lactic acid will result in noticeable muscle pain along with a very noticeable increase in respiration. The objective of this experiment was to determine the following:

1. Is the formula, anaerobic threshold heart rate = .8 x (220 – age), accurate in predicting the point at which a subject enters into anaerobic metabolism?

2. Is the presence of muscle pain and/or significant breathlessness accurate in predicting the point at which a subject enters into anaerobic metabolism?

If these predictors, which are so commonly used, are not accurate, then many people may be exercising *too hard to be healthy.*

Methods

Nineteen healthy patients who were free of disease, and who were consulting a board-certified physician in anti-aging medicine for purposes of longevity and disease prevention, were randomly selected. Ages varied from nineteen to seventy-one. Patients served as their own controls.

Oxygen consumption and carbon-dioxide production were determined using a pulmonary gas analyzer and an exercise ergometer supplied by Medical Graphics Corporation, St. Paul, MN, U.S.A. This equipment uses a mouthpiece that analyzes all of a subject's inspired and expired air for oxygen and carbon-dioxide content. Oxygen consumption and carbon-dioxide production were determined on each patient while exercising on the ergometer. The workload of the ergometer was steadily increased at varying rates, using a protocol provided by Bio-Energy Testing, LLC, Carson City, NV, U.S.A., which is based on a predicted level of fitness for each patient. The test was concluded as soon as the patient reached his anaerobic threshold.

The breath-by-breath data, consisting of oxygen consumption, carbon-dioxide production, and heart rate, were analyzed by a patented computer-driven algorithm, Bio-Energy Testing, provided by Bio-Energy Testing, LLC. Anaerobic threshold was determined by this algorithm to occur when the rate of oxygen consumption is exceeded by the rate of carbon-dioxide production. The point at which the rate of oxygen consumption is exceeded by the rate of carbon-dioxide production is generally accepted as the most accurate determination of anaerobic threshold. (5) The heart rate, when the anaerobic threshold was reached, was then reported as True Anaerobic Threshold Heart Rate (TATR).

The patient's age was then used to estimate the heart rate at which anaerobic threshold would be reached according to the formula, anaerobic threshold heart rate = .8 x (220 – age). This heart rate was reported as Estimated Anaerobic Threshold Heart Rate (EATR).

Results

Full results are shown in Table 1. Among nineteen patients tested, sixteen (84 percent) had a TATR which was significantly below EATR. Thirteen (68 percent) had a TATR which was at least 10 percent below EATR, a point which is considered as an extremely conservative estimation of anaerobic threshold heart rate. Two (10 percent) had a TATR which was significantly above the patient's EATR.

Only in two cases did the point of anaerobic threshold coincide with the classical clinical symptoms of anaerobic threshold, such as significant breathlessness and muscle pain. This occurred only in the two patients in which the TATR was significantly above the patient's EATR.

Conclusion

Using either the predictive formula, anaerobic threshold heart rate = .8 x (220 – age), or the clinical signs of breathlessness and muscle pain to estimate anaerobic threshold heart rate was unreliable in 100 percent of patients tested. Exercise programs prescribed on the basis of this formula and these symptoms will result in 90 percent of patients exercising above their aerobic capacity, which will thus expose these patients to dangerously high levels of oxidant stress and mesenchymal acidosis. Even more ominous is the fact that when using these criteria, 68% of patients will be exercising 10 to 25 percent above their anaerobic threshold.

Discussion

That anaerobic threshold can be determined by pulmonary gas analysis is well established. (5) It occurs at the point in which lactic acid production becomes greatly accelerated due to the fact that, since energy needs can no longer be met by aerobic mechanisms, they must be met by anaerobic metabolism. In order to produce the same amount of ATP as aerobic metabolism, anaerobic metabolism must produce more than eighteen times the amount of lactic acid. Through the action of the enzyme carbonic anhydrase, the increasing levels of lactic acid are converted to carbon dioxide in order to avoid sustained metabolic acidosis. This increase in carbon dioxide can be measured in the expired pulmonary gases. Anaerobic threshold occurs when the levels of carbon dioxide exceed the rate of oxygen consumption. (6)

Although many studies have shown that increased total time exercising results in better health outcomes, there is evidence that overly intense exercise programs may be harmful. (7) This study demonstrates why. It is because the majority of people who exercise in America are not in a high enough level of fitness to perform intense exercise. For them, intense exercise, as is predicted by breathlessness and the predictive formula commonly used by exercise trainers, only results in increased oxidant stress and mesenchymal acidosis. Ironically enough, this is exactly what they are exercising to avoid. No doubt this is why the majority of people who enter into an exercise regime, either on their own or under the guidance of a fitness trainer, eventually stop the program. On some level, they realize it is not good for them.

Only two people in this study had an anaerobic threshold that was not below the predicted value. Both of these people were competitive athletes, and for them the predicted anaerobic threshold was too low. Using that model, they would not have been exercising to their maximum aerobic capacity, and thus not exercising efficiently.

Therefore, in this study of nineteen healthy subjects, the predictive formula studied was in significant error 100% of the time. We conclude that this formula is essentially useless. Furthermore, even when the more conservative formula, anaerobic threshold heart rate = .6 x (220 – age), is used, over 68% of the patients will still be exercising above their predicted aerobic capacity.

Based on this study, physicians should only be prescribing exercise programs based upon the true anaerobic threshold, as determined by individual measurement. This can be easily and accurately determined using a combination of a pulmonary gas analyzer and a computer program (Bio-Energy Testing) designed to determine the level at which carbon-dioxide production exceeds oxygen consumption.

TABLE 1

Name	Age	Estimated ATR	True ATR	TATR/EATR
Lawrence	67	130	97	–26%
Chuck	47	147	122	–18%
Miguel	19	170	136	–20%
Larry	58	137	136	n.s.
Joseph	68	129	105	–19%
Larry	60	136	115	–16%
John	71	126	109	–14%
Heinz	59	136	123	–10%
Karen	54	141	148	+4%
Alice	42	151	148	–2%
Karen	39	153	126	–18%
Maureen	50	144	135	–7%
Joy	69	128	112	–13%
Lauren	20	170	150	–12%
Alice	58	137	116	–16%
Cathie	52	142	119	–17%
Margaret	71	126	120	–5%
Susan	65	131	114	–13%
Frank	56	139	160	+15%

Highlighted TATR/EATR values represent patients who would have been exercising at least 10% over their anaerobic threshold if the estimated heart-rate formula had been applied. This is a point which is considered an extremely conservative estimation of anaerobic threshold heart rate.

References

Lee IM, Hsieh CC, Paffenbarger RS Jr, Exercise intensity and longevity in men. The Harvard Alumni Health Study. JAMA. 1995 Apr 19;273(15):1179–84.Jones TF, Eaton CB. Exercise prescription. *Am Fam Physician.* 1995 Aug;52(2):543–50, 553–5.

Harman D, 1984. Free radicals and the origin, evolution, and present status of the free radical theory of aging. *Free Radicals in Molecular Biology, Aging, and Disease,* ed. D. Armstrong et al. New York: Raven.

Levine SA, Kidd PM, *Antioxidant Adaptation—it's role in free radical pathology,* Biocurrents Division, San Leandro, CA, USA.

Pischinger A, 1975, *Matrix and Matrix Regulation,* Haug International, Brussels.

Wasserman K, Hansen JE, et al, 1999, *Principles of Exercise Testing and Interpretation,* Lippincott Williams and Wilkins.

Sherman SE, D'Agostino RB, Cobb JL, Kannel WB. Does exercise reduce mortality rates in the elderly? Experience from the Framingham Heart Study. *Am Heart J.* 1994 Nov;128(5):965.

Lee IM, Skerrett PJ. Physical activity and all-cause mortality: what is the dose-response relation? *Med Sci Sports Exerc.* 2001 Jun;33(6 Suppl):S459–71; discussion S493–4.

Shephard RJ. Absolute versus relative intensity of physical activity in a dose-response context. *Med Sci Sports Exerc.* 2001 Jun;33(6 Suppl):S400–18; discussion S419–20.

Smekal G, Pokan R, Baron R, Tschan H, Bachl N. Amount and intensity of physical exercise in primary prevention. *Wien Med Wochenschr.* 2001;151(1–2):7–12.

✳ APPENDIX C ✳

THE ENERGY DEFICIT THEORY OF AGING AND DISEASE

Frank Shallenberger, MD, HMD, ABAAM

"The world belongs to the energetic."

RALPH WALDO EMERSON, ESSAYIST & POET (1803–1882)

The well documented decline in energy production both at rest and under an exertional challenge that is uniformly seen in all aging populations has traditionally been thought to be a result of mitochondrial decay and aging. The author's research into the actual production of energy in healthy and diseased subjects of all ages refutes this concept.

A computer driven program utilizing respiratory oxygen uptake and carbon dioxide production analysis has been developed to measure energy production dynamics including ATP generation, fatty acid metabolism, and glucose metabolism. With this technology it has been possible to verify that a decrease in energy production exists *long before* any signs or evidence of mitochondrial decay or aging occurs. This early decrease in energy production is caused by two primary factors: decreased fatty acid utilization and decreased mitochondrial efficiency.

The author proposes that it is precisely this early decrease in energy production that is ultimately responsible for the observed mitochondrial decay that is associated with aging. By recognizing this early decrease in energy production and reversing or improving it to youthful levels, it is possible to delay and even reverse the processes of aging and mitochondrial decay.

Health is the presence of energy

Dorland's Medical Dictionary defines health as, "A state of optimal physical, mental, and social well-being, and not merely the absence of disease or infirmity." In other words, health is not the absence of anything, but rather is the optimal presence of something, that something being described by Dorland as "well-being".

The problem with this definition is that there is no way to objectively, scientifically, or quantitatively determine "well-being," and so the definition becomes clinically impractical. The fact that we have no effective way to measure health, whereas the measurement of disease is well established, is no doubt at the heart of why we have a disease oriented health care system rather than a wellness oriented system.

I agree that health is the optimal presence of something, and that that something is energy. Specifically energy as it is stored in ATP. Every single aspect of physical, mental, and emotional functioning is 100% dependent on ATP production. Combine this with the fact that ATP production decreases *long before* any sign or symptom of either aging or disease (discussed below), and you will understand that optimal health and optimal mitochondrial function are one in the same thing.

An article which appeared in 2000 by Wilson, TM & Tanaka H, entitled "Meta-analysis of the age associated decline in maximal aerobic capacity in men: relation to training status" dramatically demonstrates the relationship between health and mitochondrial function. (1)

In the article, using pulmonary gas analysis the researchers determined optimal mitochondrial function as defined by aerobic capacity. Aerobic capacity refers to the maximum amount of ATP production that can be produced without going into lactic acidosis. Thus, aerobic capacity is a measurement of optimal mitochondrial function.

According to the authors, "Maximal aerobic capacity is an independent risk factor for cardiovascular disease, cognitive dysfunction, and *all cause mortality.*"

When they addressed the subject of aging in particular, they went on to say that although most aspects of aging could be trained away in health conscious endurance trained men, "there continued to be a significant decline in aerobic capacity" in these very same men.

In other words, there is no better assessment of aging than optimal mitochondrial function as it is determined by aerobic capacity. All of the other aspects of aging such as insulin resistance, body mass composition, bone density, cardiovascular function, etc. can be reversed by training, and hence are simply measurements of conditioning, not aging per se. On the other hand, mitochondrial function cannot be trained away, and is therefore the best candidate for both health and aging measurement.

In another article, the researchers assayed the skeletal muscle mitochondrial function in 29 subjects aged 16–92 years, and noted a significant and consistent decline in mitochondrial function associated with age. (2)

The literature is replete with studies demonstrating the integral role that decreased mitochondrial function plays in the aging process. Specifically mentioned are

cellular processes affected by decreased mitochondrial function including detoxification, repair systems, DNA replication, osmotic balance, and higher order processes such as cognitive function.(3, 20)

Mitochondrial function and aging

There are two particular studies that have recently been published that rather dramatically identify mitochondrial dysfunction as the primary cause of aging. In the first study mice were genetically manipulated to develop four times more mutations in their mitochondrial DNA than the control mice. This resulted in a greatly accelerated reduction in mitochondrial function over their lifespan. The genetically altered mice had a significantly reduced lifespan compared to controls.

In addition, and perhaps even more to the point, they developed a premature onset of age-related phenotypes such as lean body mass loss, alopecia, kyphosis, anemia osteoporosis, reduced fertility, and cardiomegaly.

The authors concluded that the results provided a clear causative link between decreased mitochondrial function and aging.(4)

In a second study, using NMR technology the resting mitochondrial function was determined in a cohort of mice, and the mice were followed over the course of their lifespan.

A very significantly positive association between resting mitochondrial function and lifespan was noted, such that the mice in the upper quartile of resting mitochondrial function lived *36% longer* than the mice in the lowest quartile.(5)

Thus, it appears that the connection between optimal mitochondrial function, health, and aging is overwhelmingly clear, and that the primary goal towards optimizing health and decelerating aging is to maintain optimal mitochondrial function as we grow older. It is the single most consistent and predictable marker of aging.

Are you healthy for your age, or are you healthy?

Which brings us to the next question. What is aging? When used in the medical sense, aging is a term that refers to the progressive physical and mental deterioration that occurs as we get older. Although it certainly is associated with getting older, aging per se is a measurement of biological function, and as such is not the same as getting older.

For example, when a person goes from being 20 years old to being 30, although he has become 10 years older, from the medical perspective he has not aged because he has not undergone any physical or mental deterioration. Similarly, when he becomes 40, he is still said not to have aged for the same reason. So aging and getting older are not synonymous, they are only associated because as we get older, we develop decreased energy production secondary to decreased mitochondrial function.

Although getting older is not synonymous with aging, mitochondrial function is. In fact, nothing is as consistent and as predictable as the gradual, linear decline in energy production seen in all aging populations.(6)

And, as has already been pointed out, every aspect of biological function is directly dependent on mitochondrial function, which makes mitochondrial function the most *global* parameter of health.

Additionally, mitochondrial function not only influences all biological function, but it is also influenced by every single biochemical and physiological event. Virtually any defect that occurs in human physiology or biochemistry will affect mitochondrial function. Thus it is also arguably the most *sensitive* parameter of health possible.

Thus, it seems probable that only to the extent that it is possible to initiate therapies that can successfully maintain youthful mitochondrial function in patients as they become older, is it possible to stop or slow down the aging process.

While ultimately aging is inevitable, the dramatic rate and extent of aging that is commonly seen today may not be. This is why monitoring a patient's mitochondrial function is so important. Because more than anything else, the rate and extent of aging appears to be dependent on it.

What are diseases?

According to the dictionary, diseases are the names that are given to various "pathological conditions of the body" in which the organs and regulating systems become dysfunctional. Study after study has demonstrated that these systems become dysfunctional as a direct result of decreased mitochondrial function.

This is particularly true of the degenerative diseases of the neurological system, but is also true of liver disease, diabetes, cancer, and cardiovascular disease. So the single best way to help patients avoid degenerative disease is to initiate therapies that maximize energy production.(7, 8, 9, 10, 11, 12, 13)

One disease—One treatment

So in effect, no matter whether one is dealing with aging or disease prevention, one is by necessity dealing with mitochondrial function to such a degree that it may be said, "There is only one disease—decreased mitochondrial function, and there is only one treatment - maximizing mitochondrial function."

This statement reveals the potential appeal of objectively measuring a patient's mitochondrial function, because it is then possible to both diagnose the "one disease," and to monitor the "one treatment."

Majid Ali, MD, noted author, teacher, and physician, emphasizing the importance of disease prevention has frequently commented, "I measure the efficacy of a doctor's treatment more by how the patient is five years from now than how the patient is now." In this regard, perhaps nothing is more important than monitoring each patient's mitochondrial function in order to be sure that the treatment recommended is optimizing it.

Mitochondrial functional analysis

Using an FDA approved pulmonary gas analyzer, a bio-impedance body fat analyzer, a heart rate monitor, a computerized ergometer, and computer software it is possible to determine a patient's mitochondrial efficiency. By that is meant, how much ATP a patient's mitochondria are capable of producing, and whether it is being produced from fat or glucose.

The heart and soul of the testing procedure is the information received from the pulmonary gas analyzer, which determines two measurements: how much oxygen is being metabolized, and how much carbon dioxide is being produced.

When analyzed correctly, these two parameters can be used to determine a patient's mitochondrial functional dynamics, including:

1. Total Resting ATP production.
2. Resting ATP production from fatty acid metabolism.
3. Maximal ATP production from fatty acid metabolism.
4. Maximal aerobic ATP production (aerobic capacity).

Early onset mitochondrial dysfunction (EOMD)

Using mitochondrial functional analysis, 50 subjects were studied as they randomly presented to one of several clinics in Carson City, NV; Los Angeles; Grand Junction, CO; and Singapore. Each subject selected was between the ages of 20–40, asymptomatic, and health conscious enough to want to have their mitochondrial function checked for preventive reasons.

The results were as follows:

* 54% (27) had normal mitochondrial function.
* 46% (23) had decreased mitochondrial function.
* 36% (18) had < 90% of predicted mitochondrial function.
* 26% (13) had < 80% of predicted mitochondrial function.
* 12% (6) had < 60% of predicted mitochondrial function, and fell within the diagnostic category of severe dysfunction.

The results of this pilot study validate what I routinely see in my medical clinic. Close to half of these healthy, asymptomatic, young, health conscious subjects had decreased mitochondrial function. A quarter of them had less than 80% of predicted. An amazing 12% of them were in the diagnostic category of severe dysfunction, and could have been diagnosed as having chronic fatigue syndrome, and were eligible for disability had they been symptomatic.(15, 16, 17)

These patients were much too young to have mitochondrial decay or any of the other effects of the aging process, and they were much too healthy to have cardio-pulmonary disease. And yet almost half of them had evidence of mitochondrial dysfunction. This led me to my very first observation concerning mitochondrial function and health: **Aging and**

degenerative disease are *preceded* by a decrease in mitochondrial function which can often be severe and asymptomatic.

I have coined the term Early Onset Mitochondrial Dysfunction (EOMD) to refer to this condition. EOMD refers to a deterioration of mitochondrial function in the absence of actual mitochondrial decay.

Furthermore, while mitochondrial decay is irreversible, subsequent treatment of the subjects mentioned in the above study revealed that EOMD is completely reversible. While mitochondrial decay is a function of the aging process itself, EOMD is not.

Although further investigation has revealed that the incidence of EOMD increases with age, it occurs even in young subjects without any evidence of aging. Could it be that EOMD is what causes mitochondrial decay and aging? The answer to this question is discussed below.

Decreased fat metabolism and EOMD

But what causes this decrease in energy production in seemingly healthy people. To answer this question I began to carefully examine the breath by breath data files of all of the test results to look for a pattern which occurred in all those who tested out poorly and which did not show up in those few who tested out well.

Finally, a pattern began to emerge. *Every subject* with EOMD also had decreased ATP production from fat. They derived most of their ATP from glucose metabolism. This was markedly different from the 27 patients who had normal mitochondrial function. Of this group only 7% had decreased ATP production from fat.

Thus the common denominator noted in 100% of the EOMD group was that they were metabolizing very little fat as an energy substrate. In fact, while I had observed that the high ATP producers derived at least 75% or more of their resting energy from fat, the EOMD group often produced less than 20% of their resting energy from fat. Furthermore, the subjects with the lowest maximal ATP production also produced the lowest amount of ATP from fat both under resting and maximal conditions.

I even found some patients with extremely low levels of ATP who essentially burned *no fat at all* in a resting state. In contrast to this was the observation that those patients who had the highest levels of ATP production usually produced greater than 75% of their resting energy from fat. In addition, what was even more striking, in fact what amounted to 93% concordance, was the fact the really high energy producers also produced a much greater amount of ATP from fat while they were exerting as well.

The statistics were so striking that I was able to predict with 100% accuracy who would be the highest energy producers simply from examining how much ATP they produced from fat.

This then led me to my second observation about EOMD and energy production in general: **Total aerobic ATP production is 100% dependent on fat metabolism, such that the more efficiently ATP is produced from fat, the higher will be the total aerobic ATP production, and the less efficiently ATP is produced from fat, the lower will be the total aerobic ATP production.** Keep in mind that total aerobic ATP production refers to aerobic capacity, which is associated with aging, degenerative disease, and all cause mortality.

What causes EOMD?

The literature is replete with evidence to support a number of events which cause a pathological increase in free radical production leading to the irreversible mitochondrial damage referred to as mitochondrial decay. (19) It is mitochondrial decay which ultimately leads to organ degeneration and disease. In fact, there is a well-known and accepted theory of aging, the mitochondrial theory of aging, which alludes to these facts, and asserts that the very process of aging itself is simply the end result of mitochondrial decay.(2, 3, 4, 5, 20)

Pathological uncoupling leading to a proton leak across the mitochondrial membrane resulting in free radical damage to mitochondrial structures has long been considered the major factor leading to mitochondrial decay, but the presence of EOMD indicates that there is more to the story. Specifically, because there is a measurable decrease in mitochondrial function that occurs long before mitochondrial decay, it seems possible that EOMD is what causes mitochondrial decay. And, if EOMD causes mitochondrial decay, if it is corrected in time, it just might be possible to prevent or delay mitochondrial decay altogether.

So, what are the factors that can lead to EOMD? I have identified nine:

1. Decreased fat metabolism.
2. Nutritional deficiencies.
3. Sleep deprivation.
4. Hormonal deficiencies.

5. Toxicity.

6. Hypoxia.

7. Decreased methylation.

8. Ischemia.

9. Decreased fitness.

EOMD secondary to decreased fat metabolism

As mentioned above, a decrease in fat metabolism, both resting and maximal, appears to be the most common single characteristic of patients with EOMD. A decrease in ATP production from fat results in a corresponding decrease in total ATP production because other than during an occasional brief period of exertion, fat is the major substrate for ATP production. The fact that fat metabolism plays the key role in mitochondrial function is emphasized in a 2002 paper demonstrating that restoration of the "key mitochondrial enzyme carnitine acetyltransferase," which is solely involved in fat metabolism, "restores mitochondrial function, thus delaying mitochondrial decay and aging".(21)

The major cause of decreased fat metabolism, even in otherwise healthy young people is the excessive ingestion of carbohydrate. Let me offer a very graphic case example to make my point.

A 42 year-old movie actor presented to my clinic to have his mitochondrial function analyzed. He was an avid exerciser, and took an array of supplements as part of an anti-aging/preventive medicine program. He had no complaints, and his physical and routine laboratory examination was within normal limits other than a modest elevation of his serum triglyceride levels. Indeed, on casual observation, this young man looked like the epitome of health. Looks can be deceiving however, especially in health.

When tested, this man had a greater than 40% reduction in his total aerobic ATP production. This placed him in a category of severe EOMD. Additionally, in a resting state, his ATP production from fat was zero. This remarkable shift from fat to glucose metabolism which is so commonly seen in my young patients is undoubtedly setting them up for metabolic syndrome. I have learned not to be too surprised by such findings, and I immediately asked him about his diet. He confessed that every day for the previous two months he had been ingesting 2–3 milk shakes blended with cookies at a popular fast food restaurant.

I asked him to continue everything he was currently doing except to avoid the milk shakes along with all other carbohydrates including grains, fruit, legumes, and sugars. In three weeks he repeated his mitochondrial functional analysis and was happy to discover that his total aerobic ATP production had now climbed to 30% greater than predicted for a man two years younger. This represented a net improvement in mitochondrial function of greater than 70% simply from decreasing dietary carbohydrate. Not surprisingly, this second test revealed that his resting ATP production from fat was now maximal. Cases such as this one form the majority of what I see on a daily basis in my clinic.

It is important to reiterate here that excessive carbohydrate ingestion though it is the most common cause of decreased fat metabolism is not the only cause. Deficiencies of the thyroid hormones T4 and T3, the adrenal hormones cortisol and DHEA, and the anabolic hormones HGH, progesterone, DHEA, and testosterone also play a significant role. Other commonly encountered factors include insulin resistance, sleep deprivation, excessive dietary intake of trans fatty acids, and deficiencies of essential fats, amino acids, magnesium, B-vitamins, chromium, lipoic acid, coenzyme Q10, and l-carnitine. All of these nutrients are especially likely to be deficient in patients who eat excessive amounts of carbohydrates.

EOMD secondary to nutritional deficiencies

What nutritional imbalances and deficiencies could directly result in decreased mitochondrial function? In terms of the needed cofactors in the Krebs cycle and the electron chain system, the most worrisome deficiencies would be the B-vitamins, CoQ_{10}, magnesium, anti-oxidant vitamins (especially C and E), and the essential amino acids. Contrary to what is often preached, there is substantial evidence in the literature to suggest that many of our patients, especially those who are elderly, ill, or who are vegetarian commonly have less than optimal essential amino acid profiles.(22, 23, 24)

Due to their critical importance in metabolic methylation, a deficiency of the vitamins folinic acid and methylcobalamin would play a particularly important role in total ATP production because both ADP and phosphocreatine are methylation dependent. Using genomics, researchers are discovering that very common genetic variations cause certain individuals to require much higher than normal dietary intake of these vitamins in order to maintain optimal methylation.

Dietary fats are also critical for energy production. The entire electron chain rests on the inner mitochondrial membrane, which is composed completely of unsaturated essential fats. A deficiency of the essential fats omega 3 and 6 is quite common, and has been shown to result in defective membrane transport and fluidity.(25, 26) Additionally, hydrogenated and partially hydrogenated fats have been reported to act as uncoupling agents apparently due to their negative effect on the mitochondrial membrane function. (13, 27)

EOMD secondary to sleep deprivation

Another cause of EOMD is sleep deprivation, either self-inflicted or in the category of sleep disorders. In the 1950's the American Cancer Society conducted a very large study in an attempt to try and determine the major lifestyle factors that caused cancer and decreased lifespan in general. The study examined sleep habits as well as smoking, diet, cholesterol levels, blood pressure, exercise, etc. Over one million Americans were surveyed over a six-year interval, and the habits of those who had died during this period were identified. Out of all the factors studied, the amount of sleep time was the best predictor of mortality. The highest death rates for all ages were for those who slept four hours or less per night, and the lowest rates were for those who regularly slept eight hours.

Other investigators have published studies revealing similar outcomes. One study in particular looked at 1,600 adults between the ages of 36–50 and found that compared to good sleepers, poor sleepers were 6.5 times more likely to have any one of a variety of health problems. (28)

Dr. William Dement, founder and director of the Stanford University Sleep Research Center, and one of the original pioneers in the study of sleep states it very clearly and succinctly in his excellent book on sleep entitled, The Promise Of Sleep: "Healthful sleep has been empirically proven to be the single most important factor in predicting longevity, more influential than diet, exercise, or heredity. And yet we are a sleep-sick society, ignorant of the facts of sleep and the price of sleep deprivation."

According to a 1997 article in the *New York Times Magazine,* many sleep researchers believe that sleep deprivation is reaching "crisis proportions." This is a problem not just for serious insomniacs, but for the populace at large, the article said, and added: "People don't merely believe they're sleeping less; they are *in fact* sleeping less - perhaps as much as one and a half hours less each night than humans did at the beginning of the century - often because they choose to do so."

Several published studies have documented that lack of adequate sleep decreases fat metabolism, resting energy production, and exertional energy production.(29, 30, 31, 32) Many indications are that these effects of sleep deprivation are mediated through a combination of a deficient hormone and neurotransmitter production.

EOMD secondary to hormone deficiencies

Since anabolic hormones such as testosterone, progesterone, and growth hormone stimulate the utilization of ATP for protein synthesis and other cell regulative activities, in so doing they increase the levels of ADP. Elevated levels of ADP are a primary stimulator of mitochondrial function. Conversely, low levels of ADP act to decrease mitochondrial function.

Catabolic hormones such as cortisol, T4, and T3 also stimulate mitochondrial function by their direct effect on the nucleus of the cell. T3 in particular is also critical for optimal functioning of physiological uncoupling, which is also responsible for the increased mitochondrial production of heat and is a major stimulant of mitochondrial function

Finally, it should be noted that estrogen exerts a negative effect on both T3 and T4 by increasing the levels of thyroid hormone binding globulin, and hence creates a decrease in mitochondrial activity. This is precisely why women have a lower level of mitochondrial function than men, and also explains why it is so important in men to keep estrogen levels as low as possible, and in women to replace estrogen only in the smallest doses necessary to do the job.

EOMD secondary to toxicity

Heavy metals and pesticides are immediately lethal in a high enough dose, but even in low doses they have two toxic effects. One is as a direct source of oxidant stress, and the other is because both of these classes of toxins has been shown to increase pathological uncoupling which leads to a decrease in mitochondrial function.

Combined with the rather well established fact that modern man commonly has abnormally elevated levels of both pesticides and heavy metals such as arsenic, lead, and cadmium, it is not hard to imagine that many patients with EOMD are suffering from an increased toxic burden.

In addition to the toxins mentioned above are the toxic by-products of many of the bacteria and fungal organisms that reside in the gastrointestinal tract. Some of these ferments, for example tartaric acid, have been found to block certain steps in the Krebs cycle. (33) The overgrowth of these organisms is the result of deficient and damaged immune systems combined with the overuse of industrial and medical antibiotics. The World Health Organization has established that mycotoxins are a major source of disease and disability throughout the world.

EOMD secondary to hypoxia

Hypoxia refers to a decreased level of oxygen in the blood, and it is much more common than is often considered. Obviously since all mitochondrial function is oxygen dependent, hypoxia results in a significant decrease in mitochondrial function.

Hypoxia is one of those causes of decreased mitochondrial function which can occur even in young people. Smoking, for example, results in significant hypoxia. And for those who don't smoke, there is always the issue of passive exposure.

Another source of hypoxia is even more insidious, and that is decreased ambient oxygen levels associated with pollution and the greenhouse effect created in urban environments. In these environments ambient oxygen levels are decreased from the activity of combustion engines and not replenished due to an absence of adequate vegetation. Urban environments have been found to have significant decreases in ambient oxygen concentration in comparison to rural environments. (34)

Yet another quite common and perhaps underestimated source of decreased ambient oxygen is encountered in the construction of new energy efficient homes, offices, and apartment buildings. These constructions are often so airtight that very little outside air is able to enter the building. In the larger office and apartment buildings the ambient air is often re-circulated to the point that ambient oxygen levels become deficient. This is especially an issue in colder climates wherein it is in the interest of energy conservation to minimize the amount of fresh air being introduced into the system. Many people live and work on a continuous basis in such environments.

Sleep apnea is a very common cause of clinical hypoxia. Sleep apnea occurs secondary to upper airway obstruction either as a result of weight gain, alcohol, medications, or allergies. Sleep apnea can also be mediated from the central nervous system.

One more often overlooked source of hypoxia comes from low-level carbon monoxide exposure. The legal limit for occupational carbon dioxide exposure over a forty hour work week has been set at 9 ppm, but based on the amount of individual variation in hemoglobin structure this amount may be excessive for many.

Additionally, many homes, especially those in colder climates, have ventilation/pressure issues that actually draw carbon monoxide into the home, often resulting in clinical carbon monoxide poisoning.(36, 37, 38) I am aware of one case in particular of a fifteen year-old girl who developed symptoms that were diagnosed as lupus. For two years she was treated for this condition by her physicians, only to have it resolved when quite accidentally it was discovered that her home had excessive ambient levels of carbon monoxide. The most interesting aspect of the case was that the other members of her household did not seem to be affected.

Asthma is a disorder that has demonstrated a consistently increasing incidence for many years now. Moreover, studies have shown that sub-clinical reactive airway with mild brocho-constriction is often not diagnosed, especially in those who don't exercise. I routinely assess the O2 saturation of my patients, and I often find O2 sats less than 93% in patients who were not complaining of dyspnea on exertion and were not aware that they had a pulmonary disorder.

This has led me to believe that yet another source of hypoxia is undiagnosed, sub-clinical reactive airway disorder stemming from allergic reactions to molds, pesticides, food additives, petrochemical outgassing, etc.

Lastly is the issue of decreased oxygen dissociation. In this condition, oxygen fails to be released from the hemoglobin molecule, and as a result, even though it is being delivered to the capillary bed, it fails to be taken up by the mitochondria and metabolized into energy.

Two factors initiate the release of oxygen from hemoglobin. The first is an acid pH. Because acid in the forms of CO2 and lactate are the byproducts of our everyday metabolism, as oxygen demands increase with exertion and/or stress more acid is produced. This results in a decreasing pH in the capillary environment. Since hemoglobin loses its affinity for oxygen in a low pH environment, the lower pH stimulates the release of more O2 from hemoglobin to satisfy the increased demands.

Unfortunately however, this mechanism can be adversely affected by alkaline salts, which neutralize the physiological decrease in the capillary pH that occurs with increasing energy requirements. The infrequent use of such salts cannot be considered much of a problem. Chronic usage, however, such as occurs in persons routinely taking antacids, or those who constantly drink alkaline water to supposedly "remove the acid from the body," may lead to decreased mitochondrial function.

The second factor that results in decreased oxygen dissociation may be even more pervasive, and that is a decrease in the molecule 2,3,di-phoshoglycerate (2,3,DPG). 2,3 DPG is produced in the red cell in the pentose phosphate pathway as a result of glucose being metabolized to lactate. This reaction is catalyzed by oxidation, and therefore the levels of 2,3 DPG are typically much lower in persons who do not regularly exercise.

EOMD secondary to decreased methylation

There are three sources of ATP in the body. Two of them have already been discussed; that is ATP derived aerobically in the mitochondria, and ATP derived anaerobically in the cytosol. The third source is from a molecule called phosphocreatine. Phosphocreatine is formed in the cytosol when ATP transfers high energy phosphate to creatine. Phosphocreatine is able to store this high energy phosphate until an energy demand is created, at which time it will transfer it back to ADP to form ATP. Thus, phosphocreatine serves as a third source of ATP.

When phosphocreatine is converted to creatine as ADP is converted to ATP, since creatine is alkaline, the pH in the tissues is shifted toward an alkaline state. This alkaline shift causes the enzyme carbonic anhydrase to convert CO2 to HCO3, thus lowering the level of CO2. The decrease in CO2 is readily detected during mitochondrial functional analysis. This decrease will be maintained until the stores of phosphocreatine are exhausted, at which time CO2 levels will begin to climb in a linear fashion. By measuring the length of time of this initial depression of CO2, it is possible to quantify phosphocreatine.(18) But why is this important?

Creatine is synthesized when the amino acid S-adenosylmethionine (SAM) methylates guanidinoacetate to form creatine and

S-adenosylhomocysteine. About 70% of all methylation in the body is devoted to this critical reaction to create creatine.(40) Therefore, the amount of phosphocreatine in the body is directly correlates with the process of methylation. To the extent that there is a phosphocreatine deficiency in the body, there is a concomitant methylation deficiency. Thus, mitochondrial functional analysis provides a way to easily diagnose and quantify methylation disorders.

But methylation is not only critical for the formation of ATP through the above mentioned reaction, it is equally critical in energy production because of its importance in adenosine production. Adenosine is the base from which ATP (adenosine triphosphate) is produced. Adenosine is produced when S-adenosylhomocysteine is hydrolysated to adenosine and homocysteine. Note that unless SAM is converted to S-adenosylhomocysteine through the methylation of guanidinoacetate to form creatine, no adenosine will be formed. Such a deficiency of adenosine will result in a depletion of ADP, ultimately resulting in the kind of pathological mitochondrial uncoupling that shuts down and eventually destroys the mitochondria.

But these observations are not just interesting academic perusings, they are in fact clinically useful. I refer to the initial depression of CO2 that is seen during mitochondrial functional analysis as the "methylation curve". The length and the depth of the methylation curve can be used to quantify an individual's ability to methylate.

What is uniformly observed is that the subjects with the highest levels of ATP production, are also those with the longest and deepest methylation curves, indicating an optimally functioning methylation process. Likewise, the subjects with lower levels of ATP production unvaryingly demonstrate little to no methylation curve, indicating both sub-optimal methylation, and an inability to produce phosphocreatine secondary to deficient ATP production.

Those who are familiar with methylation disorders will recognize that they often occur as a result of mercury toxicity, casein allergy, and genetic predisposition. Furthermore, methylation disorders can often be corrected with the orthomolecular administration of folinic acid, trimethylglycine, pyridoxine, and methycobalamin. It is interesting to note that when subjects with EOMD who also show a depressed or absent methylation curve are given these substances, they often rather dramatically show a substantial improvement in both measurements.

EOMD secondary to ischemia

Ischemia refers to a decrease in the delivery of blood to the capillary bed. This leads to decreased oxygen delivery to the cells, and causes the same kind of decrease in energy production observed with hypoxia. Ischemia however, has a much greater negative effect on mitochondrial function than hypoxia. This is because with ischemia there is not only decreased oxygen delivery, but also decreased delivery of all the cofactors of oxygen metabolism such as vitamins, mineral, fats, and glucose. Additionally, ischemia causes decreased removal of carbon dioxide.

Perhaps the single most common cause of ischemia in today's society is from decreased cardiac output secondary to sedentary lifestyle. Using the mitochondrial functional analysis protocol it is possible to estimate cardiac output with some precision. I rarely find that a subject with decreased mitochondrial function has a normal cardiac output.

A much more significant cause for ischemia would be stress and the resultant increase in vasoconstriction from increased sympathetic tone. There is a lot of published data on the vaso-constrictive effects of stress on circulation. (41, 42, 43, 44) These studies clearly verify that perceived stress such as simply hearing bad news can immediately create detectable ischemia in both heart and finger tissues. Similarly, the stress from chronic pain or other stressful symptoms can create ischemia.

Another cause of ischemia is atherosclerosis. The level of atherosclerosis can be quite considerable in patients over the age of forty even in the absence of clinical symptoms such as claudication or angina. In most cases, ischemia due to atherosclerosis will be subclinical, and will only be picked up by stress testing such as occurs with mitochondrial functional analysis.

Another cause of systemic ischemia in many patients comes secondary to an immune system activation of the coagulation cascade as described in a brilliant paper by David Berg, L.H. Berg, and J. Couvaras entitled, "Is CFS/FM due to an undefined hypercoagulable state brought on by immune activation of coagulation."(45) Ischemia from abnormal coagulation secondary to chronic inflammation is a very common cause of decreased mitochondrial function.

Ischemia can also be caused by decreased endothelial function at the level of the capillary wall. The decreased function of the endothelial cells which makeup the capillary wall results in edema of these cells with a resultant decrease in circulation and perfusion. This condition has been well described by Manfred von Ardenne is his book *Oxygen Multi-Step*

Therapy. According to Dr. von Ardenne, decreased endothelial function as a cause for decreased mitochondrial function is altogether common in many presumably healthy people.(46) Not surprisingly, I have often found that the mitochondrial dysfunction in patients whom I suspected had this disorder improves significantly using Dr. von Ardenne's stepped oxygen exercise protocol.

Lastly, please reflect on the fact that many of the same conditions that create hypoxia can also result in ischemia. Thus it is not unreasonable to assume that in many patients the two conditions coexist and act synergistically to appreciably impair energy production.

EOMD secondary to decreased fitness

Many people mistakenly assume that early onset decreases in mitochondrial function are simply a matter of decreased fitness resulting in decreased cardiac output and decreased lung function. While fitness level is certainly a factor in the EOMD so commonly detected in the individual who is over fifty years old, it can hardly explain the EOMD observed in the young and health conscious. It should also be noted that a significant number of my patients of all ages who demonstrate EOMD are already regularly exercising. A recent publication helps to illustrate the point that EOMD is not simply a function of fitness.

The authors performed a meta-analysis of mitochondrial function studies in aging men, and compared the incidence of EOMD in exercisers with highly trained marathon runners. The authors underlined the increasing frequency of EOMD in men as they became older. They also pointed out that EOMD

"is an independent risk factor for cardiovascular disease, cognitive dysfunction, and all cause mortality." Additionally, they demonstrated that even highly trained marathon runners consistently had significant EOMD, clearly indicating that there are other factors affecting mitochondrial function than fitness.(1)

The above caveat having been expressed, there is certainly no doubt that exercise does indeed play a major role in mitochondrial function. Irrcher et al. in a 2003 article on the subject point out that a program of regular endurance exercise improves mitochondrial function, induces mitochondrial generation (biogenesis), and delays the progression of aging.(47) Other studies document the beneficial role of exercise in the heart and the brain (48, 49, 50)

But not all exercise is equivalent. Statistical studies are repeatedly showing that moderate exercise seems to have a more beneficial effect than intense exercise, secondary to the excessive free radical activity induced when subjects with EOMD exercise beyond their aerobic capacity.(51) I have already published one paper on this subject which demonstrated that due to the commonality of EOMD, the majority of persons exercising today are doing so at levels which exceed their mitochondrial capacity.(52)

Nevertheless, when properly performed, exercise improves mitochondrial function, increases anti-oxidant buffering capacity, decreases oxidant stress, and increases longevity in both humans and animals.(53)

Chapter Five - EOMD, through the combined action of increased free radical formation and decreased anti-oxidant buffering capacity is the primary cause of mitochondrial decay, aging, and degenerative disease.

Mitochondrial decay induced by excessive free radical activity is known to be the intrinsic cause of aging and degenerative disease. This forms the central basis for the Free Radical Theory of Aging.(2, 3, 4, 5, 19, 54) EOMD occurs in the young, before any signs or evidence of mitochondrial decay. The evidence is strong that EOMD is the primary cause of mitochondrial decay, and hence the ultimate cause of aging and degenerative disease. The implication of this statement is important, because EOMD is preventable and even reversible, and if EOMD causes mitochondrial decay then mitochondrial decay, aging, and degenerative disease can be minimized by measuring and treating EOMD.

EOMD causes mitochondrial decay by initiating a viscous cycle chain of reactions as follows: 1. a decline in mitochondrial function caused by the nine factors mentioned in the last chapter; 2. a resultant increase in the production of free radicals as a result of the "functional hypoxia" induced by 1; 3. an accumulation of mitochondrial DNA mutations; 4. a further increase in the oxidative damage to DNA, protein, and lipids (particularly the inner mitochondrial membrane which houses the entire electron transport chain); 5. a subsequent decrease in the capacities of oxidatively damaged proteins and other critical macromolecules further impairing mitochondrial function. 6. an increase in the turnover rate of anti-oxidant buffering enzymes as a result of increased free radical production combined with a decrease in the production of these enzymes as a result of impaired mitochondrial function. The result of this cycle of events is a simultaneous increase in free radical production with a decrease in free radical buffering capacity.(55)

This viscous cycle is really brought home in an article entitled, "Oxidative damage and mutation to mitochondrial DNA and age-dependent decline of mitochondrial respiratory function." In this article the authors are depicting EOMD when they describe the "gradual impairment of respiratory function" which increases with age. They go on to state, "An immediate consequence of such gradual impairment of the respiratory function is the increase in the production of the reactive oxygen species (ROS) and free radicals in the mitochondria through the increased electron leak of the electron transport chain. Moreover, the intracellular levels of anti-oxidants and free radical buffering enzymes are gradually altered. These two compounding factors lead to an age-dependent increase in the fraction of the ROS and free radical that may escape the defense mechanism and cause oxidative damage to various biomolecules in tissue cells." They conclude by stating that it is these two processes, decreased oxidant buffering capacity and increased ROS production, which are responsible for the age-dependent process of mitochondrial decay.(56)

It is important to note here that the ROS mentioned above are formed in direct proportion to the proton gradient formed across the mitochondrial membrane as part of the function of the electron transfer chain. The greater the gradient, the more ROS are formed. Of course one very obvious way to decrease the gradient and to thereby limit the production of ROS is to allow the protons to re-enter the mitochondria through complex five, which converts ADP to ATP. As long as there is a significant amount of ADP complex five will function very well in this manner. However, four of the factors leading to EOMD mentioned in the last chapter, methylation disorders, nutritional deficiencies, hormonal deficiencies, and decreased levels of fitness, also result in the decrease of available ADP, resulting in greater ROS formation.

Another way to reduce the proton gradient and thus decrease ROS formation is through uncoupling proteins. These are proteins that are on the mitochondrial membrane which allow protons to re-enter the mitochondria without the need for ADP. The most active of these uncoupling proteins is activated by the thyroid hormone triiodothyronine, and it is via this method of decreasing the mitochondrial proton gradient that this critical thyroid hormone serves to prevent mitochondrial decay. The point here is that many of my patients with EOMD, even those with values for serum TSH, T3, and T4, which are in range, show a decrease in their resting ATP production as well as a decrease in maximal ATP production.

The most common cause for a decrease resting ATP production is hypothyroidism. Additionally, hypothyroidism is also a cause of decreased maximal ATP production. This observation has made me believe that sub-clinical hypothyroidism is much more common than it is currently thought to be, and may be a particularly onerous component of EOMD. It also serves to explain why one recently published animal study demonstrated that mice in the upper quartile of resting ATP production lived 36% longer than those in the lowest quartile.(5)

Levine and Kidd in their classic text Antioxidant Adaptation—Its Role In Free Radical Pathology emphasize that free radical pathology is an inherent result of hypoxia. On page 133 they state, "an oxygen deficit can be toxic to the cell by exacerbating free radical generation in membranes housing electron transfer assemblies." This free radical generation destroys the mitochondrial membranes housing the electron transfer assemblies, which decreases mitochondrial function while at the same time increasing the electron leak through the membranes. The increased electron leak leads to a further increase in free radical generation, all of which ultimately results in mitochondrial decay.

They go on further to state that, "The patterns of cellular damage from ischemic/hypoxic insult, which have been well studied, parallel those seen following inhibition of cellular ATP production....". Inhibition of cellular ATP production is what we are seeing in EOMD, and Levine and Kidd state that from a pathological perspective it is tantamount to classical hypoxia. On page 136 they further clarify this inhibited state of ATP production when they equate classical hypoxia to impaired oxygen utilization using the term "functional hypoxia," "Cellular hypoxia can result from deficiency of oxygen delivery (ischemia/hypoxia) or impaired oxygen utilization (functional hypoxia)."(57)

In essence, the terms "impaired oxygen utilization," "functional hypoxia," and "EOMD" are identical in implication. They all describe the same pathological mechanisms that exist in classical hypoxia, all of which lead to mitochondrial decay. The proposed mechanism by which EOMD causes mitochondrial decay, aging, and degenerative disease is pictured in Figure 1 (see following page).

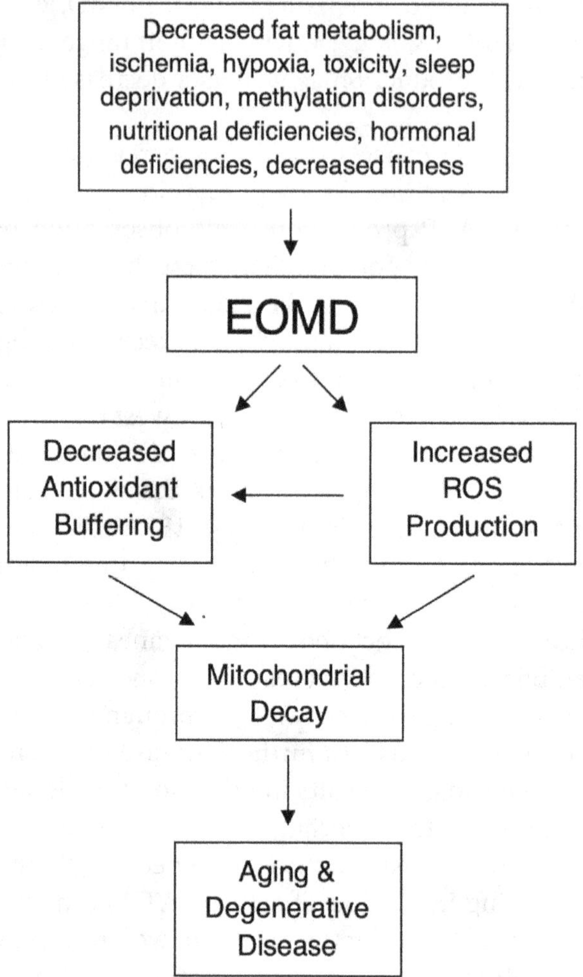

Chapter Six—The Energy Deficit Theory of Aging and Disease

After reflecting on the above observations, I made the following postulations, which I have called the Energy Deficit Theory of Aging and Disease.

1. Degenerative disease and aging are *preceded* by early onset mitochondrial dysfunction (EOMD), which occurs *long before* actual mitochondrial decay, and commonly occurs in the young and asymptomatic. The presence and extent of EOMD can be determined by mitochondrial functional testing.

2. EOMD results from two commonly occurring states:
   * Decreased pre-mitochondrial fat metabolism, which leads to
   * Decreased mitochondrial function, which is further compromised by ischemia, hypoxia, toxicity, sleep deprivation, methylation disorders, nutritional deficiencies, hormonal deficiencies, decreased fitness.
3. EOMD creates a state of "functional hypoxia," which through the combined action of increased free radical formation and decreased anti-oxidant buffering capacity is the primary cause of mitochondrial decay, aging, degenerative disease.
4. The processes causing EOMD, and hence the processes causing aging and degenerative disease can be decelerated and even reversed by altering these two states to improve mitochondrial function. The degree of success or failure in this endeavor can be documented using mitochondrial functional testing.

Energy Deficit Theory not the same as Mitochondrial Theory

The Energy Deficit Theory is not just the Mitochondrial Theory repackaged into different terminology. The Mitochondrial Theory looks at energy deficit states exclusively in terms of mitochondrial decay as a result of oxidative damage to mitochondrial DNA. The Mitochondrial Theory states that aging occurs as a result of mitochondrial decay and as such is not reversible. The Energy Deficit Theory offers a unique slant on how this happens and what comes first.

Like the Energy Deficit Theory, the Mitochondrial Theory recognizes that there is a steady, linear, and predictable decrease in energy production associated with aging. But unlike the Energy Deficit Theory, the Mitochondrial Theory assumes that this decrease in energy production is purely a result of aging, and as such is after the fact. The Energy Deficit Theory states that the observed decrease occurs *long before* aging has occurred, and hence is the root cause of aging. More importantly, the Energy Deficit Theory states the factors causing this decrease in energy production, and hence what can be done to retard and reverse it.

For the past 3000 years the Chinese have utilized a system of medicine that determines energy production by a subjective evaluation of pulses and physical findings. They use the word "chi" to refer to energy production. They hypothesized that all disease proceeds from a decrease in chi, and that health is best maintained over time by increasing chi through various exercises, acupuncture, dietary protocols, and medications. The Energy Deficit Theory is directly allied to this basic concept, and further describes in scientific terms the factors that lead to a decrease in chi. Let's look at how this can be done.

The man behind the curtain

The pulmonary gas analyzer measures the real time breath by breath consumption of oxygen and production of carbon dioxide, and the computer then records all the readings. Due to the effects of coughing, sighing, and other forms of irregular breathing which are virtually always encountered during any form of pulmonary testing, there are a significant number of artifacts in the recorded readings which do not accurately reflect true oxygen and carbon dioxide levels. The computer program identifies these artifacts and eliminates them.

It then takes the remaining readings, averages them, and uses them to calculate ATP production using the various algorithms described in the sections below.

Measuring aerobic ATP production

Almost all of the oxygen that is consumed in the human body is consumed in the mitochondria to produce energy. Although a small percentage is used as part of the oxidative burst of the activated immune system and also as part of the P450 detoxification systems in the liver, as long as the subject's immune system is not actively fighting an infection, and as long as there is no acute toxicity, it can be safely assumed that in a fasting individual all oxygen consumed is being consumed in the mitochondria.

Thus, ATP can be measured as a function of oxygen uptake as follows:

$$\text{Fatty Acid} + 23O2 \rightarrow 16CO2 = 16H2O + 130ATP$$
$$\text{Glucose} + 6O2 \rightarrow 6CO2 + 6H2O + 36ATP$$

Thus when fatty acids are metabolized by oxygen, there is a ratio of 5.6 (130/23) molecules of ATP produced per molecule of oxygen consumed. By measuring oxygen consumption, the amount of ATP being produced can be easily determined by multiplying this amount by 5.6.

In the case of glucose, there is a ratio of six molecules of ATP being produced per molecule of oxygen being consumed (36/6). Again, simply measure oxygen consumption and you can quickly determine ATP production by multiplying this amount by 6. Note also that glucose results in 7% more ATP production per molecule of oxygen than fat, which is why glucose metabolism is said to be a more efficient form of energy production than fat metabolism.

Fat or glucose?

The only problem with this particular scenario is that because glucose and fat produce different amounts of ATP per O2, in order to determine total ATP production with any degree of accuracy, it is at all times necessary to know whether the oxygen being consumed is metabolizing glucose or fatty acids. Fortunately, the above equations can also be used to solve this problem since the substrate being metabolized by oxygen can easily be determined by the amount of carbon dioxide being simultaneously produced.

For example, when glucose is being metabolized there is a one to one ratio of carbon dioxide produced to oxygen consumed. Since the pulmonary gas analyzer measures CO2 production as well as O2 consumption, it can be determined that oxygen is metabolizing exclusively glucose when the recorded ratio is one.

Likewise, since when fatty acids are being metabolized there is a ratio of .7 molecules of CO2 produced for every molecule of O2 being consumed, it can be determined that oxygen is metabolizing exclusively fatty acids when the ratio of CO2 to O2 is .7.

When the ratio of CO2 to O2 is between .7 and 1, an easy mathematical formula can determine the exact proportions of fat and glucose being metabolized since the relationship between .7 and 1 turns out to be linear. Thus, when all calculations are performed, it is possible to determine with great accuracy how much ATP is being produced from each source, and hence the total amount of ATP can be accurately calculated.

Resting ATP production

Resting ATP production can be determined in a subject by measuring the oxygen consumption and the carbon dioxide production while he is quietly resting in a relaxed, reclined position. The measurements should be made when the patient's heart rate is within 5 beats of his heart rate when he first wakes up from sleep, thus insuring a basal reading.

Measured Resting ATP Production (MR-ATP) is determined using the following variation of the Lusk formula: (14)

$$\text{MR-ATP} = \{5.676(\text{ARO2}) + 1.584(\text{ARCO2})\} \times C$$

Where: ARO2 = Average Resting O2 Consumption
ARCO2 = Average Resting CO2 Production
C is a constant, relating oxygen consumed to ATP produced.

Predicted Resting ATP Production (PR-ATP) can be estimated using a variation of the classic Harris-Benedict formulas for basal metabolic rate as follows:

$$\text{PR-ATP Men} = \frac{\{66.473 + 13.7616(\text{weight}) + 1.8496(\text{height}) - 4.6756(\text{age})\} \times C}{6.95}$$

$$\text{PR-ATP Women} = \frac{\{655.095 + 9.536(\text{weight}) + 1.8496(\text{height}) - 4.6756(\text{age})\} \times C}{6.95}$$

Where C is a constant, relating oxygen consumed to ATP produced.

Using the above formulas, it is then possible to obtain a percent predicted determination of resting ATP production as follows:

$$\text{Resting ATP production} = \frac{(\text{MR-ATP}) \times 100}{\text{PR-ATP}}$$

Two additional factors should come into play when making these calculations. The first is age. Since from an anti-aging and disease prevention perspective we are looking to maintain youthful levels of ATP production as the patient gets older, it does not make sense to evaluate energy production as a factor of age. In other words, we want our patients to be healthy, not "healthy for their age".

There is general agreement in the anti-aging, exercise physiology, and longevity literature that for all practical purposes, the effects of aging do not begin to become appreciable until after the age of forty. Hence, a reasonable benchmark for ATP production when looking to maintaining youthful levels would be those levels that are typical of a forty year-old individual.

Therefore, when calculating the resting mitochondrial function of a person over the age of forty, the default age of forty is used. Thus in the case of an individual older than forty, no matter what his age is, his resting mitochondrial function will reflect what would be considered normal and expected for a forty year-old of the same sex, weight, and height. Persons younger than forty are compared to their own age group.

The second factor that must be taken into consideration for the calculation of resting mitochondrial function is percent body fat. Notice that ATP production using the above variation on the Harris-Benedict equations is positively correlated with weight. The more a person weighs the higher the predicted ATP production.

But excess stored fat is metabolically inert tissue. Thus, using the Harris-Benedict equations as they are classically used would result in unreasonably higher predicted levels of ATP production in persons who have an excess of body fat. This will cause them to have a falsely depressed reading for resting mitochondrial function secondary to the artifact of excessive body fat.

Thus, to account for this potential inaccuracy, the weight used in determining predicted resting ATP production is corrected using a body fat analysis as follows:

* The weight of overweight men is corrected to a weight based upon an ideal body fat of 18%.
* The weight of overweight women is corrected to an ideal body fat of 22%.

Resting ATP production from fatty acids (rATP- FA)

To repeat what was already mentioned above, when glucose is being metabolized, there is a one to one ratio of carbon dioxide produced to oxygen consumed. When fat is being metabolized the ratio is .7. Since the pulmonary gas analyzer measures CO_2 production as well as O_2 consumption, the percentage of fat being metabolized can be determined by examining this ratio.

Based upon my own measurements and those published, a healthy person should be able to produce at least 75% of his total ATP production while at rest from fatty acids. (15, 16, 17)

Less than that indicates impaired fatty acid metabolism. A calculation of resting ATP production from fatty acids (rATP-FA) is formulated which determines the percentage of ATP being produced from fatty acids in the subject while at rest. The formula for this calculation is as follows:

rATP-FA = 283.52 – (Average resting CO2/O2 ratio) x 235.29

* A rATP-FA greater than 100 indicates that the subject is producing at least 75% of his resting ATP from fat, which points to optimal resting fat metabolism.
* A rATP-FA less than 100 indicates that the subject is progressively producing less than 75% of his resting ATP from fat, which points to less than optimal resting fat metabolism.
* A rATP-FA of 50 indicates that the subject is not producing any resting ATP at all from fat, which points to a severe impairment of resting fat metabolism.

rATP-FA and carbohydrate intake

There is an inverse linear relationship between carbohydrate intake as a percentage of total caloric intake and resting fatty acid metabolism.(18) The physiological reasons behind this observation are numerous but basically have to do with pre-mitochondrial factors affecting lypolysis, fatty acid mobilization, beta-oxidation of fatty acids, and fatty acid transportation into the mitochondria. These factors are sole and separate from mitochondrial function per se, and they will be discussed in detail in a later section. In its most simple terms the finding can be explained by the reasoning that when presented with dietary carbohydrate the body will elect to metabolize that carbohydrate rather than to store it for later use and in the meantime rely on fatty acid metabolism. Thus, the greater the intake of carbohydrate as a percentage of total calories, the lower will be the rATP-FA.

As one would expect, this inverse relationship is quite individual. There are some subjects who can have a relatively high intake of carbohydrates and yet still maintain an optimal rATP-FA, whereas my observation is that the majority of persons must maintain a very modest intake of carbohydrates in order to avoid an impaired rATP-FA. For these reasons, the clinical implications of rATP-FA primarily have to do with carbohydrate intake, and are as follows:

* A C-Factor greater than 100 indicates that the subject is eating an optimal amount of carbohydrate for his genetics and lifestyle.

* A C-Factor less than 100 indicates that the subject's intake of carbohydrates is excessive and is progressively impairing his rATP-FA.
* A C-Factor of 50 indicates that the subject's intake of carbohydrates is so excessive that it is completely suppressing his rATP-FA. In this case the subjects resting ATP production is resulting completely from glucose metabolism.

It is important to also note that besides the pre-mitochondrial effects of carbohydrate intake, rATP-FA is also influenced by factors which specifically affect mitochondrial function such as hormones, ADP availability, toxicity, specific nutrients, sleep habits, methylation, fitness, etc. However, because the demand for ATP is so minimal in a resting state, these factors usually exert a negligible effect on rATP-FA compared to the carbohydrate effect. Additionally, because these factors play a very significant role in maximal ATP production from fatty acids (see mATP-FA below) than they do in resting fat metabolism, they can be excluded as causes of a decreased rATP-FA in the event that the mATP-FA measurement is adequate.

So in summary, a decreased rATP-FA is almost always an indicator of excessive dietary carbohydrate intake. Sometimes the amount of dietary carbohydrate required to optimize rATP-FA is quite small. In fact, after observing the rATP-FA of hundreds of patients, I can report that there are a great many people who seem to be genetically programmed such that in order to produce an optimum rATP-FA they must eat almost no carbohydrate at all!

When both the rATP-FA and the mATP-FA are decreased, not only is dietary carbohydrate consumption in excess, but any combination of the other factors mentioned above are also at play.

Maximal ATP production from fatty acids mATP-FA

Once the resting energy production readings have been determined, the mitochondrial function analysis protocol calls for exercising the subject on a specialized stationary bicycle called an ergometer. The resistance on the ergometer is programmed by the computer to steadily increase according to a rate that is compatible with the subject's level of strength and fitness.

As the subject begins to increasingly exert, the rising energy demands cause him to metabolize increasing amounts of fat into ATP.

However, since fat metabolism is not as fast and as energy efficient as glucose metabolism, as the energy demands continue to escalate increasing amounts of glucose are mobilized into ATP.

Finally, a level of exertion is arrived at wherein the maximal amount of fat that the subject is able to metabolize is reached. Beyond this point, due to the steadily increasing energy demands, the subject will metabolize progressively more glucose and less fat to meet the rising ATP needs. This point occurs when the ratio of carbon dioxide produced to oxygen consumed is .85. Thus when the CO_2/O_2 ratio reaches .85, the subject is producing the maximal amount of ATP from fat that he is capable of. Beyond this point, as exercise intensity steadily increases, the subject will be metabolizing progressively less fat and more glucose until at some point he will be metabolizing no fat at all. At this second point, all ATP production will come entirely from glucose.

Based upon my own measurements and those published, a healthy person should be able to produce at least 60% of his total aerobic ATP production from fat.(18) Less than that indicates impaired fat metabolism. This is usually a consequence of both pre-mitochondrial factors such as excessive carbohydrate intake, impaired lipolysis, impaired fatty acid mobilization, impaired beta-oxidation of fatty acids, and impaired fatty acid transportation into the mitochondria, and mitochondrial factors such as hormone deficiencies, ADP deficiency, toxicity, nutrient deficiencies, sleep deprivation, impaired methylation, decreased fitness, etc.

Thus, mATP-FA refers to the maximal amount of ATP that the subject's mitochondria are able to produce from fatty acids, and therefore serves as a cross check of the factors mentioned in the previous paragraph. It is a percentage calculation, which compares the predicted maximal ATP production from fat in a subject with what is actually measured. The formula for mATP-FA is as follows:

$$\text{mATP-FA} = \frac{(\text{ATP Max Fat}) \times C \times 100}{(\text{PM-ATP}) \times .6}$$

Where: ATP Max Fat = O_2 consumption when the ratio of CO_2 produced to O_2 consumed = .85

PM-ATP = Predicted Maximal ATP Production

C is a constant, relating oxygen consumed to ATP produced.

Predicted Maximal ATP Production (PM-ATP) can be estimated

using a variation of the Wasserman-Hansen-Sue formulas
for predicted peak oxygen uptake as follows:

PM-ATP Men = {weight x (50.72 - .372 x age)} x C

PM-ATP Women = {(weight + 43) x (22.78 - .17 x age)} x C

Where C is a constant, relating oxygen consumed to ATP produced.

* An mATP-FA greater than 100 indicates that the subject is able to produce at least 60% of his maximal predicted ATP production from fat. This points to optimal fat metabolism.
* An mATP-FA less than 100 indicates that the subject is progressively producing less than 60% of his maximal predicted ATP production from fat. This points to less than optimal fat metabolism.
* An mATP-FA less than 70 indicates that the subject is producing less than 30% of his maximal predicted ATP production from fat. This points to a severe impairment of fat metabolism.

Maximal aerobic ATP production (maxATP)

Maximal aerobic ATP production can be established by measuring O2 consumption under exertional conditions. It is important to note here that maximal aerobic ATP refers to ATP that is produced entirely from glucose metabolism. No fat metabolism is involved at all. This is because at this maximal level of exertion it is not possible to adequately generate ATP from fat because fat cannot be mobilized as quickly as glucose and fat cannot produce as much energy per molecule of oxygen as can glucose. Therefore, at this point of exertion it is not necessary to use CO2 production in the equations to determine fat metabolism.

maxATP is a percentage calculation, which compares the expected or predicted maximal aerobic ATP production in a subject with what is actually measured. The formula for maxATP is simple:

$$\text{maxATP} = \frac{\text{(Measured Maximal ATP Production)}}{\text{Predicted Maximal ATP Production}} \times 100$$

Measured Maximal ATP Production (MM-ATP) is determined using
the following formula:

MM-ATP = (Average Maximal O2 Consumption) x C

Where C is a constant, relating oxygen consumed to ATP produced.

Predicted Maximal ATP Production (PM-ATP) can be estimated using a variation of the Wasserman-Hansen-Sue formulas for predicted peak oxygen uptake as follows:

PM-ATP Men = {weight x (50.72 - .372 x age)} x C

PM-ATP Women = {(weight + 43) x (22.78 - .17 x age)} x C

Where C is a constant, relating oxygen consumed to ATP produced.

The additional factors of excessive body fat percentage and age, which I described above in the section on resting ATP production also come to play when determining maxATP. Therefore, in all calculations of maxATP the patient's real age is only used when he is younger than forty. When calculating the maxATP of a person over the age of forty, the default age of forty is used. Similarly, excess body fat is corrected for using body fat analysis.

Correcting for anaerobic ATP production

In a resting state, the primary fuel for oxidation in the healthy individual is fat, and the ratio of CO2 produced to O2 consumed is around .7. As the subject begins to increasingly exert, since fat metabolism is not as fast and as energy efficient as glucose metabolism, progressively more glucose is mobilized to meet the rising energy demands. As this occurs the ratio of CO2 produced to O2 consumed begins to steadily increase in a linear fashion until a level of exertion has been reached that can only be met by glucose metabolism.

This point is noted when the ratio of CO2 produced to O2 consumed is equal to one. It represents the point at which ATP production from oxygen has reached its maximum. Until this point has been reached the amount of anaerobic ATP production is minimal and need not be accounted for.

However, once the aerobic production of ATP has reached its maximum, as the subject continues to progressively increase his exertion level beyond this point, he will begin to produce ATP anaerobically. At this point two factors about anaerobic ATP production come to play:

* Lactic acid is an essential byproduct of anaerobic ATP production.

* In order to produce the same amount of ATP anaerobically that is produced aerobically, nineteen times as much acid is produced in the form of lactic acid.

As a result of the carbonic anhydrase enzyme system, which the body uses to buffer blood pH, this excessive lactic acid is immediately converted to CO2:

Lactic Acid + HCO3 → H2O + CO2

Therefore, the point at which the anaerobic production of ATP occurs can be determined by a sudden acceleration in the previously linear rate at which the ratio of CO2 produced to O2 consumed had been increasing.

When the subject eventually reaches this point, the computer determines it and ends all calculation of ATP production, and the exercise portion of the test is concluded. Therefore, the amount of ATP that is recorded does not reflect any anaerobic ATP production. It only reflects ATP produced in the mitochondria.

In mitochondrial functional analysis anaerobic ATP production is not measured because it is produced in the cytosol of the cell and does not reflect mitochondrial production. Additionally, from the standpoint of health, aging, and disease, the ability to produce anaerobic energy is not important. Only aerobic ATP production has been shown to be correlated with degree of aging and with all cause mortality. Anaerobic ATP production has no similar correlation.

This is a very important distinction because many patients who score low maxATP values may in fact state that they exercise and feel as though they have much more energy than mitochondrial functional analysis gives them credit for. What they don't appreciate is that when they produce energy under exertion, although they may be able to produce an adequate amount of total energy, their mitochondria are not functioning optimally, and they are producing an unacceptable amount of energy anaerobically.

This shift from aerobic to anaerobic energy production is one of the primary causes of aging and chronic disease. More importantly, the shift will steadily increase over the years, often without producing any significant symptomatology until mitochondrial function has already become irreversibly compromised.

How old are you really?—"Biological Age"

Using an algorithm which averages the values for resting ATP production, rATP-FA, mATP-FA, and maxATP, wherein the maxATP is double weighted, the computer program compares the subject's overall ATP production efficiency to that predicted of sex, height, and weight matched subjects of various ages. This calculation can be used to determine the subject's "biological age" based on how efficiently he produces ATP.

Alas, aerobic ATP production steadily decreases with age. This decline results in diminished function in every single cell, tissue, and organ in the body, and is the primary cause behind the symptoms and diseases of aging (19). Since the brain, the liver, and the heart are the largest consumers of energy in the body, it is these organs that are the most affected. But no part of the body is spared.

An accurate, reliable, objective, scientifically based formulation for biological age not only reassures the treating physician that his recommended anti-aging/preventive medicine program is in fact really working, but it also has a tremendous motivational value for patients for long-term compliance. If the patient's biological age is less than his chronological age, he can be reassured that all the time, energy, sacrifices, and money that he has spent and continues to spend to keep strong and healthy is really doing what it's supposed to do.

If the patient's biological age is greater than his chronological age, this is also reassuring. Because instead of continuing a lifestyle or supplement program that isn't serving him well, both the patient and his physician are now armed with the information needed to make all the changes that will optimize his health and improve his biological age. Furthermore, repeat mitochondrial functional analysis will be able to confirm that his new program is effective.

We should all remember that no matter how many candles they stick in the birthday cake, our biological age may well be the best indicator how old we *really* are!

References

(1) Wilson TM, Tanaka H. Meta-analysis of the age associated decline in maximal aerobic capacity in men: relation to training status. Am. J. Physiol. Heart Circ. Physiol. Vol. 278: 829–834, 2000

(2) Trounce I, Byrne E, Marzuki S. Decline in skeletal muscle mitochondrial respiratory chain function: possible factor in ageing. *Lancet*. 1989 Mar 25;1(8639):637–9.

(3) Hagen TM, Ingersoll RT, et al: Acetyl-L-carnitine fed to old rats partially restores mitochondrial function and ambulatory activity. Proc Natl Acad. Sci. USA 1998, August 4; 95 (16):9562–6.

(4) Trifunovic A, Wredenberg A, et al. *Premature ageing in mice expressing defective mitochondrial DNA polymerase*. Nature. 2004 May 27;429(6990):417–23.

(5) Speakman JR, Talbot DA, et al. Uncoupled and surviving: individual mice with high metabolism have greater mitochondrial uncoupling and live longer. *Aging Cell*. 2004 Jun;3(3):87–95.

(6) Dean W. *Biological Aging Measurement*. 1988, second edition, The Center for Bio-Gerontology, Los Angeles, CA.

(7) Caldwell SH, Chang CY, Nakamoto RK, Krugner-Higby L. *Mitochondria in nonalcoholic fatty liver disease*. Clin Liver Dis. 2004 Aug;8(3):595–617.

(8) Duchen MR. *Mitochondria in health and disease: perspectives on a new mitochondrial biology*. Mol Aspects Med. 2004 Aug;25(4):365–451.

(9) Beal MF. *Mitochondria, oxidative damage, and inflammation in Parkinson's disease*. Ann N Y Acad Sci. 2003 Jun;991:120–31. Review.

(10) Krieger C, Duchen MR. *Mitochondria, Ca2+ and neurodegenerative disease*. Eur J Pharmacol. 2002 Jul 5;447(2–3):177–88. Review.

(11) Wenzel U, Nickel A, Daniel H. *Increased carnitine-dependent fatty acid uptake into mitochondria of human colon cancer cells induces apoptosis*. J Nutr. 2005 Jun;135(6):1510–4.

(12) Lesnefsky EJ, Hoppel CL. *Ischemia-reperfusion injury in the aged heart: role of mitochondria*. Arch Biochem Biophys. 2003 Dec 15;420(2):287–97. Review.

(13) Lamson DW, Plaza SM. *Mitochondrial factors in the pathogenesis of diabetes: a hypothesis for treatment*. Altern Med Rev. 2002 Apr;7(2):94–111. Review.

(14) Lusk G. J.Biol. Chem., 59, p41 1924.

(15) Cheney PR, Davidson M, et al., *Bicycle ergometry with gas exchange analysis and neurendocrine responses to exercise in chronic fatigue syndrome*. Albany, New York.

(16) Daly J. *The ventilatory response of exercise in CFS*, The Third Annual Conference on Chronic Fatigue Syndrome and the Brain, Bel-Air, California, April 24–26, 1992.

(17) Stevens SR. *Using exercise testing to document functional disability in CFS*. Journal of Chronic Fatigue Syndrome, Vol. 1: No. ¾, p 127–9, 1995.

(18) Wasserman K, Hansen J, Sue D, et al. *Principles of exercise testing and interpretation.* Third Addition., Lippincott Williams & Wilkins, Baltimore, MD, 1999.

(19) Shigenaga MK, Hagen TM, Ames BN. *Oxidative damage and mitochondrial decay in aging.* Proc. Natl. Acad. Sci. USA, Vol. 91, 10771–78, Nov. 1994.

(20). Hagen TM, Liu J, et al. *Feeding acetyl-L-carnitine and lipoic acid to old rats significantly improves metabolic function while decreasing oxidative stress.* Proc Natl Acad Sci USA. 2002 Feb 19; 99:1870–5.

(21) Liu J, Atamna H, Kuratsune H, Ames BN. *Delaying brain mitochondrial decay and aging with mitochondrial antioxidants and metabolites.* Ann N Y Acad Sci. 2002 Apr;959:133–66.

(22) Milne AC, Potter J, Avenell A. *Protein and energy supplementation in elderly people at risk from malnutrition.* Cochrane Database Syst Rev. 2005 Apr 18;(2): CD003288. Review.

(23) Wengreen HJ, Munger RG, West NA, Cutler DR, Corcoran CD, Zhang J, Sassano NE. Dietary protein intake and risk of osteoporotic hip fracture in elderly residents of Utah. *J Bone Miner Res.* 2004 Apr;19(4):537–45.

(24) Waldmann A, Koschizke JW, Leitzmann C, Hahn A. *Dietary intakes and lifestyle factors of a vegan population in Germany: results from the German Vegan Study.* Eur J Clin Nutr. 2003 Aug;57(8):947–55.

(25) Vognild E, Elvevoll EO, Brox J, Olsen RL, Barstad H, Aursand M, Osterud B. Effects of dietary marine oils and olive oil on fatty acid composition, platelet membrane fluidity, platelet responses, and serum lipids in healthy humans. *Lipids.* 1998 Apr;33(4):427–36.

(26) Cartwright IJ, Pockley AG, Galloway JH, Greaves M, Preston FE. *The effects of dietary omega-3 polyunsaturated fatty acids on erythrocyte membrane phospholipids, erythrocyte deformability and blood viscosity in healthy volunteers.* Atherosclerosis. 1985 Jun;55(3):267–81.

(27) Corps AN, Pozzan T, Hesketh TR, Metacalfe JC. *cis-Unsaturated fatty acids inhibit cap formation on lymphocytes by depleting cellular ATP.* J Biol Chem. 1980 Nov 25;255(22):10566–8.

(28) Dement WC. *The Promise Of Sleep.* 1999 Dell publishing, 1540 Broadway, NY, NY 10036.

(29) Van Cauter E, Plat L, Leproult R, Copinschi G. *Alterations of circadian rhythmicity and sleep in aging: endocrine consequences.* Horm Res. 1998;49(3–4):147–52. Review.

(30) Sturis J, Polonsky KS, Mosekilde E, Van Cauter E. *Computer model for mechanisms underlying ultradian oscillations of insulin and glucose.* Am J Physiol. 1991 May;260(5 Pt 1):E801–9. Review.

(31) Altman J. *Weight in the balance.* Neuroendocrinology. 2002 Sep;76(3):131–6. Review.

(32). Gerver WJ, De Bruin R, Delemarre VD, Waal HA, Aldewereld B, Theunissen P, Westerterp KR. *Effects of discontinuation of growth hormone treatment on body composition and metabolism*. Horm Res. 2000;53(5):215–20.

(33) Mahler H, Cordes E. *Biochemistry*. Harper and Row, NY, 1966, p 525–553. ambient oxygen reference p. 22.

(34) Schwela D. *Air pollution and health in urban areas*. Rev. Environ Health. 2000 Jan-Jun; 15 (1–2): 13–42.

(35) Ferrand Robson, DDS. Lecture. Orthomolecular Health-Medicine, Feb 27–29, 2004, San Francisco, California.

(36) Stevenson KJ. *Measurements of carbon monoxide and nitrogen dioxide in British homes using unflued heating or cooking appliances*. Tokai J Exp Clin Med. 1985 Aug;10(4):295–301.

(37) Howell J, Keiffer MP, Berger LR. *Carbon monoxide hazards in rural Alaskan homes*. Alaska Med. 1997 Jan-Mar;39(1):8–11.

(38) Kelley JS, Sophocleus GJ. *Retinal hemorrhages in subacute carbon monoxide poisoning. Exposures in homes with blocked furnace flues*. JAMA. 1978 Apr 14;239(15):1515–7.

(39) Viebahn R, Rilling S. *The Use Of Ozone In Medicine*. Revised edition, December, 1994. Biologica Medicina, 2937 NE Flanders St., Portland, OR 97232.

(40) Pangborn, J, Baker S. *Autism: effective biochemical treatments*. Available from the Autism Research Institute, 4182 Adams Ave., San Diego, CA 92116, p280.

(41) Martinez RM, Saponaro A, Dragagna G, Santoro L, Leopardi N, Russo R, Tassone G. *Cutaneous circulation in Raynaud's phenomenon during emotional stress. A morphological and functional study using capillaroscopy and laser-Doppler*. Int Angiol. 1992 Oct-Dec;11(4):316–20.

(42) Meerson FZ, Arkhipenko IuV, Rozhitskaia II, Kagan VE. *Damage to the Ca2+-transport system of cardiac sarcoplasmic reticulum during emotion-pain stress*. Biull Eksp Biol Med. 1981 Apr;91(4):405–6.

(43) Hasegawa R, Daimon M, Toyoda T, Teramoto K, Sekine T, Kawata T, Watanabe H, Kuwabara Y, Yoshida K, Komuro I. *Effect of mental stress on coronary flow velocity reserve in healthy men*. Am J Cardiol. 2005 Jul 1;96(1):137–40.

(44) Bacon SL, Ring C, Hee FL, Lip GY, Blann AD, Lavoie KL, Carroll D. *Hemodynamic, hemostatic, and endothelial reactions to psychological and physical stress in coronary artery disease patients*. Biol Psychol. 2005 June 13.

(45) Berg D, Berg L.H., and Couvaras J. *Is CFS/FM due to an undefined hypercoagulable state brought on by immune activation of coagulation*. Accepted for presentation: American Association Chronic Fatigue Syndrome, Oct, 98. http://www.hemex.com/publications/csf_fm_hyperstate.php

(46) von Ardenne M. *Oxygen Multi-Step Therapy*. George Thieme Verlag Publishing, January 1, 2000.

(47) Irrcher I, Adhihetty PJ, Joseph AM, Ljubicic V, Hood DA. *Regulation of mitochondrial biogenesis in muscle by endurance exercise*. Sports Medicine, 2003;33(11):783–93.

(48) Brechue WF, Pollock ML. *Exercise training for coronary artery disease in the elderly*. Clin Geriatr Med 12: 207–229, 1996.

(49) Radzewitz A, Miche E, et al. *Exercise and muscle strength training and their effect on quality of life in patients with chronic heart failure*. Eur J Heart Fail 4: 627–634, 2002.

(50) Colcombe SJ, Erickson KI, Raz N, et al. *Aerobic fitness reduces brain tissue loss in aging humans*. J Gerontol A Biol Sci Med Sci 58: M176-M180, 2003.

(51) Cooper CE, Vollaard NB, et al. *Exercise, free radicals, and oxidative stress*. Biochem Soc Trans 30: 280–285, 2002.

(52) Shallenberger, F. *Is Your Patient Exercising Too Hard To Be Healthy?* Townsend Letter For Doctors, August-September, 2004.

(53) Navarro A, Gomez C, Lopez-Cepero J, Boveris A. *Beneficial effects of moderate exercise on mice aging: survival behavior, oxidative stress, and mitochondrial electron transfer*. Am J Physiol Regul Integr Comp Physiol. 286: R505-R511, 2004.

(54) Sastre J, Pallardo FV, Vina J. *The role of mitochondrial oxidative stress in aging*. Free Radic Biol Med. 2003 Jul 1;35(1):1–8.

(55) Lee HC, Wei YH. *Mitochondrial alterations, cellular response to oxidative stress and defective degradation of proteins in aging*. Biogerontology. 2001;2(4):231–44.

(56) Wei YH, Lu CY, Lee HC, Pang CY, Ma YS. *Oxidative damage and mutation to mitochondrial DNA and age-dependent decline of mitochondrial respiratory function*. Ann N Y Acad Sci. 1998 Nov 20;854:155–70.

(57) Levine SA, Kidd PM. *Antioxidant Adaptation—Its Role In Free Radical Pathology*. 1985, Biocurrents Division, Allergy Research Group, 400 Preda St., San Leandro, CA 94577.

ACKNOWLEDGMENTS

Special thanks to my beautiful wife, Judy, who has taken good care of the business part of my life. Anyone who knows me can tell you that I have less than a sufficient interest in the matter of making a living. And without Judy running things, I am sure that this book and the time and energy that it took to put it together would have never happened. She has always had my back. Marrying a woman like Judy is the single most important thing a man can do—even more important than having optimal mitochondrial function.

ENDNOTES

CHAPTER TWO

National Academies Press, "Dietary Reference Intakes for Energy, Carbohydrate, Fiber, Fat, Fatty Acids, Cholesterol, Protein, and Amino Acids," National Academies of Sciences, Engineering, and Medicine (2005), 1.

Dariush Mozaffarian et al., "Trans Fatty Acids and Cardiovascular Disease," *New England Journal of Medicine* 354, no. 15 (April 2006): 1601–13.

A. Etzioni et al., "Systemic Carnitine Deficiency Exacerbated by a Strict Vegetarian Diet," *Archives of Disease in Childhood* 59, no. 2 (February 1984): 177–79.

K. A. Lombard et al., "Carnitine Status of Lactoovovegetarians and Strict Vegetarian Adults and Children," *American Journal of Clinical Nutrition* 50, no. 2 (August 1989): 301–306.

R. De Schrijver and O. S. Privett, "Energetic Efficiency and Mitochondrial Function in Rats Fed Trans Fatty Acids," *Journal of Nutrition* 114, no. 7 (July 1984): 1183–91.

F. A. Kummerow, "Dietary Effects of Trans Fatty Acids," *Journal of Environmental Pathology, Toxicology, and Oncology* 6, no. 3–4 (March–April 1986): 123–49.

R. Blomstrand et al., "Influence of Dietary Partially Hydrogenated Vegetable and Marine Oils on Membrane Composition and Function of Liver Microsomes and Platelets in Rats," *Lipids* 20, no. 5 (May 1985): 283–95.

G. Ravaglia et al., "Effect of Micronutrient Status on Natural Killer Cell Immune Function in Healthy Free-Living Subjects Aged >/=90 Years," *American Journal of Clinical Nutrition* 71, no. 2 (February 2000): 590–98.

E. G. Bliznakov et al., "Coenzyme Q Deficiency in Aged Mice," *Journal of Medicine* 9, no. 4 (1978): 337–46.

CHAPTER THREE

Ronald Klatz and Robert Goldman, *Stopping the Clock* (New Canaan, CT: Keats Publishing, Inc., 2002), 19.

T. M. Wilson and H. Tanaka, "Meta-Analysis of the Age-Associated Decline in Maximal Aerobic Capacity in Men: Relation to Training Status," *American Journal of Physiology Heart and Circulatory Physiology* 278, no. 3 (March 2000):829–34.

I. Trounce, E. Byrne, and S. Marzuki, "Decline in Skeletal Muscle Mitochondrial Respiratory Chain Function: Possible Factor in Ageing," *Lancet* 1, no. 8639 (March 1989): 637–39.

T. M. Hagen et al., "Acetyl-L-Carnitine Fed to Old Rats Partially Restores Mitochondrial Function and Ambulatory Activity," *Proceedings of the National Academy of Sciences in the United States of America* 95, no. 16 (August 1998): 9562–66.

T. M. Hagen et al., "Feeding Acetyl-L-Carnitine and Lipoic Acid to Old Rats Significantly Improves Metabolic Function While Decreasing Oxidative Stress," *Proceedings of the National Academy of Sciences in the United States of America* 99, no. 4 (February 2002): 1870–75.

Aleksandra Trifunovic et al., "Premature Ageing in Mice Expressing Defective Mitochondrial DNA Polymerase," *Nature* 429, no. 6990 (May 2004): 417–23.

John R. Speakman et al., "Uncoupled and Surviving: Individual Mice with High Metabolism Have Greater Mitochondrial Uncoupling and Live Longer," *Aging Cell* 3, no. 3 (June 2004): 87–95.

S. H. Caldwell et al., "Mitochondria in Nonalcoholic Fatty Liver Disease," *Clinic for Liver Disease* 8, no. 3 (August 2004): 595–617.

Michael R. Duchen, "Mitochondria in Health and Disease: Perspectives on a New Mitochondrial Biology," Molecular Aspects of Medicine 25, no. 4 (August 2004): 365–451.

M. Flint Beal, "Mitochondria, Oxidative Damage, and Inflammation in Parkinson's Disease," *Annals of the New York Academy of Sciences* 991 (June 2003): 120–31.

Charles Krieger and Michael R. Duchen, "Mitochondria, Ca2+ and Neurodegenerative Disease," *European Journal of Pharmacology* 447, no. 2-3 (July 2002): 177–88.

Uwe Wenzel, Alexander Nickel, and Hannelore Daniel, "Increased Carnitine-Dependent Fatty Acid Uptake into Mitochondria of Human Colon Cancer Cells Induces Apoptosis," *Journal of Nutrition* 135, no. 6 (June 2005): 1510–14.

Edward J. Lesnefsky and Charles L. Hoppel, "Ischemia-reperfusion Injury in the Aged Heart: Role of Mitochondria," *Archives of Biochemistry and Biophysics* 420, no. 2 (December 2003): 287–97.

Davis W. Lamson and Steven M. Plaza, "Mitochondrial Factors in the Pathogenesis of Diabetes: A Hypothesis for Treatment," *Alternative Medicine Review* 7, no. 2 (April 2002): 94–111.

Frank Shallenberger, *Practicing Anti-Aging Medicine in the New Millennium*, First International Learning Conference on Anti-Aging Medicine in Monte Carlo, Monaco (June 24, 2000).

CHAPTER FOUR

M. Simonoff, "Chromium Deficiency and Cardiovascular Risk," *Cardiovascular Research* 18, no. 10 (October 1984): 591–96.

A. S. Abraham, M. Sonnenblick, and M. Eini, "The Effect of Chromium on Cholesterol-Induced Atherosclerosis in Rabbits," *Atherosclerosis* 41, no. 2-3 (February 1982): 371–79.

S. M. Horner, "Efficacy of Intravenous Magnesium in Acute Myocardial Infarction in Reducing Arrhythmias and Mortality. Meta-Analysis of Magnesium in Acute Myocardial Infarction," *Circulation* 86, no. 3 (September 1992): 774–79.

M. Fenech, "Chromosomal Damage Rate, Aging, and Diet," *Annals of New York Academy of Sciences* 20, no. 854 (November 1998): 23–36.

E. J. Schaefer et al., "Lipoprotein(a) Levels and Risk of Coronary Heart Disease in Men," *Journal of the American Medical Association* 271, no. 3 (1994): 999–1003.

B. Cantin et al., "Lipoprotein(a) Distribution in a French-Canadian Population and Its Relation to Intermittent Claudication (The Quebec Cardiovascular Study)," *American Journal of Cardiology* 75 (1995): 1224–28.

D. Gavish et al., "Lipoprotein(a) Reduction by N-Acetylcysteine," *Lancet* 337 (1991): 203–204.

J. M. Gaziano et al., "Fasting Triglycerides, High-Density Lipoprotein, and Risk of Myocardial Infarction," *Circulation* 96, no. 8 (October 1997): 2520–25.

M. H. Frick et al., "Helsinki Heart Study: Primary-Prevention Trial with Gemfibrozil in Middlel-Aged Men with Dyslipidemia. Safety of Treatment, Changes in Risk Factors, and Incidence of Coronary Heart Disease," *New England Journal of Medicine* 317, no. 20 (November 1987): 1237–45.

M. Zucker, *User's Guide to Coenzyme Q10* (North Bergen, NJ: Basic Health Publications, 2002).

"WHO Cooperative Trial on Primary Prevention of Ischaemic Heart Disease with Clofibrate to Lower Serum Cholesterol: Final Mortality Follow-Up. Report of the Committee of Principal Investigators," *Lancet* 2, no. 8403 (September 1984): 600–604.

"WHO Cooperative Trial on Primary Prevention of Ischaemic Heart Disease with Clofibrate to Lower Serum Cholesterol: Final Mortality Follow-Up. Report of the Committee of Principal Investigators," *Lancet* 2, no. 8191 (August 1980): 379–85.

B. M. Rifkind, "Lipid Research Clinics Coronary Primary Prevention Trial: Results and Implications," *American Journal of Cardiology* 54, no. 5 (August 1984): 30C–34C.

D. J. Maron et al., "Initial Invasive or Conservative Strategy for Stable Coronary Disease," *New England Journal of Medicine* 382 (2020): 1395–1407.

E. Guadagnoli et al., "Variation in the Use of Cardiac Procedures After Acute Myocardial Infarction," *New England Journal of Medicine* 333, no. 9 (August 1995): 573–78.

Daniel B. Mark et al., "Use of Medical Resources and Quality of Life after Acute Myocardial Infarction in Canada and the United States," *New England Journal of Medicine* 331, no. 17 (October 1994): 1130–35.

S. Banerjee et al., "Magnitude and Consequences of Error in Coronary Angiography Interpretation (the ACRE study)," *American Journal of Cardiology* 85, no. 3 (February 2000): 309–14.

D. C. Wallace, "Mitochondria and Cancer: Warburg Addressed," *Cold Spring Harbor Symposia on Quantitative Biology* 70 (2005): 363–74.

Tim J. Schulz et al., "Induction of Oxidative Metabolism by Mitochondrial Frataxin Inhibits Cancer Growth: Otto Warburg Revisited," *Journal of Biological Chemistry* 281, no. 2 (January 2006): 977–81.

M. Isidoro et al., "Alteration of the Bioenergetic Phenotype of Mitochondria is a Hallmark of Breast, Gastric, Lung and Oesophageal Cancer," *Biochemistry Journal* 378, no. 1 (February 2004):17–20.

R. D. Jackson et al., "Calcium Plus Vitamin D Supplementation and the Risk of Fractures," *New England Journal of Medicine* 354, no. 7 (February 2006): 669–83.

C. R. Paterson, "Calcium Requirements in Man: A Critical Review," *Postgraduate Medical Journal* 54, no. 630 (April 1978): 244–48.

M. T. Cantorna et al., "Vitamin D Status, 1,25-Dihydroxyvitamin D3, and the Immune System," *American Journal of Clinical Nutrition* 80, no. 6 (December 2004): 1717S–20S.

E. Giovannucci et al., "Calcium and Fructose Intake in Relation to Risk of Prostate Cancer," *Cancer Research* 58, no. 3 (February 1998): 442–47.

E. J. Mayer-Davis et al., "Intensity and Amount of Physical Activity in Relation to Insulin Sensitivity: the Insulin Resistance Atherosclerosis Study," *Journal of the American Medical Association* 279, no. 9 (March 1998): 669–74.

CHAPTER FIVE

J. Liu et al., "Delaying Brain Mitochondrial Decay and Aging with Mitochondrial Antioxidants and Metabolites," *Annals of the New York Academy of Science* 959 (April 2002): 133–66.

CHAPTER SIX

M. J. Vimy and F. L. Lorscheider, "Serial Measurements in Intra-oral Air Mercury: Estimation of Daily Dose from Dental Amalgam," *Journal of Dental Research* 64, no. 8 (August 1985): 1072–75.

D. W. Eggleston, "Effect of Dental Amalgam and Nickel Alloys on T-Lymphocytes: Preliminary Report," *Journal of Prosthetic Dentistry* 51, no. 5 (May 1984): 617–23.

CHAPTER SEVEN

T. M. Hagen et al., "Feeding Acetyl-L-Carnitine and Lipoic Acid to Old Rats Significantly Improves Metabolic Function while Decreasing Oxidative Stress," *Proceedings of the National Academies of Science in the United States of America* 99, no. 4 (February 2002): 1870–75.

CHAPTER EIGHT

K. Vullo-Navich et al., "Comfort and Incidence of Abnormal Serum Sodium, BUN, Creatine and Osmolality in Dehydration of Terminal Illness," *American Journal of Hospice and Palliative Care* 15, no. 2 (March–April 1998): 77–84.

Ronald M. Lawrence, MD, PhD, and Martin Zucker, *Preventing Arthritis* (Berkeley Publishing Group, 2001).

http://www.yale.edu/ynhti/curriculum/units/1993/5/93.05.06.x.html#j

United States Environmental Protection Agency, "Lead and Your Drinking Water," June 1993.

CHAPTER NINE

Verlyn Klinkenborg, "Awakening to Sleep," *New York Times Magazine*, January 5, 1997.

A. M. Williamson and A. M. Feyer, "Moderate Sleep Deprivation Produces Impairments in Cognitive and Motor Performance Equivalent to Legally Prescribed Levels of Alcohol Intoxication," *Occupational and Environmental Medicine* 57, no. 10 (October 2000): 649–55.

K. Spiegel, R. Leproult, and E. Van Cauter, "Impact of Sleep Debt on Metabolic and Endocrine Function," *Lancet* 354, no. 9188 (October 1999): 1435–39.

CHAPTER TEN

National Research Council, "Diet, Nutrition, and Cancer," Committee on Diet, Nutrition, and Cancer, Assembly of Life Sciences, National Research Council, National Academy Press, Washington, DC, 1982.

D. E. Lawson et al., "Relative Contributions of Diet and Sunlight to Vitamin D State in the Elderly," *British Medical Journal* 2, no. 6185 (August 1979): 303–305.

G. B. Brookes, "Vitamin D Deficiency and Otosclerosis," *Otolaryngology–Head and Neck Surgery* 93, no. 3 (June 1985): 313–21.

E. Giovannucci et al., "Calcium and Fructose Intake in Relation to Risk of Prostate Cancer," *Cancer Research* 58, no. 3 (February 1998): 442–47.

C. Garland et al., "Dietary Vitamin D and Calcium and Risk of Colorectal Cancer: A 19-Year Prospective Study in Men," *Lancet* 1, no. 8424 (February 1985): 307–309.

William Campbell Douglas II, MD, *Into the Light* (Rhino Publishing, 2003). www.rhinopublish.com

CHAPTER ELEVEN

S. Cadenas et al., "Vitamin E Protects Guinea Pig Liver from Lipid Peroxidation without Depressing Levels of Antioxidants," *International Journal of Biochemistry and Cell Biology* 27, no. 11 (November 1995): 1175–81.

S. Krishnamurthy, T. George, and N. Jayanthi Bai, "Effect of Dietary Coconut Oil and Casein and Megadoses of Vitamin A or C on Tissue Lipid Peroxidation and Hemolysis in Vitamin E Deficiency," *Acta Vitaminologica et Enzymologica* 5, no. 3 (1983): 165–70.

T. K. Basu, "High-dose Ascorbic Acid Decreases Detoxification of Cyanide Derived from Amygdalin (Laetrile): Studies in Guinea Pigs," *Canadian Journal of Physiology and Pharmacology* 61, no. 11 (November 1983): 1426–30.

CHAPTER TWELVE

D. Majchrzak et al., "B-Vitamin Status and Concentrations of Homocysteine in Austrian Omnivores, Vegetarians and Vegans," *Annals of Nutrition and Metabalism* 50, no. 6 (September 2006): 485–91.

Michelle Roberts, "Children 'Harmed' by Vegan Diets," BBC News (health report), Washington DC.

Gene and Monica Spiller, *What's with Fiber?*, (Laguna Beach, CA: Basic Health Publications, 2005).

M. Duran et al., "Secondary Carnitine Deficiency," *Journal of Clinical Chemistry and Clinical Biochemistry* 28, no. 5 (May 1990): 359–63.

A. Etzioni et al., "Systemic Carnitine Deficiency Exacerbated by a Strict Vegetarian Diet," *Archives of Disease in Childhood* 59, no. 2 (February 1984): 177–79.

K. A. Lombard et al., "Carnitine Status of Lactoovovegetarians and Strict Vegetarian Adults and Children," *American Journal of Clinical Nutrition* 50, no. 2 (August 1989): 301–306.

E. Larque et al., "Dietary Trans Fatty Acids Alter the Compositions of Microsomes and Mitochondria and the Activities of Microsome Delta6-Fatty Acid Desaturase and Glucose-6-Phospatase in Livers of Pregnant Rats," *Journal of Nutrition* 133, no. 8 (August 2003): 2526–31.

T. Ide et al., "Activities of Liver Mitochondrial and Peroxisomal Fatty Acid Oxidation Enzymes in Rats Fed Trans Fat," *Lipids* 22, no. 1 (January 1987): 6–10.

P. Flachs et al., "Polyunsaturated Fatty Acids of Marine Origin Upregulate Mitochondrial Biogenesis and Induce Beta-Oxidation in White Fat," *Diabetologia* 48, no. 11 (November 2005): 2365–75.

Michelle D. Holmes, MD, DrPH, et al., "Association of Dietary Intake of Fat and Fatty Acids with Risk of Breast Cancer," *JAMA* 281 (1999): 914–20.

G. A. Boissonneault, C. E. Elson, and M. W. Pariza, "Net Energy Effects of Dietary Fat on Chemically Induced Mammary Carcinogenesis in F344 Rats," *Journal of the National Cancer Institute* 76, no. 2 (February 1986): 335–38.

CHAPTER THIRTEEN

R. S. Pafferbarger et al., "Physical Activity, All-Cause Mortality, and Longevity of College Alumni," *New England Journal of Medicine* 314, no. 10 (March 1986): 605–13.

S. N. Blair et al., "Physical Fitness and All-Cause Mortality. A Prospective Study of Healthy Men and Women," *JAMA* 262, no. 17 (November 1989): 2395–401.

M. Pahor et al., "Physical Activity and Risk of Severe Gastrointestinal Hemorrhage in Older Persons," *JAMA* 272, no. 8 (August 1994): 595–99.

J. A. Laukkanen et al., "Cardiovascular Fitness as a Predictor of Mortality in Men," *Archives of Internal Medicine* 161, no. 6 (March 2001): 825–31.

C. B. Pinnock, A. M. Stapleton, and V. R. Marshall, "Erectile Dysfunction in the Community: a Prevalence Study," *Medical Journal of Australia* 171 (1999): 353–57.

M. Babyak et al., "Exercise Treatment for Major Depression: Maintenance of Therapeutic Benefit at 10 Months," *Psychosomatic Medicine* 62, no. 5 (September–October 2000): 633–38.

R. Nelson, "Exercise Could Prevent Cerebral Changes Associated with AD," *Lancet Neurology* 4, no. 5 (May 2005): 275.

E. B. Larson et al., "Exercise Is Associated with Reduced Risk for Incident Dementia among Persons 65 Years of Age and Older," *Annals of Internal Medicine* 144, no. 2 (January 2006): 73–81.

Sharon M. Arkin, PsyD, "Student-led Exercise Sessions Yield Significant Fitness Gains for Alzheimer's Patients," *American Journal of Alzheimer's Disease and Other Dementias* 18, no. 3 (2003): 159–70.

CHAPTER FIFTEEN

D. Rudman et al., "Effects of Human Growth Hormone in Men Over 60 Years Old," *New England Journal of Medicine* 323, no. 1 (July 1990): 1–6.

B. E. Henderson, A. Paganini-Hill, and R. K. Ross, "Decreased Mortality in Users of Estrogen Replacement Therapy," *Archives of Internal Medicine* 151, no. 1 (January 1991): 75–78.

S. T. Page et al., "Exogenous Testosterone (T) Alone or with Finasteride Increases Physical Performance, Grip Strength, and Lean Body Mass in Older Men with Low Serum T," *Journal of Clinical Endocrinology and Metabolism* 90, no. 3 (March 2005): 1502–10.

P. Marin et al., "The Effects of Testosterone Treatment on Body Composition and Metabolism in Middle-Aged Obese Men," *International Journal of Obesity and Related Metabolic Disorders* 16, no. 12 (December 1992): 991–97.

L. P. Ly et al., "A Double-Blind, Placebo-Controlled, Randomized Clinical Trial of Transdermal Dihydrotestosterone Gel on Muscular Strength, Mobility, and Quality of Life in Older Men with Partial Androgen Deficiency," *Journal of Clinical Endocrinology and Metabolism* 86, no. 9 (September 2001): 4078–88.

Uzzi Reiss and Martin Zucker, *Natural Hormone Balance for Women: Look Younger, Feel Stronger, and Live Life with Exuberance* (New York: Simon and Schuster, 2002).

B. Ettinger et al., "Reduced Mortality Associated with Long-term Postmenopausal Estrogen Therapy," Obstetrics and Gynecology 87, no. 1 (January 1996): 6–12.

B. A. Gower and L. Nyman, "Associations among Oral Estrogen Use, Free Testosterone Concentration, and Lean Body Mass among Postmenopausal Women," Journal of Clinical Endocrinology and Metabolism 85, no. 12 (December 2000): 4476–80.

Broda O. Barnes, MD, *Hypothyroidism: The Unsuspected Illness* (HarperCollins, 1976).

L. J. Valenta and A. N. Elias, "How to Detect Hypothyroidism When Screening Tests Are Normal. Use of the TRH Stimulation Test," *Postgraduate Medicine* 74, no. 2 (August 1983): 267–74.

Malcolm Carruthers, *Maximizing Manhood: How to Beat the Male Menopause,* new ed. (Thorsons, 1998).

R. Savine and P. Sonksen, "Growth Hormone—Hormone Replacement for the Somatopause?", *Hormone Research* 53, no. 3 (2000): 37–41.

Walter Pierpaoli, MD, PhD and William Regelson MD, *The Melatonin Miracle: Nature's Age-Reversing, Disease-Fighting, Sex-Enhancing Hormone* (Simon and Schuster, 2011).

D. Garfinkel et al., "Improvement of Sleep Quality in Elderly People by Controlled-Release Melatonin," *Lancet* 346, no. 8974 (August 1995): 541–44.

E. Van Cauter, R. Leproult, and L. Plat, "Age-related Changes in Slow Wave Sleep and REM Sleep and Relationship with Growth Hormone and Cortisol Levels in Healthy Men," *JAMA* 284, no. 7 (August 2000): 861–68.

D. E. Blask et al., "Melatonin-Depleted Blood from Premenopausal Women Exposed to Light at Night Stimulates Growth of Human Breast Cancer Xenografts in Nude Rats," *Cancer Research* 65, no. 23 (December 2005): 11174–84.

P. Lissoni et al., "Modulation of Cancer Endocrine Therapy by Melatonin: a Phase II Study of Tamoxifen Plus Melatonin in Metastatic Breast Cancer Patients Progressing Under Tamoxifen Alone," *British Journal of Cancer* 71, no. 4 (April 1995): 854–56.

E. S. Schernhammer and S. E. Hankinson, "Urinary Melatonin Levels and Breast Cancer Risk," *Journal of the National Cancer Institute* 97 (July 2005): 1084–87.

P. K. Verkasalo et al., "Sleep Duration and Breast Cancer: A Prospective Cohort Study," *Cancer Research* 65 (October 2005): 9595–9600.

R. M. Moretti et al., "Antiproliferative Action of Melatonin on Human Prostate Cancer LNCaP Cells," *Oncology Reports* 7, no. 2 (March-April 2000): 347–51.

G. J. Maestroni, "The Immunoneuroendocrine Role of Melatonin," *Journal of Pineal Research* 14, no. 1 (January 1993): 1–10.

D. X. Tan et al., "Chemical and Physical Properties and Potential Mechanisms: Melatonin as a Broad-spectrum Antioxidant and Free Radical Scavenger," *Current Topics in Medicinal Chemistry* 2, no. 2 (February 2002): 181–97.

Ray Sahelian, *Melatonin: Nature's Sleeping Pill* 2nd ed. (London: Penguin Group, 1996).

*

RESOURCES

American Academy of Anti-Aging Medicine
1510 W. Montana Street
Chicago, IL 60614
Ph: 1–773–528–1000
Fax: 1–773–528–5390
Website: www.a4m.com
e-mail: info@a4m.com

American College for the Advancement of Medicine
24411 Ridge Route, Suite 115
Laguna Hills, CA 92653
Ph: 1–949–309–3520 or 1–800–532–3688
Fax: 1–949–309–3538
Website: www.acam.org
e-mail: info@acam.org

Bio-Energy Testing System
Bio-Energy Testing centers are now being established throughout the United States and the world. A current list of centers using Bio-Energy Testing can be found at www.bioenergytesting.com. We invite doctors, health care practitioners, and fitness centers to inquire about offering this test for their clients.

1231 Country Club Drive, Carson City, NV 89703
Ph: 1–866–376–0610
Fax: 775–884–2202
Website: www.bioenergytesting.com
e-mail: nvcenter@nvbell.net

The Nevada Center of Alternative and Anti-Aging Medicine
1231 Country Club Drive
Carson City, Nevada, 89703
Ph: 1–775–884–3990
Fax: 1–775- 884–2202
Website: www.antiagingmedicine.com
e-mail: nicole@antiagingmedicine.com

INDEX

*

ABOUT THE AUTHOR

Dr. Shallenberger has been practicing medicine since 1973. From the very beginning he recognized that what he was taught in medical school was limited to diagnosing what goes wrong and then prescribing drugs or procedures to help with the symptoms. But he wanted to know more than just symptomatic care. He believed our bodies were created with self-healing mechanisms. It is these mechanisms that are broken down by poor lifestyle choices, false belief systems, lack of properly performed exercise, and toxins.

His passion has been to find therapies that can prevent this breakdown from happening and can repair the damage when it has already happened. The secret? Oxygen. All healing centers around the effective use of oxygen.

Dr. Shallenberger is the President of the American Academy of Ozonotherapy, and is Vice President of the Society of Orthomolecular Health Medicine and has been elected to serve as a charter member of the International Scientific Committee on ozone Therapy.

He has revolutionized the practice of anti-aging and preventive medicine by developing a method to measure mitochondrial function and oxygen utilization called Bio-Energy Testing®.

He is the developer of Prolozone®, an injection technique that has been shown to regenerate damaged joints, herniated discs, and degenerated joints, tendons, and soft tissues.

Other Books

The Principles and Application of Ozone Therapy—
A Practical Guideline for Physicians

The Ozone Miracle

The Type 2 Diabetes Breakthrough

He is also the Editor of *Second Opinion* alternative medicine newsletter.